READER'S COMMENTS

Many books describe attentional disorders and related ... the importance of adapting educational strategies for ... and similar difficulties. Very few deliver really useful, ... these students learn.

Dornbush and Pruitt have put together an encyclopedic collection of usable interventions to address very specific problems with reading comprehension, written expression, math computation, homework, notetaking, preparation of reports and social skills. These experienced educator-clinicians share the fruits of their hands-on experience in ways that can be extremely helpful to educators, clinicians and parents. Highly recommended!

Thomas E. Brown, Ph.D., Associate Director of the Yale Clinic for Attention and Related Disorders
Author: Attention Deficit Disorder: The Unfocused Mind in Children and Adults

This book is so wonderfully comprehensive that my only problem with it is how heavy it is! Perhaps we appreciative readers/users could convince the publishers to make it into a set of sectional handbooks, for surely we will want to walk around with a section at a time to address the day's (or client's) needs.

Martha Denckla, M.D., Kennedy Krieger Institute
Author: Executive Function; Interventions for Learning Disabilities; School Difficulties; Attention Deficit Hyperactivity Disorder: spectrum and mechanisms

Wow! So much work – so comprehensive. Tigers, Too is the perfect comprehensive reference guide on ADHD, OCD and Tourette syndrome for both parents and professionals. Pruitt and Dornbush tap their vast clinical, teaching, and personal experiences to provide updated scientific facts and intervention strategies to ensure success in school and life. This long-awaited book is a must for every home and professional library!

Chris A. Zeigler Dendy, M.S., Author, Speaker, and Consultant
Author: A Bird's-Eye View of Life with ADD and ADHD; Teaching Teens with ADD and ADHD

Tigers, Too is the most comprehensive resource book on key learning disabilities I have encountered in over two decades of teaching. It is a virtual library between two covers, an indispensable reference that is a concise, convenient, and superbly organized work outlining and illuminating the latest research of the most renowned theoretical and clinical authorities in their respective fields. Marilyn Dornbush and Sheryl Pruitt have performed a great service for teachers, parents, administrators, learning coaches, therapists, psychologists, psychiatrists, psychometrists, and other professionals whose responsibility it is to help affected students overcome the difficulties associated with attention deficit/hyperactivity disorder, obsessive-compulsive disorder, Tourette syndrome, and other associated neurological learning difficulties. I highly recommend Tigers, Too.

Donald Gerz, B.A., High School Composition, Literature, and Humanities Teacher (Ret.)

I am extremely honored to have been asked to review Tigers, Too. Having raised a son with Tourette syndrome, I understand the importance of learning and gaining as much information as possible when facing a disorder such as this. As a parent, it is vital to surround yourself with the best advice and support possible. Speaking from experience, Tigers, Too is an invaluable resource. It is a handbook filled with a wealth of knowledge for parents, teachers, students and medical professionals. This handbook is genius in providing clear and helpful suggestions/solutions for these problems.

It is easy to flip to a particular section and find actual problem solving ideas not only from the teacher's perspective but from the student's as well. Sherry and Marilyn have a true gift of being able to communicate their extraordinary knowledge.

Alice D. Grotnes, Parent

Dornbush and Pruitt bring their combined decades of experience and training to create a major work suitable for use as a college-level reference textbook or as a school-wide resource for teachers, parents, and students.

> *Patricia Holden, M.A., M.F.T., LRW, Learning Disabilities Specialist and Family Therapist*
> *Author: articles in AET Journal*

If you are holding this book, congratulations. You are either an exceptional teacher or dedicated parent – one who digs until s/he finds the way to reach seemingly unreachable young people. Tigers, Too is the definitive go-to resource for general and special educators… and struggling parents. Down-to-earth, clearly explained, and tirelessly assembled, Tigers, Too tailors realistic goals and objectives, offers hundreds of teaching suggestions, and provides step-by-step procedures for specific disabilities and combinations of disabilities. These powerful, individualized educational blueprints map the way out of a frightening jungle of confusion and painful failure. Dig into these pages; you won't use them all. But the ones that apply to your life will speak to you and affect the child's life immeasurably. Peruse, cherry pick, bookmark and above all, use the strategies outlined in Tigers, Too. I promise there will be fewer tears… for everyone.

> *Gail Kreher, M.Ed., 18 years in special needs classroom*

I have always considered "Teaching the Tiger" to be an indispensable resource for parents, teachers and therapists dealing with children with Tourette's syndrome (TS), one of my areas of specialty practice. While there are a variety of books about individual conditions like TS, ADHD or OCD, "Teaching the Tiger" was unique in that it dealt with the real world situation that most children experience problems that overlap among these entities and they must be viewed in an integrated fashion. "Tigers, Too" is even better! I know of no other resource that covers this behavior spectrum so well. Incredibly valuable pearls of knowledge and advice are provided on virtually every page, presented in a remarkable well-organized, straightforward and user-friendly way. If you have a child with TS, ADHD or OCD at home or in your classroom, you must have this book.

> *Roger Kurlan, MD, Professor of Neurology, University of Rochester Medical Center*
> *Author: Treatment of Movement Disorders; Handbook of Tourette Syndrome and Related Tic and Behavioral Disorders; Handbook of Secondary Dementias*

Parents and professionals who struggle with a child's ADHD… need… complete, updated, reliable, and factual information about… behavior, social challenges, academic needs, interventions, assessment and psychosocial issues. Basically, they need an 'owners manual' for this child that contains current information and field-tested approaches.

Enter Sheryl Pruitt and Dr. Marilyn Dornbush.

Sheryl and Marilyn have written a ground breaking and invaluable resource with Tigers, Too. The book is filled with information and interventions that parents and professionals will find invaluable. It is extraordinarily readable and features countless lists and dot-pointed information that the reader can use and apply immediately.

The authors' experience, sensitivity, knowledge and compassion shine through on every page. Unlike similar publications, the authors cite solid research for their suggestions and strategies. My copy of their previous book, TEACHING THE TIGER, sits dog-eared on my desk.

This book belongs on every parents' bookshelf and in every Teachers' Lounge. It provides a treasure chest of strategies, methods, research and ideas. I recommend this book enthusiastically to any parent or professional who has an ADHD child in your life. The information contained in these pages will make a tremendous impact on your child… and you.

> *Richard D. Lavoie, Executive Producer, THE F.A.T. CITY WORKSHOP*
> *Author: It's So Much Work to Be Your Friend; The Motivation Breakthrough*

In this magical and wise book, the authors provide a road map to living and working with children with neurodevelopmental disorders. Comprehensive, up to date, brain based, and wise and respectful, this book is full of practical advice for children, parents and clinicians, including a nuanced picture of what it is like to live in a brain that processes information differently. Among the many worthy books competing for attention, this is one book that should be on the desk of everyone that works with children and adolescents with neurological disorders.

John S. March, MD, MPH, Director, Division of Neurosciences Medicine, Duke Clinical Research Institute
Author: Talking Back to OCD: The Program That Helps Kids and Teens Say 'No Way' – and Parents Say 'Way to Go'; OCD in Children and Adolescents: A Cognitive-Behavioral Treatment Manual; Anxiety Disorders in Children and Adolescents;

With Tigers, Too, Dornbush and Pruitt have provided educators and parents with the kind of practical advice and ideas that they need to meet the needs of students with Tourette's Syndrome, Obsessive-Compulsive Disorder, Attention Deficit Hyperactivity Disorder, Executive Dysfunction, and memory impairment.

This reference guide belongs on every educator's bookshelf. I am delighted to have a reference I can recommend to my school district, clients, and parents of my patients.

Leslie E. Packer, Ph.D.
Co-Author: Challenging Kids – Challenged Teachers; book in progress with Woodbine House

This publication provides very good information on Tourette syndrome and associated disorders. Additionally, and what I find of more importance, are the guidance and tips that this publication provides for those afflicted with these disorders, parents and family members, as well as the key segment – our educators!

Having experienced the struggles as a parent of a child with TS and ADHD, I find very useful strategies and plans within this publication. Of equal importance, educators interested in the success of our youth can find and apply very specific strategies or tactics that will be of great benefit to the student.

Lorne W. Perrin, CHA, President, Tourette Syndrome Foundation of Canada, Board of Directors

At first glance Tigers, Too is overwhelming, but everything a parent would want to know is in the book. Sherry Pruitt and Marilyn Dornbush have once again created a useful guide for parents and teachers and a single source for the academician on the subject of ADHD, and associated neurological disorders. I can see how easy it will be to use this reference when both first learning of your child's challenges and when needing extra help in their later developmental years.

Debbie Scott, GMS, Parent

This comprehensive book is packed with information for all school professionals who work with youngsters with ADHD, Tourette Syndrome and Obsessive-Compulsive Disorder. The authors' vast knowledge and clinical wisdom brings hope and optimism for parents and teachers who are looking to understand and help these youngsters through their day-to-day struggles. Full of practical how-to strategies, Tigers, Too will be a wonderful and valuable resource for professionals that will be referenced time and again.

Aureen P. Wagner, Ph.D., University of Rochester School of Medicine
Author: What To Do When Your Child Has OCD; Worried No More: Help and Hope for Anxious Children; Feeling Thermometer; Up and Down the Worry Hill; Treatment of OCD in Children and Adolescents: A Cognitive-Behavioral Therapy Manual

TIGERS, TOO

Tigers, Too

Executive Functions/Speed of Processing/Memory

Impact on Academic, Behavioral, and Social Functioning of Students With ADHD, Tourette Syndrome, and OCD

Modifications And Interventions

Marilyn P. Dornbush, Ph.D.
Sheryl K. Pruitt, M.Ed., ET/P

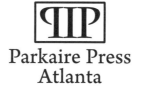

Parkaire Press
Atlanta

Copyright © 2008 by Marilyn P. Dornbush and Sheryl K. Pruitt

All rights reserved. No part of this book may be reproduced, translated, stored in a retrieval system, or transmitted, in any form or by any means, electronic, mechanical, photocopying, microfilming, recording, or otherwise, without written permission from the Publisher, except brief quotations used in a review.

Notice: This book is designed to provide information regarding subject matter covered. It is sold with the understanding that the authors and publisher are not engaged in rendering medical, psychiatric, psychological, legal, or other professional services to the reader. If such are required, the services of a competent professional in the appropriate field should be sought.

Every effort has been made to make this book as complete and accurate as possible. It contains only the information available to the authors at the time of printing. However, there may be mistakes both typographical and in content. Therefore, the text should be used only as a source of general information. Specifics relating to an individual should be obtained from the services of a professional.

The purpose of this book is educational. Neither the authors nor the publisher shall have or accept liability or responsibility to any person or entity with respect to loss or damage or any other problem caused or alleged to be caused directly or indirectly by information covered in this book.

Parkaire Press, Inc.
4939 Lower Roswell Road, Building C
Marietta, Georgia 30068-4328
www.parkairepress.com

Publisher's Cataloging-in-Publication
(Provided by Quality Books, Inc.)

Dornbush, Marilyn Pierce, 1933-
    Tigers, too : executive functions/speed of processing/memory : impact on academic, behavioral, and social functioning of students with attention deficit hyperactivity disorder, Tourette syndrome, and obsessive-compulsive disorder : modifications and interventions / Marilyn P. Dornbush, Sheryl K. Pruitt.
    p. cm.
    Includes bibliographical references and index.
    LCCN 2009927652
    ISBN-13: 978-0-9818643-3-4
    ISBN-10: 0-9818643-3-3

    1. Attention-deficit-disordered children--Education--United States. 2. Attention-deficit hyperactivity disorder--United States. 3. Tourette syndrome in children--United States. 4. Obsessive-compulsive disorder in children--United States.   I. Pruitt, Sheryl K., 1944- II. Title.

LC4713.4.D675 2009   371.94
                              QBI09-600072

Cover designed by Mayapriya Long, Bookwright Press, Inc.

Photograph of Julianna by Shari Zellers Photography, Atlanta. Other photos by Istockphoto.com. All of the children on the cover are models. Use of their photos is not intended to suggest that they have any of the disorders discussed in this guide.

1 10 9 8 7 6 5 4 3

Printed in the United States of America

This book is homage to our wonderful families. Writing a book is a mammoth undertaking and has a major impact on loved ones. To our families who have endured this twice and have always been supportive and encouraging – Dan and Terry; our children – Darin, Jory, Laura, Kirk, and Claire; and our grandchildren – Julianna, Alexandra, Allison, Laura Caroline, Amelia, Hunter, and Lauren – we thank you for all that you do to enrich our lives.

It does not get any better than this!

ACKNOWLEDGEMENTS

We had the encouragement of so many individuals to write a new book addressing the problems associated with executive functions, processing speed, and memory that we would like to acknowledge them.

We first want to thank all the students who generously shared their struggles and triumphs and helped us understand the disorders from their point of view. Many of the recommendations were derived from their personal experiences and insights and those of their parents and teachers. We are especially indebted to our family members who have these disorders. They have given us a deeper understanding of what it is like to live day in and day out with these disorders and which strategies are helpful and which are not.

To say this book is thorough is an understatement. We were privileged to have professionals who were willing to read and comment on this book: Thomas Brown, Ph.D.; Martha Bridge Denckla, M.D.; Chris Zeigler Dendy, M.S.; Don Gerz, B.A., Patricia Holden, M.A., M.F.T., Richard Lavoie, M.A., M.Ed.; Gail Kreher, M.Ed.; Paul Kreher, B.S.; Roger Kurlan, M.D.; John March, M.D.; Leslie Packer, Ph.D.; Lorne Perrin, CHA; and Aureen Wagner, Ph.D. We are also indebted to Robbyn Laufer, OTR/L, Danielle Moore, M.S.Ed., Florence Cannon, M.S., CCC-SLP, and Elisabeth Wiig, Ph.D., who read sections relating to their fields of expertise, were also willing to answer numerous questions and furnish critical assistance within the specific content areas.

This book would not be possible without numerous other colleagues who have reviewed the manuscript, provided invaluable feedback, and shared their knowledge and skills. Mary Jane Trotti, M.A., edited the entire text and made important contributions. Gayle Born, M.Ed., and Laura Kirk, M.Ed., offered editorial advice and suggested many unique interventions.

A special thanks goes to parents who read and provided useful critiques: Kellie Gilpin, Ivie Graiser, Alice Grotnes, Jennifer Musser, Debbie Scott, and Julie Solomon.

This book would not have been completed without the dedication of Dan Pruitt, CPCC, PCC, our publisher, webmaster, graphic artist, layout genius, and renaissance man who did all that we asked and all that we did not know we needed to ask. He has devoted much of the year to our project without complaint, even when we made changes over and over again.

Throughout the writing of this book we have had the unfailing support and assistance of our administrative staff, Jewell McClure and Judi Anderson. We also want to thank our illustrator, Mayapriya Long for her cover illustrations and patience with our input.

We also are grateful to David E. Comings, M.D., and Hope Press for their willingness to publish our first book. It remains a useful book for all individuals working with children with ADHD, TS, and OCD.

Finally, we are most grateful to the numerous researchers who have provided updated information which has increased our knowledge of the underpinnings of the disorders and formed the basis of many of the interventions and management approaches.

To those colleagues and friends whose names and contributions have been overlooked, we apologize but offer our sincere gratitude.

I've come to the frightening conclusion that I am the decisive element in the classroom. It's my personal approach that creates the climate. It's my daily mood that makes the weather. As a teacher, I possess a tremendous power to make a child's life miserable or joyous. I can be a tool of torture or an instrument of inspiration. I can humiliate or humor, hurt, or heal. In all situations, it is my response that decides whether a crisis will be escalated or de-escalated and a child humanized or dehumanized.

Ginott, H. G. (1993). <u>Teacher and Child: A Book for Parents and Teachers</u>. New York, NY: Collier Books. (pp. 15-16)

TABLE OF CONTENTS

Acknowledgements vii
List of Tables xviii
List of Figures. xix
Forward xxi
Preface xxiv

Section I. Awareness   1

    Chapter 1. Attention-Deficit/Hyperactivity Disorder. 3

    Chapter 2. Tic Disorders 11
        Transient Tic Disorder 11
        Chronic Motor Or Vocal Tic Disorder 12
        Tourette Syndrome 12

    Chapter 3. Obsessive-Compulsive Disorder 19

    Chapter 4. Arousal/Processing Speed/Attention/Inhibition. 27

    Chapter 5. Executive Functions 29
        Problem Solving 30
            Goal Setting. 30
            Planning 30
                Proposal/Analysis 30
                Prioritization 30
                Organization/Sequencing. 31
                Time Management 31
        Flexibility 31
        Initiation/Execution 32
        Self-Monitoring. 32
        Use of Feedback 32
        Self-Correction 32

    Chapter 6. Memory 35
        Short-Term Memory. 35
            Immediate Memory 35
            Working Memory. 35
        Long-Term Memory 38
            Encoding/Consolidation (Learning) 38
            Retrieval (Recalling) 38
            Semantic Memory 39
            Episodic/Autobiographical Memory 39
            Procedural Memory 39
            Prospective Memory. 39
            Strategic Memory. 39
            Metamemory. 39

Section II. Resources   41

Chapter 7. Medication/Therapeutic Interventions/Educational and Community Resources . 43

    Medication 43
    Awareness Education 43
    Counseling And Therapeutic Interventions 44
        Anxiety Management 44
        Cognitive-Behavioral Therapy 44
        Comprehensive Behavioral Intervention for Tics 45
        Child/Adolescent Psychotherapy. 46
        Group Therapy 46
        Family Therapy 46
        Parent Support Groups 46
    Educational Resources 47
        Administrators. 47
        Educational Support Team (EST) 47
        Learning Disability Teachers (LD) 47
        Speech and Language Pathologists (SLP) 47
        Occupational Therapists (OT). 47
        School Counselors 47
        School Psychologists 48
        Assistive Technology Consultants 48
        Academic Mentors/Assistants 48
        Home-School Case Managers 48
    Community Resources 49
        Pediatric (Child) Neuropsychologists. 49
        Educational Consultants/Educational Therapists 49
        Tutors. 49
        Coaches 49
        Social Skills Trainers. 50
        Computer Consultants 50
        Advocates 50

Section III. Interventions   51

Chapter 8 Classroom Modifications/Accommodations 53

Chapter 9. Student Interventions. 61

Chapter 10. Underarousal/Slow Cognitive Processing Speed 71

    Sleep disorders 74

Chapter 11. Anxiety/"Storms"/Overarousal 79

    Anxiety 79
    "Storms"/Overarousal 81

Chapter 12. Inattention/Impulsivity/Hyperactivity. 97

    Inattention 97
    Impulsivity 103
    Hyperactivity 105

Chapter 13. Executive Dysfunction 107

Impaired Problem Solving (Tasks/Activities/Situations) 108
Difficulty Setting Goals 110
Difficulty Planning 111
Difficulty Proposing or Generating Ideas/Strategies/Solutions 111
Difficulty Prioritizing 112
Difficulty Organizing 114
Difficulty Sequencing 118
Difficulty Managing Time 119
Inflexibility (Cognitions/Behaviors/Emotions) 122
Initiation/Execution Difficulties (Tasks/Activities) 125
Impaired Self-Monitoring/Use of Feedback/Self-Correction 127
Difficulty Self-Monitoring 127
Difficulty Using Feedback 129
Difficulty Self-Correcting 130

Chapter 14. Memory Problems 131

Short-Term Memory Problems 131
Difficulty with Immediate Memory (Sensory Register) 131
Difficulty with Working Memory 132
Long-Term Memory Problems 136
Difficulty Encoding or Consolidating (Learning) 136
Difficulty Retrieving (Recalling) 144
Difficulty with Procedural Memory 145
Difficulty with Prospective Memory 146
Difficulty with Strategic Memory 147
Difficulty with Metamemory 147

Section IV. Academic Interventions   149

Chapter 15. Oral Expression 151
General Recommendations 151

Chapter 16. Listening Comprehension 153
General Recommendations 153
Underarousal/Slow Cognitive Processing Speed 156
Inattention/Impulsivity/Hyperactivity 157
Executive Dysfunction 158
Impaired Problem Solving (Tasks/Activities/Situations) 158
Difficulty Setting Goals 160
Difficulty Planning 160
Impaired Self-Monitoring/Use Of Feedback/Self-Correction 162
Memory Problems 163
Difficulty with Working Memory 163

Chapter 17. Basic Reading Skills 165
General Recommendations 166
Underarousal/Slow Cognitive Processing Speed 167
Inattention/Impulsivity/Hyperactivity 169
Executive Dysfunction 170

    Difficulty Sequencing.. 170
    Initiation/Execution Difficulties... 171
    Impaired Self-Monitoring/Use Of Feedback/Self-Correction 171
  Memory Problems.. 172
    Difficulty with Working Memory.. 172
    Difficulty Encoding (Learning) 173
    Difficulty Retrieving (Recalling) 175

Chapter 18. Reading Comprehension.. 177
  General Recommendations.. 177
  Underarousal/Slow Cognitive Processing Speed 179
  Inattention/Impulsivity/Hyperactivity.. 180
  Executive Dysfunction 181
    Impaired Problem Solving.. 181
    Inflexibility 191
    Initiation/Execution Difficulties... 193
    Impaired Self-Monitoring/Use Of Feedback/Self-Correction 193
  Memory Problems... 195
    Difficulty with Working Memory.. 195
    Difficulty Encoding/Consolidating (Learning) 197
    Difficulty Retrieving (Recalling) 198

Chapter 19. Written Expression/Long-Term Reports 199
  General Recommendations.. 200
  Underarousal/Slow Cognitive Processing Speed 204
  Inattention/Impulsivity/Hyperactivity.. 204
  Executive Dysfunction 205
    Impaired Problem Solving (Tasks/Activities/Situations) 205
    Initiation/Execution Difficulties... 213
    Impaired Self-Monitoring/Use of Feed Back/Self-Correction 214
  Memory Problems... 219
    Difficulty with Working Memory.. 219
    Difficulty Retrieving (Recalling) 220

Chapter 20. Math Computations... 221
  General Recommendations.. 221
  Underarousal/Slow Cognitive Processing Speed 223
  Inattention/Impulsivity/Hyperactivity.. 224
  Executive Dysfunction 225
    Impaired Problem Solving.. 225
    Inflexibility 230
    Initiation/Execution Difficulties... 231
    Impaired Self-Monitoring/Use Of Feedback/Self-Correction 231
  Memory Problems... 235
    Difficulty With Working Memory.. 235
    Difficulty Encoding/Consolidating (Learning) 236
    Difficulty Retrieving (Recalling) 238

Chapter 21. Math Reasoning 241
    General Recommendations 241
    Underarousal/Slow Cognitive Processing Speed 242
    Inattention/Impulsivity/Hyperactivity 243
    Executive Dysfunction 244
        Impaired Problem Solving 244
        Inflexibility 249
        Initiation/Execution Difficulties 250
        Impaired Self-Monitoring/Use Of Feedback/Self-Correction 250
    Memory Problems 252
        Difficulty with Working Memory 252
        Difficulty Encoding/Consolidating (Learning) 253
        Difficulty Retrieving (Recalling) 255

Section V. Study Skills   257

Chapter 22. Notetaking 259
    General Recommendations 259
    Underarousal/Slow Cognitive Processing Speed 260
    Inattention/Impulsivity/Hyperactivity 261
    Executive Dysfunction 261
        Difficulty Prioritizing 261
        Difficulty Organizing/Sequencing 262
        Initiation/Execution Difficulties 263
    Memory Problems 264
        Difficulty with Working Memory 264
        Difficulty Encoding/Consolidating (Learning) 266

Chapter 23. Homework 267
    General Recommendations 267
    Underarousal/Slow Cognitive Processing Speed 269
    Inattention/Impulsivity/Hyperactivity 271
    Executive Dysfunction 275
        Impaired Problem Solving 275
        Initiation/Execution Difficulties 283
        Impaired Self-Monitoring/Use Of Feedback/Self-Correction 285
    Memory Problems 286
        Difficulty with Working Memory 286

Chapter 24. Test Preparation 287

Section VI. Tests   291

Chapter 25. Tests 293
    General Recommendations 293
    Nonstandardized/Teacher-Prepared Tests 296
    Standardized Tests 296

Chapter 26. Test-Taking Strategies **299**
    Test Review 302

Section VII. Social Competence   305

Chapter 27. Social Skills Interventions **307**
    General Recommendations 309
    Underarousal/Slow Cognitive Processing Speed 315
    Inattention/Impulsivity/Hyperactivity 316
    Executive Dysfunction 322
        Impaired Problem Solving (Tasks/Activities/Situations) 322
        Inflexibility 327
        Initiation/Execution Difficulties 330
        Impaired Self-Monitoring/Use of Feedback/Self-Correcting 332
    Memory Problems 337
        Difficulty with Working Memory 337
        Difficulty Retrieving Information (Recalling) 338

Section VIII. References   339

  References 341

Section IX. Appendix   369

    Definitions of Comorbid Disorders 371
    GET A CLUE Visual Organizer Template 374
    PLAN Visual Organizer Template 375
    The Story of Mother Vowel 376
    Dolch Basic Sight Vocabulary 377
    Story Organizer Template 379
    Problem/Solution Template 380
    Sequence Template 381
    Information/Description Mind Map Template 382
    Main Ideas/Facts Chart Template 383
    Compare and Contrast 2 Circle Venn Diagram Template 384
    Compare and Contrast 3 Circle Venn Diagram Template 385
    Opinions/Facts Chart Template 386
    Cycle of Events Template 387
    Cause and Effect Template 388
    Revision Checklist for Narrative Writing Template 389
    Revision Checklist for Expository Writing Template 390
    Proofreading Checklist Template 391
    Addition Facts Strategies Chart Template 392
    Multiplication Facts Strategies Chart 393
    Editing Strips Templates 394
    Dirty Marvin Smells Bad Template 395
    Math Editing Checklist Template 396
    Math Words And Corresponding Symbols Chart 397

Ready the Plane for the Math's 4 C's Template 398
Math Editing Checklist for Word Problems 399
Class Notes Template 400
Shorthand Symbols For Notetaking Chart 401
Feeling Words Chart 402
Feeling Thermometer Template 403
Sleep Survey - Parent Reporting Form 404
Organizational Skills Survey - Parent Reporting Form 405
Homework Survey - Parent Reporting Form Template 406
Organizations/Web Sites 407
Reading/Media Resources 409

Section X. Index   423
Index 425

LIST OF TABLES

Table 1.1. Comorbidity of Students with ADHD Compared to Students in General Population 7

Table 1.2. Academic Deficits of Clinic-Referred Students with ADHD Compared to Students in Control Group 7

Table 1.3. School Functioning Deficits of Clinic-Referred Students with ADHD Compared to Students in Control Group 8

Table 1.4. Comorbidity of Adolescents with ADHD Compared to Adolescents in General Population 8

Table 1.5. Comorbidity of Adults with ADHD in Community Follow-Up Study Compared to Adults in General Population 10

Table 2.1. Comorbidity of Clinic-Referred Students with TS Compared to Students in General Population With and Without TS 16

Table 3.1. Comorbidity of Clinic-Referred Students with OCD Compared to Students in General Population 24

Table 3.2. Comorbidity of Clinic-Referred Adolescents with OCD Compared to Adolescents in General Population 25

Table 3.3. Comorbidity of Clinic-Referred Adults with OCD Compared to Adults in General Population 26

Table of Contents

LIST OF FIGURES

Figure 1.1. ADHD Diagnostic Criteria 3

Figure 2.1. Transient Tic Disorder Diagnostic Criteria 11

Figure 2.2. Chronic Motor or Vocal Tic Disorder Diagnostic Criteria 12

Figure 2.3. Tourette Syndrome Diagnostic Criteria 12

Figure 3.1. Obsessive-Compulsive Disorder Diagnostic Criteria 19

Figure 5.1. Example of Intact Executive Functioning 33

Figure 8.1. My Shell – Written by the brother of student with Tourette syndrome 53

Figure 11.1. Is It Naughty or Neurological? – Approaches to treating behavior 86

Figure 11.2. Feeling Thermometer 91

Figure 13.1. GET A CLUE – Cognitive strategy for teaching academic, behavioral, and social skills 109

Figure 13.2. PLAN – Cognitive strategy for teaching academic, behavioral, and social skills 109

Figure 14.1. Mother Vowel's House – Visual cognitive cue for positioning letters in space 135

Figure 14.2. Learning Pyramid – Activities that increase learning 138

Figure 14.3. Recall During Lesson – Information recalled at beginning, middle, end of lesson . . . 139

Figure 14.4. Elapsed Time and Review Following Lesson – Passage of time on retention of information, with and without review. 143

Figure 16.1. GET A CLUE – Cognitive strategy used with student who had difficulty with listening comprehension 159

Figure 16.2. PLAN – Cognitive strategy used with student who had difficulty with listening comprehension 160

Figure 18.1. GET A CLUE – Cognitive strategy used with student who had difficulty with reading comprehension 182

Figure 18.2. PLAN – Cognitive strategy used with student who had difficulty with reading comprehension 183

Figure 19.1. Written Expression Sample – Written by student with ADHD, tics, OCD, depression, and executive dysfunction 199

Figure 19.2. GET A CLUE – Cognitive strategy used with student who had difficulty with written expression 206

Figure 19.3. PLAN – Cognitive strategy used with student who had difficulty with written expression 207

Figures 19.4. Mind Map – Visual cognitive strategy for brainstorming, organizing, outlining ideas. 208

Figure 19.5. Revision Checklist for Narrative Writing 215

Figure 19.6. Revision Checklist for Expository Writing 216

Figure 19.7. Written Expression Editing Strip 217

Figure 19.8. Proofreading Checklist – Checklist to assist with editing. 218

Figure 20.1. GET A CLUE – Cognitive strategy used with student who had difficulty with computation. 226

Figure 20.2. PLAN – Cognitive strategy used with student who had difficulty with computation. 227

Figure 20.3. Math Editing Cue 231

Figure 20.4. Use of Graph Paper 232

Figure 20.5. Multiplication Carrying Strategy 233

Figure 20.6. Long Division Cognitive Strategies 233

Figure 20.7. Alignment of Division Problem 234

Figure 20.8. Math Editing Checklist for Computations 234

Figure 21.1. GET A CLUE – Cognitive strategy used with student who had difficulty solving word problems 245

Figure 21.2. PLAN – Cognitive strategy used with student who had difficulty solving word problems 246

Figure 21.3 Math Editing Checklist for Word Problems 251

Figure 21.4. The Hand Trick – Visual cognitive strategy for converting liquid measures 254

Figure 21.5. Slope – Visual cognitive strategy depicting different slopes. 254

Figure 23.1. Example of Homework Contract 274

Figure 23.2. GET A CLUE – Cognitive strategy used with student who had difficulty completing homework. 276

Figure 23.3. PLAN – Cognitive strategy used with student who had difficulty completing homework 277

Figure 27.1. Impact of ADHD on Social Functioning 307

Figure 27.2. GET A CLUE – Cognitive strategy used with student who had difficulty with social interactions 323

Figure 27.3. PLAN – Cognitive strategy used with student who had difficulty with social interactions 324

Figure 27.4. Feeling Thermometer 335

FOREWORD

American culture can be fascinating to observe and analyze. Each month national magazines print columns and feature articles on what is currently "in" and "out". Clothing, movies, televisions shows, restaurants, celebrities are valued and celebrated for a period of time… only to fall out of favor months later. Nehru Jackets. Wide lapels. Short skirts. Disco. Fusion restaurants. Bell-bottoms. Hula-Hoops……

This phenomenon is illustrated by the concept of "political correctness". Jokes, stories and language that had been deemed socially acceptable previously are suddenly viewed as forbidden and insensitive. For the record, I feel that "correctness" is largely a positive movement as it eliminates language that can be derogatory or hurtful.

But one aspect of political correctness has always fascinated and troubled me. Many, many topics and subjects are currently viewed as verboten and are no longer fodder for late night comedians and water cooler humor. Handicaps. Race. Gender issues. I say, "Bravo".

But there are three topics that seem to have escaped the filter of political correctness. Inexplicably, these topics continue to be the subject of comedic routines, television skits and punch lines. People who struggle daily with these challenges are the subject of derision, mockery and ridicule.

Those three challenges are: Attention Deficit Disorder, Tourette syndrome, and Obsessive-Compulsive Disorder.

What is funny about a student who is gifted and cannot pass his school courses because he cannot pay attention? What is funny about a high school student with TS who is on a date but gets thrown out of a movie for making vocal noises? What is funny about a middle school student who is writing a report but needs to tear it up and start over every time a mistake is made? Or, what is funny about a student who is accused of not trying and being lazy after staying up late to finish a written assignment and is unable to turn it in because it is not perfect?

Not much. I know many students and their loved ones who have struggled with all three of these disabilities. Not funny at all.

I have worked with hundreds of students whose lives have been complicated and compromised by these disorders and the neurological deficits associated with them. Their grades suffer. Their relationships are impacted. They are often confused, bemused and distressed by their inability to focus their attention, regulate their actions, and control their thoughts. Later in life they are often unemployed or underemployed.

No, not funny at all.

Another aspect of ADHD/TS/OCD that troubles me is the enormous "cottage industry" of instant cures that has developed in the media and on the Internet. These untested strategies are marketed to desperate and despairing parents who are frustrated with their child's daily behavior, progress and performance.

So, simply, these disorders are neither funny nor simple. They are complex and pervasive disorders that impact on nearly every aspect of a student's behavior and performance. They often occur with other co-morbid psychological and physiological disorders. This complicates and compromises the progress, performance, and potential of academic, behavioral, and social competence.

In *Tigers, Too*, Marilyn Dornbush and Sheryl Pruitt approach ADHD, TS, and OCD and related disorders in a serious, scientific and sound manner. I am pleased that they have asked me to write this

Foreword. They offer sound, scientific rationales for their strategies and techniques. Their innovative hypotheses concerning underarousal/overarousal, executive dysfunction, and memory problems enable the reader to better understand these disorders.

Tigers, Too will explain what Attention Disorders, Tourette syndrome, and Obsessive-Compulsive Disorder ARE. Perhaps the best service that I can provide in this Introduction is to explore what the disorders ARE NOT by discussing the most common myths and misconceptions that are currently held. Unfortunately, the media often promulgates these misconceptions. As I travel throughout North America, I find these long-disproved myths still exist in our schools… and they often prevent students from receiving the services and the assistance that they need and deserve.

Myth #1 – ADD is the "syndrome-of-the-week" and is a recently invented American disorder that is being promoted as an excuse for poor parenting and ineffective teaching.

Detailed descriptions of this syndrome have appeared in pediatric journals since the middle of the nineteenth century. However, it was not until the 1980's that professionals began to recognize the tremendous impact that attentional problems can have on a child's progress and performance in the classroom and in social situations.

Research and surveys throughout Europe, Asia and Australia indicate that attentional disorders occur in similar percentages of the population regardless of culture, race or socioeconomic conditions.

ADHD is recognized as a legitimate disorder by the National Institutes of Health, the United States congress, the Office of Civil Rights and the American Medical Association.

Myth #2 – ADD represents normal – albeit immature – childhood behavior. The child will eventually outgrow it.

Certainly, all children occasionally display symptoms of hyperactivity, distractibility and immaturity. However, with the child with ADHD, the behaviors are chronic, persistent and long lasting. The child is unable to conduct himself in an age-appropriate manner in most settings.

Often, the adolescent or young adult appears to have outgrown the disorder because she has developed strategies to compensate.

Many children with ADHD continue to have marked difficulty with focus, time management and organizational skills as adults. These difficulties, impact on their careers and relationships.

Myth #3 – ADHD is caused by poor parenting.

Although thoughtful, sensitive, effective parenting can be of assistance in improving the child's behavior, there is absolutely no evidence that ineffective parenting is a causal factor in ADHD. In my experience, many ADHD children have siblings who are well behaved and responsive. This would appear to disprove the myth of poor parenting.

Myth #4 – Attentional problems impact primarily on boys

Although most studies indicate that ADHD are more common among boys, girls tend to exhibit attentional problems without hyperactivity (e.g., distractibility, inattention) and they are often not identified. Boys' behavior, on the other hand, is often disruptive and boys are referred for assistance and intervention.

Myth #5 – Attentional and related disorders are greatly over-identified

Certainly, some professional may be overly eager to place the ADHD label on a disruptive child. However, there are also thousands of students with attentional problems (particularly of the inattentive type) that go undiagnosed and untreated.

There are myriad reasons why an individual may struggle with attention, including learning problems, trauma, depression, anxiety or modality difficulties. Medical professional must work closely with parents and educators to make a complete and thorough diagnosis and treatment plan.

Myth #6 – Medications can cure Attentional Disorders, Tourette syndrome, and Obsessive-Compulsive Disorder

There are a wide variety of psychotropic/stimulant medications that can temporarily moderate the effects of the disorders by improving the child's ability to concentrate, focus and reflect, control tics, and negate obsessions and compulsions. A reduction in aggressive, hyperactive and disruptive behaviors is also noted.

However, the medications will not eliminate the deficits and must be supplemented by specialized academic, social and behavioral supports in order to enable the child to reach fullest potential.

Myths also exist that claim that stimulant drugs often lead to drug abuse and addiction. Actually, the opposite is true. If left untreated, individuals with ADHD are at a significant risk for substance abuse. The rate of abuse/addiction for persons receiving prescribed stimulant medications is considerably lower than similar populations. There is no proven correlation between prescribed psychotropic medications and drug addiction.

Myth #7 – Everyone who has Tourette syndrome curses.

This is what some people call TV Tourettes. Regular kids with TS who have the most common tic or motor movement have excessive eyeblinking. This would be of little interest to most TV audiences so the vast majority of children and adolescents with tics do not curse and would be boring to watch on TV.

Myth # 8 – Myth - Everyone with OCD acts like the TV character, Monk

This is again the televised version of OCD. Monk is displaying obsessions and compulsions that many people with OCD experience. This behavior is very unusual and, therefore, very interesting for viewers to watch. The obsessions and compulsions of students with TS plus OCD are often quite different. These students are less concerned about cleanliness and more concerned about having things "just right."

****

In *Tigers, Too*, the authors provide detailed information about the nature and needs of children who struggle daily with ADHD, TS, and OCD and related disorders. They also provide specific, field-tested strategies and methods to use with these students in several academic areas. This combination of theoretical information and specific techniques makes *Tigers, Too* unique and supremely useful. My "manuscript copy" of this book sits dog-eared on my desk. I find myself referring to the book constantly when I am designing curriculum or preparing an assessment. The authors are to be commended for their pragmatic and positive approach to this problem. Children who struggle with these disorders – and those of us who serve them – are in their debt.

Richard D. Lavoie, M.A., M.Ed.

Author, It's So Much Work to Be Your Friend: Helping the Child with Learning Disabilities Find Social Success

The Motivation Breakthrough: 6 Secrets to Turning On the Tuned-Out Child

Preface

Students with Attention Deficit Hyperactivity Disorder (**ADHD**), Tourette syndrome (**TS**), and Obsessive-Compulsive Disorder (**OCD**) are more likely to experience school-related problems than their peers. Many of the challenges are due to the associated disorders of executive dysfunction, impaired processing speed, and memory disorders.

- **ADHD** is often the primary source of learning deficits in the classroom.
  - *Over one-half of the students with **TS** and one-third of students with **OCD** have **ADHD**.*
- Approximately one-third of students with **ADHD** and **TS plus ADHD** repeat a grade.
- Many of these students require extra academic help.
- More than one-third of students with **ADHD**, **TS**, and/or **OCD** attend special classes.
- School-related problems persist into adolescence.
- **ADHD** significantly impacts adult educational, occupational, and social outcomes.

Over the last decade and since the publication of our first book, Teaching the Tiger, understanding of the impact of executive dysfunction, impaired processing speed, and memory problems on academic, behavioral, and social competence has increased substantially. It is essential that school professionals, clinicians, and parents responsible for the cognitive, social, and emotional development of students be knowledgeable about the influence these disorders can have on functioning. Thus, we felt there was a need for a book that addresses these disorders and provides modifications and interventions that are congruent with each student's unique needs.

This handbook is based on a review of the literature, clinical and teaching experience with these students, and consultations and interactions with school personnel and parents. In addition to research findings, this book provides clear, concise, and comprehensive suggestions for ameliorating the effect of these problems on performance and for helping students and teachers be successful.

The book has been divided into seven sections. The first part reviews current research. Arousal, processing speed, attention, disinhibition, executive functions, and memory are defined. An overview of what is considered age-appropriate functioning is provided.

The second section discusses various treatment alternatives. This part gives brief summaries of medication, awareness education, counseling and therapy, and educational and community resources which are available to improve the cognitive and emotional development of students.

The third section of the book is devoted to classroom modifications, individual student interventions, and general recommendations for ameliorating specific deficits associated with executive dysfunction, impaired processing speed, and memory problems.

The fourth and fifth sections provide intervention strategies to circumvent the effect these disabilities have on reading, writing, math, and study skills (note taking, homework, and studying for tests).

The sixth section addresses testing. It offers recommendations for creating teacher-prepared tests, preparing for standardized testing, and teaching test-taking strategies.

The final section of the book is devoted to social skills.

The concerned reader does not necessarily have to start at the beginning and read sequentially to the end of the book. It is recommended to quickly scan through the book, look at the headings and subheadings, and get an overview of what is provided. Before reading a specific academic chapter or the social skills section, the third part should be read as this section offers general recommendations that are not included in the individual chapters. Some of the text has been <u>underlined</u> or **bolded** to make locating specific information easier.

Tigers, Too, like *Teaching the Tiger*, is useful for teachers, clinicians, and parents of students with ADHD, TS, and OCD and for all individuals working with students who experience difficulties associated with executive dysfunction, impaired processing speed, and memory problems..

 The recommendations in this handbook represent good teaching practices for all students.

SECTION I
AWARENESS

REVIEW OF THE ADHD/TS/OCD LITERATURE, PROCESSING SPEED, EXECUTIVE FUNCTIONS, MEMORY

ADD/ADHD is often more complex than most people realize! When you think of attention deficit disorder, visualize an iceberg with only one-eighth of its mass visible above the water line. As is true of icebergs, often the most challenging aspects of ADD and ADHD are hidden beneath the surface. ADD/ADHD may be mild, moderate, or severe, is likely to coexist with other conditions, and may be a disability for some students.

Chris A. Zeigler Dendy, M. S. (2000). <u>Teaching Teens with ADD and ADHD. A Quick Reference for Teachers and Parents</u>. Bethesda, MD: Woodbine House. (pp. 9-10)

Because most educators are never trained in rare neurological disorder such as Tourette syndrome, they often find themselves unable to manage a child's symptoms in the regular classroom and unable to find support or resources to guide them.

Leslie E. Packer, Ph.D. (1994). Educating children with Tourette syndrome: Understanding and educating children with a neurological disorder. I. Psychoeducational Implications of Tourette syndrome and its associated disorders. Albany, NY: New York State Education Department. (Preface)

Parents, teachers and even doctors often misunderstand OCD as bad habits, purposeful misbehavior or weakness of character. Instead of treatment, the prescription is tighter discipline and "better" parenting... A correct diagnosis is necessary for the right treatment. Yet, more often than not, the diagnosis of OCD can be elusive, especially for children... A child's chances of living a good life are greatly increased if OCD is diagnosed and treated both promptly and properly.

Aureen P. Wagner, Ph.D. (2006). <u>What to do when your Child Has Obsessive-Compulsive Disorder</u>. Rochester, NY: Lighthouse Press. (pp. 79-80)

CHAPTER 1

ATTENTION-DEFICIT/HYPERACTIVITY DISORDER

Attention-Deficit/Hyperactivity Disorder (ADHD) is a clinically diagnosed neurological syndrome. For the diagnosis of ADHD, the following criteria of the Diagnostic and Statistical Manual of Mental Disorders, Fourth Edition, Text Revision (DSM-IV-TR) (1) must be met:

A. Either (1) or (2):

(1) Six (or more) of the following symptoms of inattention have persisted for at least 6 months to a degree that is maladaptive and inconsistent with developmental level:

Inattention
(a) often fails to give close attention to details or makes careless mistakes in schoolwork, work, or other activities
(b) often has difficulty sustaining attention in tasks or play activities
(c) often does not seem to listen when spoken to directly
(d) often does not follow through on instructions and fails to finish school work, chores, or duties in the workplace (not due to oppositional behavior or failure to understand instructions)
(e) often has difficulty organizing tasks and activities
(f) often avoids, dislikes, or is reluctant to engage in tasks that require sustained mental effort (such as schoolwork or homework)
(g) often loses things necessary for tasks or activities (e.g., toys, school assignments, pencils, books, or tools)
(h) is often easily distracted by extraneous stimuli
(i) is often forgetful in daily activities

(2) Six (or more) of the following symptoms of hyperactivity-impulsivity have persisted for at least 6 months to a degree that is maladaptive and inconsistent with developmental level:

Hyperactivity
(a) often fidgets with hands or feet or squirms in seat
(b) often leaves seat in classroom or in other situations in which remaining in seat is expected
(c) often runs about or climbs excessively in situations in which it is inappropriate (in adolescents or adults, may be limited to subjective feelings of restlessness)
(d) often has trouble playing or engaging in leisure activities quietly
(e) is often "on the go" or often acts as if "driven by a motor"
(f) often talks excessively

Impulsivity
(g) often blurts out answers before questions have been completed
(h) often has trouble awaiting turn.
(i) often interrupts or intrudes on others (e.g. butts into conversations or games)

B. Some hyperactive-impulsive or inattentive symptoms that caused impairment were present before age 7 years.
C. Some impairment from the symptoms is present in two or more settings (e.g., at school (or work) and at home).
D. There must be clear evidence of clinically significant impairment in social, academic, or occupational functioning.
E. The symptoms do not occur exclusively during the course of a Pervasive Developmental Disorder, Schizophrenia, or other Psychotic Disorder and are not better accounted for by another mental disorder (e.g., Mood Disorder, Anxiety Disorder, Dissociative Disorders, Personality Disorder).

Code based on type:
ADHD, Combined Type: if both Criteria A1 and A2 are met for the past 6 months
ADHD, Predominantly Inattentive Type: if Criterion A1 is met but Criterion A2 is not met for the past 6 months
ADHD, Predominantly Hyperactive-Impulsive Type: if Criterion A2 is met but Criterion A1 is not met for the past 6 months.

Coding note: For individuals (especially adolescents and adults) who currently have symptoms that no longer meet full criteria, "In Partial Remission" should be specified.

Reprinted with permission from the Diagnostic and Statistical Manual of Mental Disorders, Fourth Edition, Text Revision, (Copyright 2000). American Psychiatric Association.

Figure 1.1. ADHD Diagnostic Criteria

Section I

Attention-Deficit/Hyperactivity Disorder, Predominately Hyperactive/Impulsive Type (ADHD-H/I), more common in the preschool years, is often a precursor to **Attention-Deficit/Hyperactivity Disorder, Combined Type (ADHD-C)**. (2) Although not required for diagnosis, some of the following hyperactive, impulsive, and inattentive behaviors may be exhibited by students with **ADHD-C**:

Hyperactive Behaviors (motor/vocal/cognitive/emotional/sensory)

Becoming physically uncomfortable when bored or needing more stimulation/movement	Tapping pencils/fingers/feet
	Making noises
Shifting from one uncompleted activity to another	Being hypersensitive (overreacting) to auditory/visual/tactile/olfactory (smell)/gustatory (taste) input
Having overactive/associative thoughts	Being hypersensitive to pain
Playing with objects	

Impulsive Behaviors

Acting without thinking/waiting	Failing to self-monitor vocal/motor/emotional/sensory behavior
Beginning work before directions completed	
Having difficulty following oral/written directions	Seeking immediate gratification ("I have to have it NOW!")
Rushing through assignments	Neglecting to predict consequences of behavior
Lacking skills to self-monitor classwork	
Making careless mistakes	Grabbing things from others
Talking during quiet activities	Engaging in risk-taking behaviors

Inattentive Behaviors

Being unable to sustain attention	Delaying initiation of tasks
Avoiding tasks requiring persistence (schoolwork/homework)	Having trouble following directions
	Failing to finish assignments
Having difficulty remaining on tasks considered dull/boring	Performing inconsistently on academic tasks
	Overfocusing on electronic screens (TV/phone/computer/video games)
Being distracted by auditory/visual/tactile/olfactory stimuli	

Other Behaviors

Performing like younger student	Failing to learn from experience
Not using problem-solving skills	Feeling anxious/irritable/angry
Overlooking need to use strategies to manipulate/store/retrieve information	Experiencing rapid/unpredictable mood swings
Having difficulty perceiving/expressing verbal and nonverbal social behaviors	Having low frustration tolerance
	Overreacting to situations
Having difficulty following rules	Acting aggressively towards others
Using belligerent/disrespectful language	Overlooking abstract moral principles when responding to others

- Students with **Attention-Deficit/Hyperactivity Disorder, Predominately Inattentive Type, (ADHD-I)**, particularly those with a "Sluggish Cognitive Tempo" (**SCT**), manifest different behaviors than those with **ADHD-C**.

    > *Sluggish cognitive tempo is experienced by one-fourth to one-half of students with **ADHD-I**. (2, 3)*

Behaviors

Having trouble focusing attention on tasks	Delaying initiation of tasks
Experiencing auditory/visual/tactile distractibility	Performing tasks/activities slowly
	Retrieving information slowly
Appearing tired/lethargic/sleepy	Responding slowly to questioning
Being hypoactive (underreacting) to auditory/visual/tactile input	Lacking persistence
	Being unable to finish assignments/homework/chores
Daydreaming (staring into space/free-associating)	Forgetting newly learned material
Seeming "lazy"/"unmotivated" when confronted with goal-oriented tasks/activities	Having difficulty mastering skills at automatic levels
	Displaying inconsistent learning/academic performance
Being disorganized	Underachieving
Forgetting materials needed for tasks/activities	Appearing unhappy/withdrawn/anxious/depressed
Having slow cognitive processing speed	
Forgetting to follow instructions	Being shy/socially passive

General Information

> *Estimates vary depending on the sample source (clinical or general population), number of participants, age range, sex, diagnostic criteria, and comorbidity.*

Frequency

- The overall prevalence of ADHD in large community-based samples ranges from 1% to 8.7%. (1, 4, 5, 6, 7)

- **ADHD-I** has been found in population studies to be the most common category. (3, 6, 8, 9, 10, 11, 12, 13, 14)

    ○ 4.4% – 11.4% ADHD, Inattentive Type

    ○ 1.9% – 5.4% ADHD, Combined Type

    ○ 1.7% – 3.9% ADHD, Hyperactive-Impulsive Type

- The prevalence of DSM-IV-TR subtypes is increased in clinic-referred students. (15)

    ○ 30% ADHD-I

    ○ 61% ADHD-C

    ○ 9% ADHD-H/I

- **ADHD-H/I** is more common in preschool and less common at the elementary and secondary levels. (14)

Section I

- **ADHD-C** is the most prevalent disorder in preschool and more prevalent than ADHD-H/I in elementary and secondary grades. (14)
- **ADHD-I** is more frequent in elementary and secondary school. (14)
- The incidence of adolescents with ADHD varies from 0.4% – 7.8%. (5, 16, 17)
- 2% – 8% of adults are diagnosed with ADHD. (18, 19, 20, 21)

Gender

- ADHD affects both genders and results in a similar pattern of symptoms (hyperactivity, impulsivity, inattention) and comorbidities. (22)
- ADHD is more common in males than females during both childhood and adolescence. In community samples, the ratio is approximately 3:1 and, in clinic-referred groups, 6:1 to 9:1. (6, 14, 23)
- The gender ratio in adulthood is approximately 3:2 or 1:1. (21, 24)
- Females exhibit less hyperactive, aggressive, oppositional, and disruptive behaviors. (23, 25)
- Females are two times more likely to be diagnosed with ADHD-I. (26)

Age of Onset

- Symptoms OF **ADHD-H/I** typically emerge before 7 years. However, about 20% of **ADHD-C** and 40% of **ADHD-I** do not meet the DSM-IV-TR 7 year age-of-onset criterion. (27)

Diagnosis

- There is no definitive diagnostic test for ADHD. The diagnosis relies on the student's developmental history and a description of behaviors observed by parents and teachers.
- Students with **ADHD-I** tend to be referred for evaluation 1 to 3 years later than those with **ADHD-H/I**. (9, 28) Symptoms that interfere with school performance and social competence rarely are evident until the demands for focused and sustained attention, problem solving, planning, organization, time management, and independence increase.

Comorbid (co-occurring) Disorders

- Comorbid disorders may develop during childhood, adolescence, or adulthood. If unrecognized and untreated, they lead to greater disability and poorer long-term prognosis.
  - Research suggests that approximately one-half of the students with ADHD have one or more comorbid disorders. (29)
- Comorbidity studies indicate that ADHD increases the risk for disruptive, mood, and anxiety disorders (2, 29, 30) when compared to the overall incidence of these disorders in childhood (ages 9-12). (5, 7, 31)

Table 1.1. Comorbidity of Students with ADHD Compared to Students in General Population

	ADHD	General Population
<u>Disruptive Disorders</u>		
Oppositional Defiant Disorder	45% – 65%	2.1% – 2.7%
Conduct Disorder	22% – 45%	2.6% – 3.3%
<u>Mood Disorders</u>		
Major Depression	25% – 30%	0.0% – 0.1%
Bipolar Disorder	6% – 11%	0%
<u>Anxiety Disorders</u>	25% – 35%	2.6% – 23.9%

- ○ The most commonly experienced anxiety disorders were Separation Anxiety and Overanxious Disorder.

- ○ Brief descriptions of comorbid disorders are provided in the Appendix (pp. 371 – 373).

    - 🐾 *An exacerbation of ADHD symptoms usually produces a similar increase in symptoms associated with the comorbid disorders.*

- Students with **ADHD-C** often have more severe disorders with increased rates of oppositional, conduct, and bipolar disorders than those with either **ADHD-I** or **ADHD-H/I**.

    - 🐾 *Comprehensive assessment and treatment are required.*

- A significant number of students have symptoms associated with comorbid disorders that interfere with functioning but do not meet the full diagnostic criteria.

- Clinic-referred students frequently experience impaired academic and school functioning. (2, 30, 32, 33)

Table 1.2. Academic Deficits of Clinic-Referred Students with ADHD Compared to Students in Control Group

	ADHD	Comparison Subjects
<u>Learning Disabilities</u>	24% – 70%	**% – 39%
Reading	18% – 34%	2% – 4%
Basic Reading Skills	**% – 20%	**%
Reading Comprehension	**% – 20%	**%
Spelling	**% – 30%	6%
Math Calculation	21% – 31%	8%
Written Expression	**% – 65%	27%
** Not assessed/reported		

- 🐾 *Note that learning disabilities in written expression were <u>two</u> times more common than those in reading and math.*

- 🐾 *The incidence of learning disabilities in the general population is 5% – 10%. (34, 35)*

Section I

Table 1.3. School Functioning Deficits of Clinic-Referred Students with ADHD Compared to Students in Control Group

	ADHD	Control Group
<u>Underachievement</u>		
Repeat a grade	31% – 32%	11%
Require extra help	45% – 56%	25%
Attend special classes	32% – 45%	1%

PROGNOSIS

Adolescence

- 🐾 *No follow-up studies have been conducted on **ADHD-I**. The following information concerns the adolescent outcome of the **ADHD-C** and **ADHD-H/I** subtypes.*

- Research suggests that symptoms persist into adolescence in 50% to 85% of students diagnosed with ADHD. (19, 30, 36, 37, 38)

  - 30% – 50% continue to meet the full diagnostic criteria. (38, 39, 40)
  - 40% – 84% experience two or more symptoms that cause impairment. (39, 41)
  - 10% – 15% have complete remission of the disorder. (38, 40)
  - Remission prior to age 12 is characterized by a low rate of comorbidity, psychosocial problems, and family history of ADHD. (38)

- Hyperactivity and impulsivity tend to diminish in late childhood, but inattention persists. Academic underachievement, emotional difficulties, and impaired socialization persist. (2, 19, 38, 40, 42)

- Follow-up assessments suggest that many adolescents with ADHD (ages 13-17) meet comorbidity criteria (30, 36, 38, 43) as compared to community samples. (5, 44, 45, 46)

Table 1.4. Comorbidity of Adolescents with ADHD Compared to Adolescents in General Population

	ADHD	General Population
<u>Disruptive Disorders</u>		
Oppositional Defiant Disorder	59% – 73%	2.7% – 3.0%
Conduct Disorder	19% – 43%	2.7% – 3.3%
<u>Mood Disorders</u>		
Major Depression	25% – 45%	1.5% – 4.3%
Bipolar Disorder	18% – 23%	1.0% – 3.0%
<u>Anxiety Disorders</u>	19% – 35%	1.0% – 13.0%

- More common anxiety disorders experienced by adolescents with ADHD included: Agoraphobia, Overanxious Disorder, Simple Phobia, Social Phobia, and Separation Anxiety.
- Brief descriptions of comorbid disorders are provided in the Appendix (pp. 371–373).

- Adolescents with **ADHD-C** have been found to have higher rates of academic problems and school dysfunction. (2, 30, 36, 38, 39, 47)
    - 29% – 42% repeat a grade.
    - 56% – 85% require extra help with academic subjects.
    - 32% – 46% attend special classes.
    - 10% – 32% drop out of school.
    - 46% – 80% are suspended.
    - 10% – 13% are expelled.

- An elevated incidence of driving problems (e.g., accidents, speeding tickets, suspended or revoked licenses) is reported. (36, 48, 49, 50)

- Elevated rates of substance use and abuse are identified (e.g., cigarettes, alcohol, marijuana). (2, 51)

    Research indicates that stimulant medication does <u>not</u> lead to substance abuse in adolescence. In fact, medication reduces the risk by 50% and results in levels that are consistent with the incidence in the general population. (52, 53)

- There is an increased risk for sexual activity, pregnancy, and sexually transmitted diseases. (2, 54)

Adulthood

*No studies have been conducted on adults with **ADHD-I**. The following information concerns the outcome of adults with persistent **ADHD-C** and **ADHD-H/I** who were evaluated in clinical settings. Therefore, the rates of impairment may not be as high in the general population.*

- Symptoms of ADHD persist into adulthood in 40% – 60% of the students diagnosed with the disorder in childhood. (55, 56)
    - 41% – 44% meet the full diagnostic criteria.
    - 20% – 30% experience several symptoms that cause impairment.
    - 35% – 36% have full remission of symptoms.

- ADHD tends to be associated with comorbidity throughout the life span. Follow-up studies suggest that 33% – 80% of adults continue to have at least one comorbid disorder. Approximately one-half have two additional disorders, and one-third have three disorders. (56, 57, 58, 59, 60, 61)

Section I

Table 1.5. Comorbidity of Adults with ADHD in Community Follow-Up Study Compared to Adults in General Population

	ADHD	General Population	(21, 46)
<u>Disruptive Disorders</u>			
Antisocial Personality Disorder	10% – 18%	10%	
Oppositional Defiant Disorder	20% – 30%	9%	
Conduct Disorder	17% – 20%	10%	
<u>Mood Disorders</u>	1% – 24%	7%	
Major Depression	25% – 30%	6% – 17%	
Bipolar Disorder	6% – 11%	1% – 4%	
<u>Anxiety Disorders</u>	4% – 50%	16% – 29%	
<u>Drug/alcohol abuse/dependence</u>	6% – 34%	8% – 13%	

- Brief descriptions of comorbid disorders can be located in the Appendix. (pp. 371–373)

- Research indicates that stimulant treatment in childhood and adolescence does not precipitate substance use or abuse in adulthood. (62, 63)

- Chronic ADHD influences adult educational, occupational, and social outcomes. (2, 24, 39, 47, 59, 60, 61, 62, 63, 64, 65)

  - 17% – 32% do not graduate from high school versus only 1% – 9% of comparison subjects (12% – 50% of those receive a high school equivalency diploma). Class rankings and grade point averages are significantly lower.

  - 5% – 19% complete a bachelor's degree or higher in contrast to 26% – 41% of adults without ADHD.

  - 3% enroll in graduate school or obtain a graduate degree compared to 12% – 16% of control participants.

  - 90% are employed, although the most common occupation is skilled worker (25% versus 14%). Only 4% are employed as professionals.

  - 77% have chronic employment difficulties and change jobs frequently. Problems in the workplace include inattention, disorganization, difficulty handling daily responsibilities and large workloads, trouble managing time, and difficulty getting along with co-workers.

  - 48% impulsively quit their jobs.

  - 53% – 55% are fired from their jobs.

  - 28% are divorced/separated compared to 15% without ADHD.

  - Many have driving problems (e.g., accidents, speeding tickets, suspended or revoked licenses). (2, 19, 55, 61)

  - 72% feel that ADHD has a negative impact on adult family, social, and professional outcomes (53% versus 32% are dissatisfied with their family life, 62% versus 42% with their social life, and 78% versus 60% with their professional life).

CHAPTER 2
TIC DISORDERS

- Tics are sudden, repetitive, stereotyped movements (motor) or sounds (vocal/phonic) produced by an underlying neurological condition. They are characterized by their frequency, duration, and intensity. Tics may be brief, meaningless movements or sounds (simple tics) or slower, longer, more purposeful movements or sounds (complex tics).

- Large population-based studies indicate that up to 20% of students have tics at some time during childhood and adolescence. (1, 2, 3)

- More boys have tics than girls. (1, 4)

- 2% – 3% of adolescents have tics, suggesting a decrease in symptoms for some students during the teenage years. (3)

- Symptoms may change, move, and wax and wane in number, frequency, complexity, and severity.

- Tics may be absent during waning periods.

- Tic disorders lie on a continuum of symptomatology ranging from Transient Tic Disorder to Tourette syndrome.

Transient Tic Disorder

Transient Tic Disorder comprises the most common and mildest form of the spectrum of tic disorders. For the diagnosis of Transient Tic Disorder, the following criteria from the Diagnostic and Statistical Manual of Mental Disorders, Fourth Edition, Text Revision (DSM-IV-TR) must be met: (5)

> A. Single or multiple motor and/or vocal tics (e.g., sudden, rapid, recurrent, nonrhythmic, stereotyped motor movements or vocalizations) are present.
> B. The tics occur many times a day, nearly every day for at least 4 weeks, but for no longer than 12 consecutive months.
> C. The onset is before age 18 years.
> D. The disturbance is not due to direct physiological effects of a substance (e.g., stimulants) or a general medical condition (e.g., Huntington's disease or postviral encephalitis).
> E. Criteria have never been met for Tourette's Disorder or chronic motor or vocal tic disorder.
>
> *Reprinted with permission from the Diagnostic and Statistical Manual of Mental Disorders, Fourth Edition, Text Revision, (Copyright 2000). American Psychiatric Association.*

Figure 2.1. Transient Tic Disorder Diagnostic Criteria

- Estimates suggest that 2% – 4% of students with tics have transient tic disorders. (2, 4)

- The age of onset is typically between 3 and 10 years.

- Boys are at greater risk for developing transient tics than girls.

- Tics usually occur on the head, neck, shoulders, and/or arms.

Section I

CHRONIC MOTOR OR VOCAL TIC DISORDER

- For the diagnosis of **Chronic Motor or Vocal Tic Disorder**, the following DSM-IV-TR criteria must be met: (5)

> A. Single or multiple motor or vocal tics (e.g., sudden, rapid, recurrent, nonrhythmic, stereotyped motor movements or vocalizations), but not both, have been present at some time during the illness.
> B. The tics occur many times a day, nearly every day or intermittently throughout a period of more than 1 year, and during this period there was never a tic-free period of more than 3 consecutive months.
> C. The onset is before age 18 years.
> D. The disturbance is not due to the direct physiological effects of a substance (e.g., stimulants) or a general medical condition (e.g., Huntington's disease or postviral encephalitis).
> E. Criteria have never been met for Tourette's Disorder
>
> *Reprinted with permission from the Diagnostic and Statistical Manual of Mental Disorders, Fourth Edition, Text Revision, (Copyright 2000). American Psychiatric Association.*

Figure 2.2. Chronic Motor or Vocal Tic Disorder Diagnostic Criteria

- The prevalence of chronic motor tic disorders ranges from 0.03% – 3.5%. (1, 2, 3, 4, 6)

- Motor movements are the most common tics and tend to involve the head, neck, shoulders, and/or arms.

- Chronic vocal tic disorders have been identified in 0.26% – 0.75% of students. (1, 2, 3, 4, 6)

TOURETTE SYNDROME

Tourette syndrome (TS) is the most severe tic disorder. For the diagnosis of Tourette's Disorder, the following DSM-IV-TR criteria must be met: (5)

> A. Both multiple motor and 1 or more vocal tics have been present at some time during the illness, though not necessarily concurrently. (A tic is a sudden, rapid, recurrent, nonrhythmic, stereotyped motor movement or vocalization).
> B. The tics occur many times a day (usually in bouts) nearly every day or intermittently throughout a period of more than 1 year, and during this period there was never a tic-free period of more than 3 consecutive months.
> C. The onset is before age 18 years.
> D. The disturbance is not due to the direct physiological effects of a substance (e.g., stimulants) or a general medical condition (e.g., Huntington's disease or postviral encephalitis).
>
> *Reprinted with permission from the Diagnostic and Statistical Manual of Mental Disorders, Fourth Edition, Text Revision, (Copyright 2000). American Psychiatric Association.*

Figure 2.3. Tourette Syndrome Diagnostic Criteria

- TS usually begins as simple motor tics occurring about the face, head, and neck (eye blinking or head jerking) with a progression to the arms, legs, and body over several years.

- Vocal tics appear about 1-2 years after the onset of motor tics.

- Complex tics are rarely present without simple motor or vocal tics.

- Tic severity: 31% mild, 51% moderate, 18% severe. (7)

- Tics are often preceded by sensory sensations that result in their expression and subsequent relief. Attempts to suppress these urges lead to increasing uneasiness and tension and an intensification of the need to express the tic. Students under 10 years are usually less aware of or unable to articulate the urge to tic. (8, 9)

    > *The need to tic resembles the need to sneeze or scratch.*

- TS symptoms are different for each student and may include any movement or sound. (10)

Motor Symptoms

Abdominal jerking	Head jerking/rolling	Object twirling
Ankle flexing/moving	Hitting self/others	Obscene gesturing
Arm flailing/flapping	Hopping	Pinching
Arm flexing/jerking	Inhaling/exhaling	Scratching
Blowing on hands/fingers	Jaw/mouth moving	Shivering
Body jerking/tensing/ posturing	Joint/knuckle cracking	Shoulder shrugging
	Jumping	Skipping
Book/paper tearing	Kicking	Spitting
Clapping	Kissing hand/others	Squatting
Eye blinking	Knee/deep bending	Stepping/walking backwards
Eye rolling/squinting	Knee knocking	Stomping
Eye twitching	Leg bouncing	Stooping
Facial contorting	Leg jerking	Table banging
Facial grimacing	Lip licking/smacking	Tapping objects
Finger moving/tapping	Lip pouting	Teeth/clenching unclenching
Foot shaking/tapping	Muscle tensing/relaxing	Tongue thrusting
Hair tossing/twisting	Nose twitching	Twirling in circle
Hand clenching/unclenching	Object throwing	

  ○ The most common motor symptoms are eye blinking, head jerking, and shoulder shrugging.

Vocal Symptoms

Barking	Hissing/honking	Screeching
Belching	Humming	Shouting
Blowing	Making animal noises	Shrieking
Breathing noisily	Making "tsk," "pft" sounds	Sniffing
Calling out	Making motor/jet noises	Snorting
Clicking/clacking	Making unintelligible	Squealing
Coughing sounds	Mimicking character	Throat clearing
Gasping	Moaning	Uttering "hey hey," "ha ha"
Grunting voices	Saying "hmm," "oh," "wow," "uh," "yeah"	Whistling
Gurgling		Yelping
Hiccupping	Screaming	

Echolalia (repeating other's words)
Palilalia (repeating own words)
Unusual speech patterns (peculiarly accenting words/stammering or stuttering/using unusual vocal rhythms)
Coprolalia (uttering obscene words)

  > *Less than 15% of individuals with TS develop coprolalia. (7)*

  ○ The most common vocal symptoms are sniffing and throat clearing.

Section I

- The similarity of several motor and vocal symptoms with OCD compulsions makes the precise categorization difficult.

General Information

🐾 *Estimates vary depending on the sample source (clinical or general population), number of participants, age range, sex, diagnostic criteria, and comorbidity.*

Frequency

- Once considered to be a rare disorder, the prevalence of TS is currently estimated to be 0.1% – 4.5% during childhood. (1, 2, 6)
- The incidence of TS during adolescence varies from 0.03% – 0.26%. (3, 11, 12)

Gender

- TS is more common in males than females. (2, 4)

Age of Onset

- Onset of ADHD is often earlier than the onset of tics. (13, 14)
- Average age of TS onset is 6–7 years. (7, 15, 16, 17, 18)
  - 41% under 6 years (7)
  - 75% – 93% by the age of 11 years (7, 18)
  - 1% between ages 16 to 20 years (7)
- Motor tics are usually the first symptoms to appear. (19)
  - 50% – 70% have facial tics at onset.
  - Initial symptoms may disappear to be replaced with new symptoms.
  - Motor tics typically progress from the head, neck, and shoulders to the torso and extremities.
- Vocal tics, usually noises instead of words, appear between 8 to 15 years. (15)
- Tics develop gradually with intermittent remissions. Abrupt onset is rare.
- Obsessive-compulsive symptoms appear approximately 2-3 years after the onset of TS. (17, 19, 20)

Symptom Control

- Students often can suppress their tics for a period of time. However, when the symptoms of the disorder are severe, or the students are stressed, symptom control is difficult. Tasks and activities that require focused attention (e.g., watching TV, playing hand-held games) and fine motor control (playing sports, creating art projects) often decrease tics.
- Factors that increase symptoms often include timed tasks and tests, handwritten assignments, restricted movement, unstructured activities, holidays, birthdays, family vacations, and the beginning and ending of the school year. (21)
- Students who fear being embarrassed, teased, or humiliated by their peers may become preoccupied with controlling movements and sounds. Suppression takes intense effort and diverts attention from the tasks at hand. Schoolwork may be affected.

- Students who try to control their tics in school frequently display out of control behavior due to tic suppression. An increase in tics is noted at home.

- Anxiety, anger, excitement, fatigue, physical illness, and viral or bacterial diseases increase symptoms and reduce the ability to suppress tics. (10)

DIAGNOSIS

- There is no definitive test for Tourette syndrome. The diagnosis relies on the student's developmental history and a description of the behaviors observed by parents and teachers.

- The diagnosis of TS is frequently made several years after the onset of the disorder.

- Information about the disorder that leads to the diagnosis is often found by a family member in the media or on the Internet.

- Since students frequently are able to control their tics during office visits, professionals mistakenly consider the symptoms to be associated with nervousness, allergies, visual problems, or habits.

- The myths about coprolalia (utterance of obscene words) or intellectual deterioration are unfounded.
    - *The intelligence quotients of students with TS fall within the normal distribution of scores. (22)*

COMORBID (CO-OCCURRING) DISORDERS

- 5% – 10% of individuals have **TS-only** (no reported comorbidity). (7, 23)

- Comorbid disorders are present in 95% of students with mild to moderate symptoms and 100% with severe symptoms. (23)

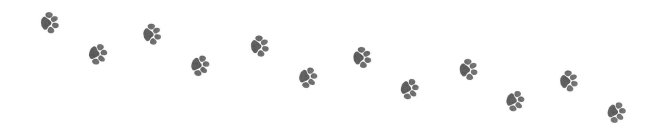

Section I

- Data from a large population-based study (1596 students, ages 9-17) suggest that students with TS are at increased risk for experiencing symptoms associated with comorbid disorders (24) as compared to unaffected subjects (1, 25). Clinic-referred students have a higher incidence of disruptive, anxiety, and mood disorders. (26)

   Table 2.1. Comorbidity of Clinic-Referred Students with TS Compared to Students in General Population With and Without TS

	TS	Clinic-Referred	General Population
<u>Disruptive Disorders</u>			
ADHD	55.6%	66%	0.9%
Oppositional Defiant Disorder	34.7%	52%	2.7%
Conduct Disorder	6.9%	16%	2.7%
<u>Mood Disorders</u>			
Major Depression	11.1%	64%	0.4%
Bipolar Disorder	0%	**	<0.1%
<u>Anxiety Disorders</u>	**	53% – 70%	2.6% – 23.9%
<u>Obsessive-Compulsive Disorder</u>	19.4%	25% – 42%	0.1%
Subclinical OCD		52%	

   ** Not assessed/reported

  - 32% of students with mild to moderate symptoms and 54% with severe symptoms have multiple (> 2) anxiety disorders. (23)

  - More commonly experienced anxiety disorders include: Overanxious Disorder, Simple Phobia, Social Phobia, and Separation Anxiety.

  - Brief descriptions of comorbid disorders are provided in the Appendix (pp. 371–373).

    - *When there is an exacerbation of the TS symptoms, there is usually a similar increase in symptoms associated with the comorbid disorders.*

- Students with **TS plus ADHD** and **ADHD-only** have been found to have an increased rate of disruptive, mood, and anxiety disorders when compared to **TS without ADHD** and normally developing students. (16, 26, 267) The combination of **TS with ADHD** is associated with a higher incidence of aggression and "storms" (pp. 81–95). (26, 28)

  - *Clinical experience suggests that students with TS plus OCD and/or TS with mood disorders also experience severe irritability, fluctuating arousal, and temper outbursts.*

- **ADHD** is the primary source for academic underachievement. (13, 27, 29, 30)

  - 12% – 30% repeat a grade.

  - 50% – 53% require extra help.

  - 12% – 40% attend special classes.

- Learning disabilities are uncommon except in the area of written expression. (30)
  - *Clinical and teaching experience indicates that the second most common academic deficit is in math calculation.*

PROGNOSIS

- The course of the disorder varies as much as the symptoms.
  - Tics are most severe between 6 and 19 years (average 10-11), followed by a gradual diminishing of symptoms during adolescence and early adulthood. (15, 31, 32)
  - **OCD** symptoms associated with TS reach their peak in the teenage years and may continue throughout adulthood.
  - **ADHD** and **OCD** symptoms often persist more than the tics. (13, 31)
- TS may remain a chronic, lifelong disorder. (15, 31)
  - 0% – 30% have complete remission of tics.
  - 34% – 78% experience a reduction of symptoms in both number and severity.
  - 4% – 55% continue to be symptomatic.
- While tic severity improves over time, a follow-up study of students through adulthood indicated that 90% of adults continued to have tics (50% were inaccurate in their assessments and considered themselves tic-free). (33)
- Tic severity does not predict the outcome of the disorder.
- An analysis of outcome studies suggested that persistent TS may affect educational, occupational, and social outcomes. (19)
  - 33% did not graduate from high school.
  - 10% completed a bachelor's degree or higher.
  - 48% were employed full time, 9% part-time, 27% – 29% unemployed. 32% were employed as professional, executives, managers; 31% as clerks and sales representatives; 20% as laborers, service providers, domestic help.
  - 39% never married, 9% were divorced or separated.

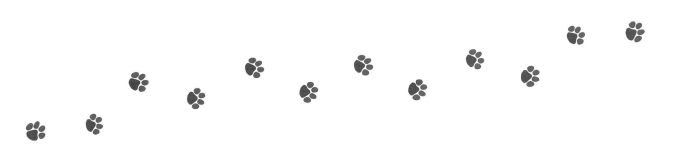

CHAPTER 3

OBSESSIVE-COMPULSIVE DISORDER

Obsessive-Compulsive Disorder (OCD) is a clinically diagnosed neurological disorder. Symptoms range on a continuum from subclinical OCD with mild and transient symptoms causing no problems to many symptoms resulting in significant impairment. For the diagnosis of obsessive-compulsive disorder, the following criteria from the Diagnostic and Statistical Manual of Mental Disorders, Fourth Edition, Text Revision (DSM-IV-TR) must be met: (1)

A. Either obsessions or compulsions:

Obsessions as defined by (1), (2), (3), and (4):
  (1) recurrent, persistent thoughts, impulses or images that are experienced, at some point during the disturbance, as intrusive and inappropriate and that cause marked anxiety or distress
  (2) the thoughts, impulses, or images are not simply excessive worries about real-life problems
  (3) the person attempts to ignore or suppress such thoughts, impulses or images, or to neutralize them with some other thought or action
  (4) the person recognizes that the obsessional thoughts, impulses, or images are a product of his or her own mind (not imposed from without as in thought insertion)

Compulsions as defined by (1) and (2):
  (1) repetitive behaviors (e.g., hand washing, ordering, checking) or mental acts (e.g., praying, counting, repeating words silently) that the person feels driven to perform in response to an obsession, or according to rules that must be applied rigidly
  (2) the behaviors or mental acts are aimed at preventing or reducing distress or preventing some dreaded event or situation; however, these behaviors or mental acts either are not connected in a realistic way with what they are designed to neutralize or prevent or are clearly excessive

B. At some point during the course of the disorder, the person has recognized that the obsessions or compulsions are excessive or unreasonable. Note: This does not apply to children.

C. The obsessions or compulsions cause marked distress, are time consuming (take more than 1 hour a day), or significantly interfere with the person's normal routine, occupational (or academic) functioning, or usual social activities or relationships.

D. If another Axis I disorder is present, the content of the obsessions or compulsions is not restricted to it (e.g., preoccupation with food in the presence of an Eating Disorder; hair pulling in the presence of Trichotillomania; concern with appearance in the presence of Body Dysmorphic Disorder; preoccupation with drugs in the presence of a Substance Abuse Disorder; preoccupation with having a serious illness in the presence of Hypochondriasis; preoccupation with sexual urges or fantasies in the presence of Paraphilia; or guilty ruminations in the presence of Major Depressive Disorder).

Reprinted with permission from the Diagnostic and Statistical Manual of Mental Disorders, Fourth Edition, Text Revision, (Copyright 2000). American Psychiatric Association.

Figure 3.1. Obsessive-Compulsive Disorder Diagnostic Criteria

- OCD symptoms frequently wax and wane and change over time.

- OCD symptoms may appear when students experience internal or external stress (e.g., strep, viral infection, divorce).

- Once symptoms are apparent, any stressor can precipitate an increase in symptoms.

Section I

Obsessions (anxiety-provoking thoughts, impulses, images) (2)

Aggressive
Being preoccupied with knives/scissors/blood/fire
Having violent thoughts/images/desires
Thinking macabre or gory thoughts
Thinking about harming self/others
Thinking about cutting self
Thinking about stealing

Contamination
Being concerned about dirt/germs/bodily waste
Worrying about sticky substances/residues

Counting
Counting letters/words/steps/objects
Focusing on special numbers
Thinking about doing things specific number of times

Doubting/Worrying
Worrying that something terrible might happen
Worrying about causing something to happen (fire, burglary, divorce, death of parent/relative)
Not trusting self/others ("I'm doing something wrong")
Worrying about others not loving them
Being afraid of losing things
Worried about having uttered insults/obscenities

Hoarding/Collecting/Saving
Focusing on collecting/saving

"Just Right" Feeling
Needing everything to feel/look/occur "JUST RIGHT" (food/clothing/appearance/events)

Perfectionism/Symmetry/Exactness
Needing everything in certain order/alignment/symmetry (words/clothing/appearance/possessions/schoolwork)
Needing to do things in a certain way/sequence

Religious/Moral
Focusing on moral issues (right/wrong/fairness)
Thinking about sacrilege/blasphemy (moral scrupulosity)

Sexual
Experiencing forbidden sexual thoughts/images/desires

Somatic
Being concerned with illness/disease

Miscellaneous
Focusing on movie/TV show/computers
Focusing on special words/colors
Over focusing on details
Focusing on sensory input (pain/fluorescent noises/texture of clothing/computer games)
Needing to know/remember things
Ruminating on one idea/action/feeling/hurt feeling/embarrassing

- Most frequently reported obsessions include:

    38% – 81% aggressive/catastrophic events, 52% – 87% contamination, 64% symmetry/exactness, 23% – 29% religious, 4% – 27% sexual, 3% – 38% somatic complaints (3, 4, 5)

- 60% – 97% have multiple obsessions. (3, 4, 5, 6)

Intrusive thoughts and images lead to impulses to perform compulsive behaviors.

Compulsions (purposeful, anxiety-reducing rituals) (2)

Checking
Checking/rechecking (doors/locks/windows/stoves)
Checking that something did not/will not cause harm to self/others
Checking that nothing terrible has happened (fire/death of parent/contamination)
Checking if mistakes were made
Checking/rechecking class work/homework until late/not turned in

Cleaning/Washing
Engaging in excessive/ritualized hand washing/bathing/showering
Engaging in excessive/ritualized tooth brushing/hair combing/grooming
Cleaning objects excessively

Counting
Counting/grouping objects repeatedly
Doing things specific number of times
Touching objects exact number of times

Hoarding/Collecting/Saving
Needing to have extensive collections
Filling room with unnecessary items
Being unable to throw things away
Creating excessive piles of items

Making Everything "Just Right"
Putting items in certain position/place
Arranging/rearranging pencils/papers/books on desk
Needing extra sharp point on pencil
Adjusting/readjusting clothing (socks/shoelaces/sleeves) until feel/look "JUST SO"
Dressing/redressing/changing clothes
Insisting on certain size of clothing
Needing to say/hear something again
Insisting on certain foods

Mental Rituals
Performing mental rituals involving counting/reciting/spelling
Playing computer/video games
Visualizing disturbing scenes repeatedly

Ordering/Arranging/Evening Up
Excessive ordering/arranging objects (desk/cubbyhole/locker)
Evening-up (socks/shoelaces/objects)
Not allowing possessions/objects to be touched to preserve exact order

Repeating
Reciting sequence of statements/series of numbers
Repeating actions (in/out door, up/down from chair)
Repeating sounds/words/numbers/music/movies to oneself
Reading/rereading words, sentences, paragraphs
Calculating/recalculating
Sharpening/resharpening pencils
Erasing/re-erasing until paper torn
Writing/rewriting until paper looks perfect
Locking/relocking combination lock

Touching
Biting/licking (nails/arms/objects/others/self)
Touching objects/self/others/wounds
Sexually touching others (breasts/buttocks/genitals)
Sexually touching self (sometimes masturbating)
Constantly rubbing cloth/objects

Miscellaneous
Avoiding certain people/objects
Having to make comments even when unnecessary/unwanted/inappropriate
Having to finish verbalization when interrupted
Needing to start task/activity over if interrupted
Needing to do/say what told not to do/say
Being unable to change to new task ("stuck" on activity)
Engaging in rituals for good luck
Needing to experience painful sensations (pinch/cut/burn)
Seeking reassurance over and over
Stealing

- Most frequently reported compulsions include:

    64% – 76% repeating rituals, 43% – 64% checking, 57% – 84% washing/cleaning, 24% – 42% counting, 40% – 62% ordering/arranging, 10% – 42% hoarding/collecting/saving. (3, 4, 5)

Section I

- 87% – 100% of children and adolescents with OCD have multiple compulsions. (3, 4, 5, 6)
- Compulsions without obsessions are more common in children than adolescents. (7)
- The OCD student may experience anxiety and have a feeling of being "stuck" while involved in obsessions and compulsions. (2)
  - Being "stuck" may include:
    - difficulty delaying gratification ("I have to have it NOW!").
    - an inability to change tasks or to let go of a subject.
    - perfectionism (erasing until tearing a hole in the paper, writing/tracing numbers and letters over and over again, spending hours making sure homework is perfect).
    - perseveration on feelings/thoughts/routines/numbers/wants/etc.
  - A student may become anxious or angry when interrupted and feel compelled to finish the task.

GENERAL INFORMATION

Estimates vary depending on the sample source (clinical or general population), number of participants, age range, sex, diagnostic criteria, and comorbidity.

FREQUENCY

- Population-based studies suggest that OCD affects approximately 0.1% – 0.17% of elementary students. (8, 9)
- A prevalence of 0.2% – 5.5% is reported in adolescence. (10, 11, 12, 13, 14)
- Approximately 1% – 3.3% of adults have OCD. (11, 15)
- 3% of clinic-referred elementary and 11% of adolescent students with **ADHD** (16) and 19% – 25% of those with **TS** (17, 18) meet the diagnostic criteria for OCD.
- 3.9% – 8.4% of adolescents have OCD symptoms which may cause impairment but do not meet the full diagnostic criteria (referred to as subclinical OCD), obsessive-compulsive behaviors (OCB), or obsessive-compulsive symptoms (OCS). (13, 14)

GENDER

- OCD is more common in boys than girls in childhood (3:2). (10, 19, 20)
- Males and females are equally affected in adolescence and adulthood. (19, 20)

AGE OF ONSET

- Onset of ADHD and other anxiety disorders may precede the onset of OCD. (4, 5)
- Age of onset may occur either in childhood (average 8-10 years) or in adulthood (21 years). (4, 5, 20, 21)
- Boys often have an earlier onset than girls. (10, 22)
- Obsessive-compulsive symptoms typically increase gradually over the course of years. Abrupt onset is rare. (4)

Symptom Control

- OCD symptoms are usually experienced throughout the day. Occasionally, an attack may occur suddenly and last several hours or days. During that time, the student cannot change focus and direct attention to academic tasks.

- Obsessions and compulsions can sometimes be suppressed or partially controlled. The severity of the disorder and psychological and environmental factors impact suppressibility.

- Students who fear being embarrassed, teased, or humiliated by peers may become preoccupied with trying to control their obsessions and compulsions. Suppression takes intense effort and diverts attention from the tasks at hand. School performance may be affected.

  - *The resulting inattentive behavior often resembles that associated with ADHD but is secondary to the suppression of obsessions and/or compulsions.*

- Excessive control can produce a build-up of symptoms which must be released. Students who suppress their symptoms at school are reported by their parents to have an explosion of symptoms when they arrive home. (22, 23)

- Anxiety, anger, excitement, fatigue, physical illness, viral or bacterial diseases, and stress increase symptoms, thereby reducing the ability to control obsessions and compulsions.

Diagnosis

- There is no definitive test for obsessive-compulsive disorder. The diagnosis relies on the student's developmental history and a description of the behaviors observed by parents and teachers.

  - *A comprehensive interview by a knowledgeable professional is frequently the most important tool for identifying obsessions and compulsions.*

- Diagnosis of OCD is often delayed 2.5 years from the onset of symptoms. (10)

  - OCD is frequently not diagnosed by professionals because they lack knowledge about OCD and do not ask questions regarding the symptoms.

  - Children often do not reveal information about their obsessions and compulsions because they feel "crazy" about having irrational thoughts and unusual behaviors.

  - Young children have limited understanding of their obsessions and compulsions and have difficulty articulating them. (5, 6)

Comorbid (co-occurring) Disorders

- Comorbidity is common in clinic-referred students with OCD. (3, 4, 5, 21)

  - 62% – 97% have comorbid disorders.

    - 34% – 97% of those students have at least one additional diagnosis.

    - 43% – 50% have two or more.

      - *Clinical experience suggests that many students with OCD have fears and phobias (e.g., dark, thunder, lighting, tornadoes, animals, insects, reptiles).*

Section I

- Research studies of clinic samples revealed an increased incidence of comorbid disorders (3, 4, 5, 6, 21, 22) as compared to community samples. (8, 9, 24)

    Table 3.1. Comorbidity of Clinic-Referred Students with OCD Compared to Students in General Population

	OCD	General Population
<u>Disruptive Disorders</u>		
ADHD	10% – 51%	1.7% – 1.9%
Oppositional Defiant Disorder	11% – 51%	2.0% – 2.7%
Conduct Disorder	2% – 7%	2.6% – 3.3%
<u>Mood Disorders</u>		
Major Depression	10% – 73%	0% – 0.1%
Mania	27%	<0%
<u>Anxiety Disorders</u>	26% – 70%	2.6% – 23.9%
<u>Tourette Syndrome</u>	1% – 25%	0.1% – 0.2%

    > *When there is an exacerbation of the OCD symptoms, there is usually a similar increase in symptoms associated with the comorbid disorders.*

    ○ Brief descriptions of comorbid disorders are provided in the Appendix (pp. 371–373).

    ○ Trichotillomania (excessive pulling out of hair), Body Dysmorphic Disorder (feeling ugly or physically repulsive), Anorexia Nervosa and Bulimia (eating disorders) share some characteristics, but important differences, with OCD and are considered obsessive-compulsive spectrum disorders.

- Students with **OCD plus ADHD** experience the academic, behavioral, and social problems associated with ADHD. (21, 25, 26)

- Approximately 25% of clinic-referred students with OCD exhibit tics, ranging from transient tics to Tourette syndrome. (3, 4, 5, 27)

- The co-existence of **OCD plus TS** is associated with a more severe disorder than either disorder alone.

    ○ Research suggests important differences between tic-related OCD and non-tic-related OCD. (28, 29, 30, 31)

Tic-related OCD

- earlier age of onset
- affects more males than females
- higher rates of comorbidity (ADHD, mood disorders, anxiety disorders, disruptive behaviors, trichotillomania, body dysmorphic disorder, substance abuse)
- inner feeling of the need to make a movement or a sound (sensory sensation) associated with TS at times preceding more tic-like compulsions
- more aggressive/violent/sexual thoughts, checking, counting, hoarding, symmetry/exactness, "Just Right" feelings

- more "tic-like" compulsions (touching, tapping, rubbing, blinking, staring)
- less contamination worries/cleaning compulsions

Non-tic-related OCD
- obsessive worries preceding compulsions
- more contamination/cleaning obsessions

- Almost half of the students with OCD have been found to have school-related problems. 27% report difficulty writing, 32% completing class assignments, 33% taking tests, and 46% doing homework. 7% repeat a grade, 48% require extra help, and 40% attend special classes. (5, 21)

PROGNOSIS

- OCD is considered for many individuals a chronic, waxing and waning, life-long disorder. The course and duration of the disorder vary as much as the symptoms. The disorder may produce unusual behaviors and negatively influence academic achievement, social relationships and activities, development of a positive self-concept, and emotional functioning.

Adolescence

- 74% – 84% of clinic-referred adolescents with OCD meet the diagnostic criteria for a comorbid disorder (6, 23, 27, 32) as compared to unaffected adolescents. (8, 33)

Table 3.2. Comorbidity of Clinic-Referred Adolescents with OCD Compared to Adolescents in General Population

	OCD	General Population
<u>Disruptive Disorders</u>		
ADHD	10% – 36%	0.4%
Oppositional Defiant Disorder	10% – 47%	3.0%
Conduct Disorder	7% – 16%	2.7%
<u>Mood Disorders</u>		
Major Depression	23% – 62%	0.6%
<u>Anxiety Disorders</u>	35% – 44%	1% – 13%
<u>Tourette Syndrome</u>	5% – 9%	0%
Alcohol abuse/dependence	2% – 24%	3.7%

  ○ Brief descriptions of comorbid disorders are provided in the Appendix (pp. 371–373).

Section I

Adulthood

- Adults with persistent OCD who are seen in the clinical settings have a higher rate of comorbidity (6, 23, 34) as compared to adults in the general population (33, 35):

  Table 3.3. Comorbidity of Clinic-Referred Adults with OCD Compared to Adults in General Population

	OCD	General Population
<u>Disruptive Disorders</u>		
ADHD	** – 26%	8.1%
Oppositional Defiant Disorder	** – 11%	8.5%
Conduct Disorder	** – 4%	9.5%
<u>Mood Disorders</u>		
Major Depression	19% – 78%	16.6%
Bipolar Disorder	** – 2%	3.9%
<u>Anxiety Disorders</u>	30% – 49%	16% – 29%
<u>Tourette Syndrome</u>	6% – 15%	**
Alcohol/substance abuse/dependence	** – 6%	14.6%

  ** Not assessed/reported

  ○ Brief descriptions of comorbid disorders are provided in the Appendix (pp. 371–373).

- A review of research studies (36) analyzing the long-term outcome of OCD which developed during childhood and adolescence revealed the following:

  ○ 60% met OCD diagnostic criteria or experienced subclinical symptoms.
  - 40% met the full OCD diagnostic criteria.

  ○ Earlier age of onset and longer duration of symptoms were associated with persistence of the disorder.

  ○ Comorbid tic and mood disorders predicted the prolonged impact of OCD symptoms.

  ○ OCD did not affect educational attainment but influenced both occupational and social outcomes.
  - 30% – 70% attended college.
  - 45% were unemployed.
  - 20% had difficulty maintaining a job.
  - 55% – 100% reported social/peer problems.
  - 52% were unmarried.
  - 30% lived with their parents as adults.

CHAPTER 4
AROUSAL/PROCESSING SPEED/ATTENTION/INHIBITION

Optimal Arousal

A student's state of arousal (alertness) significantly impacts the ability to attend, use executive skills, and learn and retrieve information. **Optimal arousal** enhances academic performance, behavioral control, and socialization.

Behaviors associated with optimal arousal:

- Being alert/available for learning
- Focusing/sustaining attention to task
- Attending to details
- Initiating assignments/tasks/activities
- Persisting on assignments/tasks/activities until completion
- Performing consistently from one day/week to the next
- Self-regulating cognitions/behaviors/emotions
- Having flexible cognitions/behaviors/emotions
- Generating ideas/plans/solutions to problems
- Organizing efficiently
- Using effective strategies
- Reasoning abstractly/drawing conclusions
- Learning/remembering information
- Solving problems
- Socializing appropriately
- Recognizing the feelings/needs of others

Cognitive Processing Speed

Processing speed refers to the pace and automaticity with which the student accumulates, assimilates, and integrates incoming information; retrieves information stored in long-term memory; and performs cognitive tasks. Processing speed influences attention, executive functions, memory, academic achievement, behavior, and social competence. Cognitive processing speed gradually increases throughout childhood and adolescence. (1, 2)

Behaviors suggestive of adequate processing speed:

- Processing oral/written information rapidly/fluently/automatically
- Sustaining attention to task
- Understanding and following instructions/explanations
- Retrieving on demand information stored in long-term memory
- Finishing tasks/activities/assignments/tests in the allotted time
- Attending to/understanding/participating in social interactions

Section I

ATTENTION

Attention is a fundamental cognitive function. Two basic components of attention – **focus** and **sustain** – are particularly relevant to the school setting.

Focus – ability to recognize and select the most important information for further processing and ignore unimportant stimuli.

Sustain – ability to maintain attention, resist distractions, and persist until task completion.

The ability to focus attention reaches maturity by 7-10 years of age. Sustained attention gradually increases until age 11 after which rapid development continues into adolescence. (3, 4)

Behaviors associated with ability to focus and sustain attention:

- Being optimally aroused
- Appearing "motivated" when confronted with goal-oriented tasks
- Screening out auditory/visual/tactile/mental distractions
- Listening to school personnel/parents/peers
- Following oral and written instructions/explanations
- Knowing/using strategies
- Remaining on-task to completion
- Taking notes/copying from board
- Reading independently
- Focusing on main ideas/important details when reading/listening
- Expressing ideas in writing
- Performing mental calculations
- Solving math calculations/word problems
- Following the sequence of math operations
- Displaying consistent academic performance
- Completing assignments/homework/long-term reports/projects independently
- Remembering materials needed for tasks/activities
- Knowing/using effective study skills
- Completing homework efficiently
- Engaging in age-appropriate social interactions

INHIBITION

Inhibition is the ability to manage or control impulsive thoughts, behavior, and emotions. Self-regulation matures between 6-8 years, with significant improvement noted until 10 years. (5)

Behaviors reflecting adequate self-control:

- Stopping/thinking before acting/speaking
- Interrupting/changing one's response/action/behavior when needed
- Suppressing/ignoring disruptive, irrelevant internal/external distractions
- Using internalized language to monitor, control, regulate thoughts/behaviors/emotional reactions
- Coping with anxiety/frustration/stress/anger
- Separating thoughts from feelings
- Delaying gratification/reinforcement

CHAPTER 5
EXECUTIVE FUNCTIONS

Executive Functions (EF) are overlapping skills that have a direct impact on school performance, behavioral control, and social interactions. There is no current consensus on the specific processes comprising executive functions. They have been variously defined as follows:

- Executive functions require "attention to the future and comprise control processes which involve inhibition and delay of responding, maintenance of anticipatory set/preparedness to act, and planning of sequences of selected actions. Efficiency and productivity are observable outcomes of these constructs." (p. 266) (1)

- EF involve "selective and sustained attention, inhibition of verbal and nonverbal responses, strategic memorization, self-monitoring, planning and sequencing of complex behaviors, and management of time and space." (p. 307) (2)

- "The executive functions consist of those capacities that enable a person to engage successfully in independent, purposive, self-serving behavior." (p. 42) (3) EF comprise four components:

    a) <u>Volition</u> – capacity to understand needs and wants, to generate a goal, and to establish an "intention" to carry out the goal.

    b) <u>Planning</u> – ability to identify and organize the steps and materials needed to carry out the goal, consider alternatives, and make decisions.

    c) <u>Purposive Action</u> – ability to put the plan into action, be flexible and shift the course of action as needed.

    d) <u>Effective Performance</u> – ability to self-monitor and self-correct.

- Executive function is "the ability to maintain an appropriate problem-solving set for attainment of a future goal. This set can involve one or more of the following:

    a) intention to inhibit a response or defer it to a later more appropriate time,

    b) strategic plan of action sequences,

    c) a mental representation of the task, including the relevant stimulus information encoded into memory and the desired future goal-state." (p. 201) (4)

- "Attention is essentially a name for the integrated operation of the executive functions of the brain . . . The management system of the brain . . . involves organizing and setting priorities, focusing and shifting focus, regulating alertness, sustaining effort, and regulating the mind's processing speed and output. It also involves managing frustration and other emotions, recalling facts, using short-term memory, and monitoring and self-regulating action." (pp. 12, 14) (5)

- Executive functions are neurological control or self-regulatory functions that organize and direct all cognitive activity, emotional response, and overt behavior when confronted with new, unfamiliar problem-solving situations. EF include "ability to initiate behavior, inhibit competing actions or stimuli, select relevant task goals, plan and organize a means to solve complex problems, shift problem-solving strategies flexibly when necessary, and monitor and evaluate behavior." (p. 1) (6)

Section I

For the purposes of this handbook, executive functions are considered to include the following:

> **Problem Solving (Tasks/Activities/Situations)**
>   **Goal Setting**
>   **Planning**
>   **Proposal/Analysis (Ideas/Solutions/Strategies)**
>   **Prioritization**
>   **Organization/Sequencing**
>   **Time Management**
> **Flexibility (Cognitions/Behaviors/Emotions)**
> **Initiation/Execution (Tasks/Activities)**
> **Self-Monitoring/Use of Feedback/Self-Correction**

- Research studies suggest that executive functions follow a developmental course that begins in childhood and continues through early adolescence. The most significant age-related development occurs in the 5-8 year range with more moderate changes during 9-12 years. Mastery of most functions is achieved by adolescence. The course of EF development is considered consistent with the maturation of the brain. (7, 8, 9, 10)

  - <u>Goal setting</u> skills gradually develop until 11-12 years.
  - Simple <u>planning</u> skills may be observed as young as 5-6 years, but continue to develop through adolescence.
  - Ability to <u>organize</u> and <u>use strategies</u> is achieved by 11-13 years.
  - <u>Flexibility</u> reaches maturity by late childhood (8-10 years).
  - Maturation of <u>self-monitoring</u> is attained by 9-12 years.

Problem Solving (Solution of Tasks/Activities/Situations) – ability to define the nature of a problem; set a goal; propose strategies; prioritize, organize, and sequence the steps/skills/materials needed to achieve the goal; and estimate and allocate the time needed to accomplish the goal.

Behaviors associated with effective and efficient problem solving:

Goal Setting
Examining/identifying/analyzing demands of task/problems/situations
Understanding what needs to be accomplished
Anticipating/foreseeing/predicting outcomes of future tasks/activities/situations
Setting realistic goals

Planning
Proposal/Analysis (Ideas/Solutions/Strategies)
  Formulating spontaneously ideas/solutions/strategies for solving tasks/problems/situations
  Identifying/predicting cause-effect/solutions to problems
  Assessing best strategy for accomplishing goals associated with tasks/activities/situations

Prioritization
  Determining importance of various ideas/tasks/activities
  Judging essential from nonessential information

Organization/Sequencing
Organizing thoughts/actions/behavior
Analyzing/breaking down/ordering steps needed to complete tasks/assignments/
  long-term projects
Using strategies to perform tasks/activities and solve problems
Following steps needed to accomplish tasks/assignments/problems
Using a structured approach when learning new information/studying
Interpreting multi-step explanations/instructions
Organizing time/space/materials/belongings

Time Management
Estimating time accurately
Recognizing how long it takes to complete assignments/tests/homework/reports/
  projects
Allocating enough time to complete assignments/reports/projects
Structuring time when confronted with numerous tasks to be completed
Knowing when to start tasks/assignments/solve problems in order to finish in the
  allotted time
Working neither too quickly nor too slowly
Accomplishing most important tasks and not wasting time on unimportant activities
Following a schedule
Using a calendar
Meeting due dates and deadlines

Flexibility – ability to adapt, change, or shift one's responses, behavior, and emotional reactions when confronted with new, unfamiliar, or unexpected tasks, activities, and situations.

Behaviors associated with a flexible response style:

Generating diverse ideas
Processing several ideas simultaneously
Analyzing task demands/problems/situations
Considering alternative responses/options in light of new information
Forming new ideas/opinions
Assessing best strategy for accomplishing goals associated with tasks/activities/situations
Reasoning abstractly
Making inferences
Identifying cause-and-effect
Envisioning or predicting outcomes
Altering plan in order to manage changing circumstances
Modifying behavior/trying new ways of reacting when confronted with frustration/problems
Generalizing from one situation to another
Adapting easily to transitions/changes in routine
Evaluating/adapting/responding appropriately to complex, unfamiliar social situations
Taking into consideration perspective of others (understanding teacher's/parent's/peer's
  point of view)

Section I

Once the **goal** has been set and the **plan** has been determined, the student must **initiate** and **execute** the plan.

Initiation/Execution – ability to begin and carry out a task or activity without prompts.

Behaviors suggestive of proper initiation/execution:

Beginning tasks/activities easily and at appropriate time
Initiating tasks/activities even when considered uninteresting or "BORING"
Finishing tasks/activities within a reasonable time frame
Understanding that tasks are not finished until all details are completed and work is turned in

Execution of the plan requires continual **monitoring, use of feedback,** and **editing** so that changes can flexibly be made as needed.

Self-Monitoring – ability to identify and evaluate one's own performance and behavior before, during, and after a task, activity, or situation.

Behaviors demonstrating the ability to self-monitor:

Recognizing/acknowledging one's own strengths and weaknesses
Identifying mistakes while completing tasks/activities/socializing
Asking for help when needed
Perceiving the impact of one's own behavior on self/others

Use of Feedback – ability to use feedback to correct mistakes and adjust behavior.

Behaviors reflecting the utilization of feedback:

Responding appropriately to positive reinforcement (rewards)
Accepting feedback from teachers/parents/peers
Altering behavior/actions in response to feedback cues
Learning from past mistakes and consequences
Using feedback to build self-confidence

Self-Correction – ability to independently correct mistakes and adjust behavior in response to monitoring and feedback.

Behaviors reflective of the ability to self-correct:

Using strategies to detect and correct mistakes
Revising/adapting responses during tasks/activities/situations
Adapting/responding appropriately to complex/unfamiliar situations

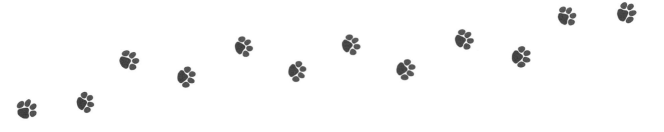

> **Goal Setting:** "What is the problem? I have difficulty recalling the steps I should use to solve division problems."
>
> **Planning:** "I need to think of a strategy that will help me remember. Which division strategy should I choose?"
>
> **Proposal/Analysis of Solutions:** "I can use 'Daddy, Mother Sister, Brother' or 'Dirty Marvin Smells Bad.' I have a hard time remembering the sequence of the first strategy so I think the best one might be 'Dirty Marvin Smells Bad.'"
>
> **Organization/Sequencing:** "First is 'Dirty' – So I Divide. Second is 'Marvin' – So I Multiply. Next is 'Smells' – I Subtract. Finally is 'Bad' – I Bring down."
>
> **Time Management:** "I need to finish the assignment in 30 minutes. That means I have 3 minutes to complete each problem."
>
> **Initiation/Execution:** "I need to get started and finish my assignment."
>
> **Self-Monitoring:** "Am I following all the steps of the strategy in the right order? Am I making any calculation errors?"
>
> **Use of Feedback:** "The last time I tried to solve division problems I made many errors. I kept adding when I should have been subtracting. I need to check."
>
> **Self-Correction:** "Oh, I added here instead of subtracting. I'll correct this error."

Figure 5.1. Example of Intact Executive Functioning

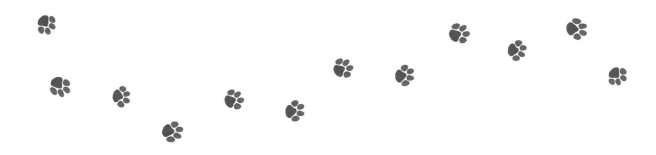

CHAPTER 6
MEMORY
SHORT-TERM MEMORY

Immediate Memory (sensory register) – brief recognition of verbal, visual, and/or tactile stimuli that lasts for only milliseconds. Any sensory information that does not attract attention disappears from immediate memory.

Information that is registered advances to working memory.

Working Memory (WM) – process by which information is temporarily held in mind while complex tasks are performed and problems solved. Working memory is often compared to the computer's Random Access Memory (RAM) that stores information "online" during processing.

- A current conceptualization of working memory posits that WM consists of four components. (1, 2, 3)

    - Verbal short-term working memory (phonological) – maintains both spoken and written materials and nameable objects. Verbal short-term memory is of limited duration (2-3 seconds) unless the information is preserved through subvocal rehearsal (whispered repetition of that which was heard or read).

    - Visual-spatial short-term memory (visual-spatial sketch pad) – temporarily stores nonverbal information.

    - Workspace or processing component (central executive) – is responsible for the coordination of attention, information in phonological and visual-spatial storage, and cognitive processing (e.g., determining what is relevant or not, forming associations, reasoning, analyzing and synthesizing information, applying strategies for encoding).

    - Integrative component (episodic buffer) – is a temporary storage space that handles the flow of information between working memory and long-term memory and is considered to also hold information not maintained in the verbal and visual stores.

- WM follows a developmental course with improvement continuing through adolescence. The development of working memory is consistent with the maturation of the brain. (4, 5, 6)

    - Recognition memory (remembering with the assistance of cues or bits of information) is fully developed by 9-10 years of age. (5, 6)

    - Verbal or phonological working memory is not fully developed until the teenage years. Subvocal rehearsal to enhance storage often is used after the age of 7-8. (6, 7, 8)

    - Visual-spatial working memory may be exhibited by students as young as 5-6 years of age, but gradually develops until early adolescence when adult levels of performance are achieved. (7, 8) Nonverbal information is increasingly changed by students into words for processing.

    - The ability to store information is age dependent. A normally developing 7-8-year-old student is able to hold in working memory 3 pieces or chunks of information, an 11-year-old 4-5 items, and a 15-year-old 7 chunks. (4, 9)

Section I

- The ability to both store and process information depends on the familiarity and complexity of the WM tasks. Performance on tasks that require minimal storage and processing (remembering and reproducing short lists of words or numbers) develops at an earlier age than on those that demand considerable maintenance and manipulation (remembering information presented in reading passages or math word problems and then summarizing the material or calculating the answers to the problems). (6, 9) The ability to store and process unfamiliar and complex tasks is not fully developed until late adolescence. (5, 6)

- Working memory is limited in <u>capacity</u>. Its resources may be diminished by either the storage or processing component. If a complex task demands effortful processing, less space is available for storage. Conversely, as more storage is required to hold information in mind, less workspace is available. Intact attention, adequate processing speed, automaticity of skills, strategy use, and speed of retrieval reduce the need to remember and enhance the capacity to perform cognitive tasks. When the amount of information exceeds capacity, any new information replaces or deletes what was originally there.

    🐾 *The amount of storage and processing space available is different for each student.*

- <u>Speed of processing</u> significantly impacts working memory performance. (4)

- The ability to hold and process complex or unfamiliar information is <u>time limited</u>. Information is stored just long enough to process or carry out a task or activity.

- Working memory is affected by the <u>type</u> of content being processed. If the student has a strength in a particular area, the student will be able to efficiently and effectively maintain and process information presented in that modality.

- WM impacts the majority of skills that comprise <u>executive functions</u>. On the other hand, executive functions significantly influence working memory skills.

    Executive functions requiring/influencing working memory:

    Analyzing task demands
    Considering the outcomes of future tasks/activities
    Setting goals
    Planning ahead
    Generating/evaluating different alternatives to achieve goals
    Considering/predicting consequences of responses/behavior
    Drawing conclusions/making decisions
    Processing/solving tasks with several parts or steps
    Using strategies
    Thinking about and responding to positive and negative feedback and adjusting
      responses/behavior accordingly
    Generalizing (carrying over) to other situations
    Being aware of the passage of time

- Working memory is a predictor of academic performance. (4) It is also crucial for social competence.

Academic skills requiring working memory:

Oral Expression
    Thinking of and organizing possible responses before speaking
    Remembering what one was planning to say
    Retrieving precise word to use

Listening Comprehension
    Following and processing ongoing conversations
    Comprehending complex, lengthy sentences
    Remembering what has been said
    Following complicated oral directions
    Remembering information heard at the beginning of a teacher's explanation/lesson while listening to the rest of it
    Retaining teacher's question, while searching for the answer
    Holding a question in mind, while waiting to be called upon
    Listening to lecture and taking satisfactory notes
    Recalling what one was sent on an errand to do

Basic Reading Skills and Reading Comprehension
    Recalling automatically and fluently sound symbol relationships when confronted with unfamiliar word
    Remembering main ideas and details
    Recalling facts/ideas read at beginning of a page/chapter, while completing reading task
    Reading lengthy selections with several parts
    Generating ideas/solutions to solve problem situations in stories
    Understanding inferences
    Envisioning/predicting the outcome of events
    Determining author's purpose and opinions
    Retelling/paraphrasing/summarizing material
    Remembering answers to questions after a reading passage

Written Expression
    Separating assignments into parts/knowing when and what to do
    Remembering the organization/sequence of the ideas generated
    Expressing ideas in writing while simultaneously retrieving from long-term memory and integrating age-appropriate vocabulary words/proper sentence structure/correct spelling/capitalization/punctuation
    Recalling most relevant ideas/omitting less important information
    Being able to write and edit simultaneously

Math Computation and Reasoning
    Computing mental arithmetic problems correctly
    Recalling details of word problem while carrying out calculation
    Remembering correct procedure (carrying/borrowing/multiplying/dividing/algebraic formula) and its steps while solving problems
    Being able to simultaneously calculate and edit
    Retrieving math facts

Miscellaneous
    Remembering what one is doing while working
    Copying from the board/book
    Remembering homework assignments/turning in completed homework

Section I

Social Competence
    Creating and carrying out successful conversations
    Adapting/responding to complex and new social situations
    Remembering words/phrases/sentences/meaning of peer's communication
    Following topic shifts during conversations
    Maintaining thoughts while listening to another speaker and waiting turn to speak
    Recalling consequences of peer interaction problems in the past and using that information to adapt current behaviors

Long-Term Memory

Long-term memory – ability to learn, store, and maintain information over an extended period of time. It is permanent, limitless in capacity, and can be accessed repeatedly. Long-term memory is the computer's hard drive that contains all the "saved" items. However, unlike the computer which saves information with a file name, information is stored in many interconnecting files.

- Long-term memory involves two important components.

  - **Encoding/Consolidation (Learning)** – acquisition, filing, storage, and consolidation of information and skills into long-term memory. Variables that impact encoding include activation and elaboration of existing knowledge, organization, and strategy utilization. Sleep, in particular the rapid-eye-movement phase (REM), plays an important role in consolidating (organizing and reorganizing) recently acquired knowledge into a more stable and enhanced form. (10)

    Behaviors associated with effective encoding:

        Relating new information to previous knowledge
        Selecting/using strategies to learn rather than relying on rote memory
        Rehearsing verbal and visual information
        Organizing/classifying information to file logically
        Using verbal/visual/cognitive strategies
        Categorizing/chunking information

  - **Retrieval (Recalling)** – accessing information stored in long-term memory quickly, automatically, and efficiently. Retrieval depends on how adequately information has been elaborated, organized, and encoded. Retrieval requires either <u>recall</u> (remembering without assistance) or <u>recognition</u> (remembering when provided cues). Forgetting may result from ineffective encoding and consolidation or retrieval problems.

    Behaviors suggestive of efficient retrieval processes:

        Responding promptly to questioning
        Recalling information on demand
        Retrieving words and facts efficiently
        Producing precise answers
        Using search strategies to aid retrieval
        Remembering today what was learned yesterday
        Completing fill-in-the-blank tests successfully

There are several types of long-term memory that are relevant to the educational setting. These are often classified as explicit and implicit memory. Explicit memories are those that are consciously encoded and include semantic and episodic memories. An explicit memory task is one in which the student is instructed to recall facts or a previous event. Free recall, recognition, and cued recall are measures of explicit memory. Implicit memories are unconsciously learned and often involve specific step-by-step procedures (procedural memory) or specific feelings and emotions. Implicit memories which are remembered automatically without conscious effort or the use of strategies to facilitate recall.

- **Semantic Memory** – memory for meaningful facts, ideas, and concepts acquired through deliberate learning (e.g., vocabulary, math facts, history dates, Pledge of Allegiance).

- **Episodic/Autobiographical Memory** – recall of past personal experiences (e.g., field trips, vacations, special occasions, traumatic events).

- **Procedural Memory** – memory of motor, perceptual, and cognitive skills or memory composed of automatic skills that are so thoroughly mastered that they no longer need to be consciously recalled (e.g., knowing how to ride a bicycle, tie shoes, read, perform math operations, organize and prepare long-term projects, write term papers, establish friendships).

- **Prospective Memory** – "remembering to remember" – remembering to carry out a planned task/activity at a future time without being told to do so (e.g., remembering to check class assignments, take books home, look at assignment book, place homework in the bookbag, return completed homework to school, be on time to school and classes, meet friends, keep appointments).

    🐾 *Prospective memory reaches maturity during adolescence. (11)*

- **Strategic Memory** – remembering to use strategies (e.g., verbal, visual, cognitive, organizational, mnemonic) to maintain information in short-term working memory and to facilitate both encoding and retrieval.

    🐾 *Early elementary students are able to attend to and apply strategies when prompted to do so, but the use of strategies is not automatic. Spontaneous and effective use of strategies to encode and retrieve information is usually attained by 12 years of age. (12, 13)*

- **Metamemory** – self-awareness, understanding, and control of one's own memory. Metamemory also includes awareness of the need to use strategies, knowledge of different strategies, evaluation of the most efficient strategy for performing various memory tasks, and how to use a particular strategy most effectively.

    🐾 *Metamemory is normally established by age 12. (7)*

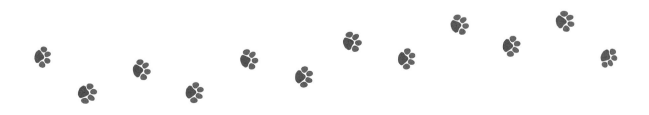

Section II
Resources

CHAPTER 7

MEDICATION/THERAPEUTIC INTERVENTIONS/ EDUCATIONAL AND COMMUNITY RESOURCES

ADHD, **TS**, and **OCD** are complex, chronic neurological disorders that often produce significant educational, behavioral, psychological, and social consequences for the student. An appropriate treatment program must be an interdisciplinary and coordinated team effort that addresses not only the symptoms associated with the disorder(s) but also the difficulties experienced in everyday functioning.

MEDICATION

Medication is often helpful for students diagnosed with **ADHD**, **TS**, and/or **OCD.** The use of medication is a decision made between the treating physician and the parents. A decision to initiate drug therapy is typically based upon the severity of the symptoms and the extent to which they are affecting the student's academic, behavioral, social, and emotional adjustment. When needed, medication often makes students neurologically available for learning and functioning in the school, home, and social environment. However, medication alone cannot remedy the academic, social, or psychological challenges of the disorder(s). (1) Currently, there is no medication that amelioriates problems associated with executive dysfunction, impaired processing speed, and memory problems.

The most definitive treatment study of children with **ADHD**, 7 to 9 years of age, indicated that, when the primary symptoms of the disorder (inattention, hyperactivity, impulsivity) were examined, medication alone was superior to other treatments. A carefully monitored and adjusted medication regime in combination with behavioral management (parent training, school consultation, participation in a summer program, classroom aide, contingency behavior management, clinical behavior therapy) was an effective intervention for treating the other problems associated with the disorder. (2) A 36-month follow-up study suggested that medication continued to relieve the symptoms of the combined-type of ADHD better than behavioral interventions alone. Regardless of the form of treatment, symptoms of the disorder improved with age but remained problematic when compared to those of the control group. (3)

 For tips on accommodating the side effects of medication consult <u>Challenging Kids, Challenged Teachers!</u> by Leslie E. Packer, Ph. D. and Sheryl K. Pruitt, M. Ed., ET/P (working title, manuscript in press. Bethesda, MD: Woodbine House)

AWARENESS EDUCATION

It is essential that students, parents, siblings, extended family members, school personnel, and peers become familiar with **ADHD**, **TS**, and/or **OCD** and the many manifestations associated with the disorder(s). These are complex neurological disorders with unusual and frequently changing symptoms. The symptoms may be affected by medication, as well as situational, emotional, and physical factors. Representatives from the local chapters of organizations such as the Children and Adults with Attention Deficit/Hyperactivity Disorder (CHAAD), the Tourette Syndrome Association (TSA), or Obsessive-Compulsive Foundation (OCF) are available to provide in-service programs designed to foster understanding and thereby reduce ineffective or inappropriate management. Advocates from local associations also present age-appropriate programs that educate peers about the symptoms of the disorders and their impact on academic and behavioral functioning so that teasing and ridicule are minimized. There are many resources (websites, DVDs, CDs, publications) that can be obtained from local and national organizations for use by schools and other groups.

Section II

THERAPEUTIC INTERVENTIONS

Anxiety Management

Approximately one-fourth to one-half of students with **ADHD, TS**, and/or **OCD** experience significant levels of anxiety. (p. 7, 16, 24) Anxiety management techniques are methods used to reduce or control anxiety. The most commonly used strategy is <u>relaxation training</u> (e.g., deep breathing, progressive muscle relaxation, visual imagery, yoga, self-statements of relaxation).

 While relaxation training can have a positive effect on anxiety levels and be used as part of a multimodal treatment plan, it does not cure the symptoms associated with the neurological disorder(s).

Cognitive-Behavioral Therapy

Cognitive-behavioral therapy (CBT) is an intervention that is regarded as the treatment of choice for students with anxiety and OCD. CBT is a combination of two types of therapy, behavioral and cognitive, that helps students understand the disorder, develop strategies to identify problem situations, and resist yielding to the obsessive thoughts and compulsive behaviors. (4)

 CBT has been demonstrated in several studies to be an effective treatment for ameliorating symptoms associated with child and adolescent OCD. (5)

- <u>Behavioral therapy</u> uses two techniques, exposure and response prevention, to change behavior and resist OCD. Initially, trained therapists and students make lists or hierarchies of the obsessions and compulsions and rank them from the most stressful to the least troubling. Intervention begins with the least anxiety-provoking situation. Homework is considered an essential component as many of the circumstances that produce obsessions and compulsions cannot be reproduced in the therapy setting. Homework provides a chance to practice new behaviors outside the clinic.

  - <u>Exposure</u> requires students to repeatedly face feared or avoided objects, thoughts, situations, or places that provoke intense anxiety. Through repeated exposure anxiety is reduced.

  - <u>Response prevention</u>, also called ritual prevention, involves having students refrain from engaging in repetitive, time-consuming compulsions. Through response prevention, students become less anxious and the compulsive rituals decrease and may be eventually eliminated.

    - *Comorbid attention, oppositional, conduct, and mood disorders interfere with treatment response due to inattention, overactivity, impulsivity, resistance, noncompliance, and/or underarousal during treatment sessions. Therefore, an assessment of comorbid conditions is essential before initiating treatment. (6, 7)*

- <u>Cognitive therapy</u> focuses on, questions the significance of, and reframes obsessive thoughts, assumptions, beliefs, and the need to perform the rituals. The trained clinician guides and encourages new, more positive patterns of thinking.

  - *A recent analysis of a large 5-year treatment program, the Pediatric OCD Treatment Study, found that combining medication with cognitive-behavioral therapy was more effective than either treatment alone. It was recommended that children and adolescents with OCD begin treatment with either CBT or a combination of CBT and medication. (8)*

- <u>Thought Stopping</u> is a technique that attempts to interrupt unwanted <u>obsessions</u>. Students forcefully utter "Stop!" and at times simultaneously snap rubber bands placed on the wrists. Once the thought has stopped, students think about something personally interesting and pleasurable. This procedure has been found to be helpful for some students with primarily obsessions and few compulsions. (9)

    > *Clinical experience suggests that <u>developmentally appropriate</u> interventions by a knowledgeable therapist can be used with some young children to interrupt and eliminate unwanted obsessions.*

Comprehensive Behavioral Intervention for Tics

Comprehensive Behavioral Intervention for Tics (CBIT) is a treatment that is used to decrease tics and nervous habits. (10) Generally, there are four components to CBIT which are taught by a trained therapist (Self-Monitoring/Awareness Training, Relaxation Training, Competing Response Training, and Contingency Management). (11, 12) Each segment is practiced separately and then combined into an integrated program.

- <u>Self-Monitoring/Awareness Training</u> is designed to promote identification, description, and knowledge of tic frequency. This is achieved through the use of mirrors or videotapes to observe the tics and of notebooks or hand-held counters to record the number of tics. Students are then taught to detect sensory sensations or internal warning signs that often precede tics so that their expression can be blocked. Students are also encouraged to identify environmental factors (persons, places, situations, or events in their everyday life) that increase and decrease symptoms.

- <u>Relaxation Training</u> utilizes anxiety management strategies (deep breathing, progressive muscle relaxation, visual imagery, relaxing self-talk statements).

- <u>Competing Response Training</u> helps students acquire socially inconspicuous muscle tensing responses which are incompatible with the tics and make them difficult to perform (e.g., pressing arm rigidly against side rather than jerking, keeping eyes tightly closed for a few seconds instead of blinking, putting clenched hand in pocket in place of touching others, breathing deeply through nose with mouth firmly closed instead of calling out). The responses must be able to be maintained for a few minutes until the need to tic dissipates.

- <u>Contingency Management</u> encourages significant others to prompt the use of competing responses and to frequently praise and reinforce successful use of awareness techniques, competing responses, and signs of improvement.

Recent research suggests that the most essential components are Self-Monitoring/Awareness Training and Competing Response Training. (13)

> *A recent review of the research using this intervention indicated that many studies contained methodological problems and addressed primarily motor tics. Based on the criteria established by the Task Force on Promotion and Dissemination of Psychological Procedures of the American Psychological Association, the investigators classified behavioral treatment as "probably efficacious." Further research is required before it can be classified as a "well-established" treatment. (14) Collaborative studies are currently being conducted at major research sites.*

Section II

Child/Adolescent Psychotherapy

Individual therapy is most beneficial when students are unresponsive to other forms of treatment (e.g., educational modifications and interventions, group therapy, social skills training) or when the emotional and behavioral problems are too serious to be handled in group therapy (e.g., severe and untreated anxiety, conduct disorder, bipolar disorder, depression). Individual therapy allows students to meet on a one-to-one basis with warm and impartial adults. The focus of therapy is to enable students to cope with feelings and conflicts caused by the disorder(s) and resolve emotional issues. Traditional insight-oriented psychotherapy does not cure the core symptoms associated with **ADHD**, **TS**, or **OCD** (inattention, impulsivity, hyperactivity, tics, obsessions, and compulsions). However, a skilled therapist who understands these neurological disorders may help students reframe and accept the disorder(s) and handle the challenges that accompany them. (1)

Traditional psychotherapy should never be the primary or only treatment for students with ***ADHD, TS,*** *and/or* ***OCD.*** *Insight-oriented therapy aimed at helping the students understand their problems by accessing unconscious thoughts and feelings is generally ineffective. Students with* executive dysfunction *(pp. 107-130) often have* difficulty prioritizing *the most important problems to be addressed, engaging in realistic* problem solving, *and* initiating *(knowing how or where to begin expressing themselves). During the therapy session, they may be* unable to self-regulate *their thoughts and feelings. While being bombarded by extraneous mental images and associations, they tend to become* disorganized, *ramble, and lose track of the issue being discussed. Additionally, students with executive deficits may* lack self-awareness *of the inappropriateness of their behavior and emotions which further limits the efficacy of this form of treatment.*

Group Therapy

Group therapy provides an environment in which students can meet with others who have similar neurological problems. Students become knowledgeable about the symptoms associated with the disorder(s) and how they are specifically affected by them. They share experiences, learn how to identify problems, and find solutions to those problems. The group setting restores a sense of normalcy and provides a safe environment to practice age-appropriate social skills and to receive realistic feedback from peers. Receiving support and acceptance often alleviates feelings of loneliness and isolation. Therapists monitor school and family functioning and intervene before situations escalate out of control. A review of research studies found that group therapy is an effective intervention for students with behavior disorders and social problems. (15)

Family Therapy

The cognitive and behavioral characteristics of the neurological disorder(s) can produce serious disruption within the family. Parents, siblings, and extended family members learn how to function as family units, manage the symptoms, handle interactions between family members, create supportive home environments, and relate more effectively.

Parent Support Groups

Parents of students with **ADHD**, **TS**, and/or **OCD** often experience higher rates of parental stress. Support groups provide settings in which parents can be heard by empathetic individuals who understand the problems associated with trying to raise neurologically challenged children. Group members offer assistance in dealing with the emotional reactions to the diagnosis of the disorder(s) (e.g., denial, anger, frustration, sorrow, depression, blame, guilt). Parents become familiar with the various manifestations of the disorder(s), learn effective parenting skills, and become knowledgeable advocates with doctors, family members, school personnel, and peers. (1)

Chat rooms are available for additional support, reassurance, and immediate response and feedback.

Chapter 7

Educational Resources

Most school systems have personnel who provide assistance or special education services when needed. These specialists are valuable assets when a classroom teacher needs recommendations for day-to-day management. (1)

Administrators

Administrators are the key to helping school personnel understand neurological disorders by scheduling in-service training and awareness workshops for teachers and peers as well as supervising the students' educational programs.

Educational Support Team (EST)

The Educational Support Team in each school meets on a regular basis to consider the needs of students having problems in the regular classroom. The EST may be composed of an administrator, one or two teachers, a special education teacher, school psychologist, counselor, and other support personnel as needed. EST members brainstorm with classroom teachers to develop modifications and strategies to help students circumvent problems and remain in the regular classes. If those modifications do not help students make sufficient progress, the team considers whether psychoeducational, neuropsychological, or other evaluations are warranted. (1)

 The EST has different names in different schools systems (e.g., Student Support Team).

Learning Disability Teachers (LD)

Learning disability teachers are trained to provide services to students experiencing academic problems. Classroom teachers often consult with LD teachers to obtain strategies for accommodating students' cognitive styles and special learning needs. Resource rooms are often made available on a flexible basis to students who require additional academic support, quiet places to finish assignments and take tests, or respite from the pressures of regular classrooms. (1)

Speech and Language Pathologists (SLP)

Speech and language pathologists evaluate and provide therapy for students who are having difficulty expressing or processing language. SLPs are trained to remediate problems with articulation, auditory processing, expressive and receptive language development, word retrieval, and pragmatic language use. SLPs also work with students who are having difficulty expressing ideas in writing due to language problems. (1)

Occupational Therapists (OT)

Occupational therapists evaluate and remediate problems affecting the motor and perceptual skills required by the activities of daily living, fine motor coordination, graphomotor functioning (handwriting), visual perception, visual-motor integration, motor planning, and sensory integration. OTs use special exercises and activities to improve deficit areas. In addition, OTs provide adaptive methods and equipment, if needed. (1)

School Counselors

School counselors are available to provide emotional support to students and to conduct social cognition and therapeutic groups. Counselors lead awareness workshops that help classmates understand the nature of handicapping condition(s) and needs of the students. In addition, they offer assistance in scheduling and programming decisions and assist in large and small group testing. (1)

Section II

School Psychologists

School psychologists are trained in the areas of assessment, academic instruction, classroom management, social interaction, family structure, and parenting. School psychologists conduct psychoeducational evaluations to determine the intellectual ability, learning styles, academic achievement, and emotional functioning of students with learning problems. The obtained information is then used to develop an appropriate educational plan. School psychologists consult with teachers, principals, and other educators and provide them with information regarding **ADHD**, **TS**, and **OCD** executive dysfunction, slow processing speed, and memory problems. (1)

Assistive Technology Consultants

Assistive technology consultants evaluate students to determine whether they are eligible for a technology device or product that can be used to increase, maintain, or improve the functional capabilities of students with disabilities. Technology consultants evaluate students' strengths and weaknesses, personal interests, and specific tasks or functions to be performed (reading, writing, math, organization, time management). They determine the most appropriate compensatory equipment and assist with the selection, acquisition, and the use of the devices. Assistive technology may include "low tech" tools, such as headphones, tape recorders, books on tape, or hand-held calculators to "high tech" equipment, such as personal computers, spell checkers, word processing programs, speech recognition systems, or converters of electronic text to synthetic speech. Assistive technology evaluations are available to students with IEPs and 504 contracts and often result in school systems providing devices that ease work production.

Academic Mentors/Assistants

Mentors, usually school personnel, provide support, structure, and strategies. Assistants meet with the students on a regular basis to set realistic academic and social goals (e.g., increase completion of assignments, follow daily and weekly schedules, inhibit aggressive responses to teasing), to develop problem solving skills, to help with organization and time management, and to evaluate performance. Assistants meet with the teachers and try to prevent academic problems before they occur.

Home-School Case Managers

Case managers establish home-school management programs that foster communication between parents and teachers. Cooperation then enables students to view their parents and teachers as respected authority figures working together for their success. Behavior management programs are developed to provide consistency between the home and the school and to teach students responsibility, the value of hard work, and respect for self and others. Rewards/privileges or consequences both at school and at home are based on work completion and appropriate behavior. (1)

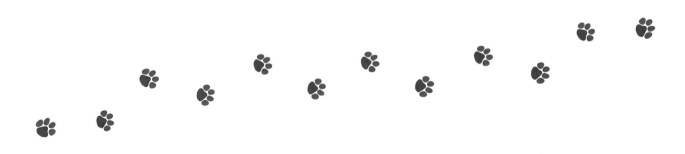

Chapter 7

COMMUNITY RESOURCES

Pediatric (Child) Neuropsychologists

Pediatric neuropsychologists are licensed psychologists with advanced degrees and specialized training and experience in understanding brain-behavior relationships. They apply knowledge pertaining to brain function and development, as well as information from other areas of psychology, to the evaluation and treatment of students with neurological disorders such as **ADHD, TS, OCD,** closed head injuries, seizure disorders, or learning disabilities. Neuropsychologists evaluate attention, intelligence, language, speed of processing, executive functions, memory, fine motor and graphomotor skills, auditory and visual processing, sensory perception, academic achievement, and emotional functioning. They analyze test results and design educational programs and treatment plans. Many pediatric neuropsychologists work closely with schools to help them provide appropriate educational programs for students with special needs. (1)

Educational Consultants/Educational Therapists

Educational consultants and therapists are professionals with specialized training in the evaluation, remediation, case management, and advocacy for students with learning problems and special needs. They offer awareness education to teachers, parents, and siblings so that the needs of the students are understood. They conduct school observations, perform educational assessments, and help design individualized educational programs (IEPs) and 504 plans. Remediation of academic deficiencies, executive dysfunction, and memory problems, is an important component of their work. Advice regarding regular, special education, or college placement options is often available.

Educational therapists are professional members of the Association of Educational Therapists (AET) who have met requirements in the academic areas of elementary and/or secondary education, child development, educational assessment, learning theory, learning disabilities, and principles of educational therapy. Many members have graduate degrees and are Professional Educational Therapists (ET/P) or Board Certified Educational Therapist (BCET).

 Educational consultants have different specialties. It is important to locate a consultant with specific training and interest in the disorders and areas needed.

Tutors

Tutors are private instructors who remediate various academic deficits, executive dysfunction, and memory problems. Some are credentialed professionals. Others are high school and college students who are proficient in specific subjects. Tutors help students understand academic materials, complete classwork, and study for tests.

Coaches

Coaches are professionals who are knowledgeable about **ADHD, TS, OCD, EDF**, and working memory; understand their challenges; and guide the development of problem solving skills and coping strategies. Coaching is a pragmatic, behavior-oriented intervention that involves a supportive, ongoing relationship between "coaches" (trusted adults - not parents or therapists) and students. Coaches help students increase self-awareness of strengths; establish realistic goals; identify obstacles to achieving those goals; and delineate practical, specific strategies for achieving the goals. Typically a coaching session consists of reviewing the goals and plans made at the previous session; evaluating whether they were met; determining what needs to be accomplished before the following meeting; and providing support, encouragement, and motivation.

Section II

Social Skills Trainers

Students with **ADHD**, **TS**, and/or **OCD** may not acquire age-appropriate social skills. Failure to successfully develop and maintain social relationships often results from impaired executive functions (pp. 107-130). Difficulty expressing ideas and feelings, understanding and responding to the feelings of others, recognizing the effect and consequence of behavior, and resolving conflict situations impacts social competence. Social skills training programs are highly structured, follow a set curriculum that is also recommended to teachers and parents, and are taught and practiced in small group settings.

Computer Consultants

Many students with **ADHD**, **TS**, and/or **OCD** have graphomotor (handwriting) problems. In addition, students with TS may have hand and arm tics that interfere with writing. Students with OCD may have compulsions to write, erase, and rewrite words. Direct instruction in computer skills, word processing, and/or use of voice-activated programs is a necessity. (1)

Advocates

Advocates are qualified and experienced attorneys, other professionals, or interested individuals who are knowledgeable about local, state, and federal education laws and policies. These experts understand the rights of the student with special needs, inform parents of the accommodations and services available to their child, and assist and support parents as they work with the school system. They help parents determine whether appropriate diagnostic testing has been completed, suggest referrals to other services if needed, develop individual education plans (IEP) and 504 plans, and ensure that the remediations, accommodations, and modifications detailed in the IEP are being provided to meet the academic, behavioral, and social goals.

SECTION III
INTERVENTIONS

> Children do well if they can.
> If they can't, we need to figure out why, so we can help.
>
> Ross W. Greene, Ph.D. (1998). <u>The Explosive Child</u>.
> New York, NY: Harper Collins (p.325)

CHAPTER 8
CLASSROOM MODIFICATIONS/ACCOMMODATIONS

Appropriate classroom modifications can create an environment that allows students with neurological disorders to succeed. Success promotes positive self-esteem. Consistency in structure, routines and limits, decrease stress and unacceptable behaviors.

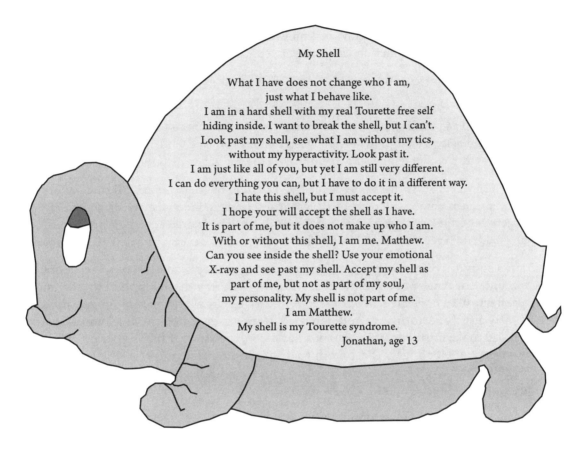

Figure 8.1. My Shell – Written by the brother of student with Tourette syndrome

- Provide awareness training for the school staff including an understanding of the complexity, unpredictability, internal and external factors, stress, and impact of medication on symptoms.

   🐾 *Peer education programs for students with TS are infrequently provided. (2)*

Section III

- Request teacher and peer education (disability awareness). Understanding diversity is important for all students. (1)

    - Promote empathy by having classmates act out symptoms associated with the disorder(s). For example, ask the teachers or peers to solve ten math problems and, each time signaled, stand up and change positions at the desk; try to read a passage for a few minutes and, when indicated, blink their eyes five times; or copy five sentences but erase each word twice and try to make it neater. This allows others to experientially feel the stress and frustration caused by a need for movement, an eyeblinking tic, or a compulsion.

    - Invite guest speakers to discuss individual similarities/differences and a variety of disorders (e.g., ADHD, allergies, asthma, autism, diabetes, epilepsy, learning disabilities, OCD, TS).

    - Utilize the health curriculum to teach students about neurological disorders.

    - Help classmates understand and accept the need for modifications. For example, some students cannot see well and need glasses; others cannot hear well and need to sit at the front of the room; some have difficulty reading and need to listen to books on tape; and others have poor handwriting and need to use a computer. Be sure to emphasize the special contributions each student can make.

    - Teach the concepts of "fairness" and "equality." Fair does not mean equal. All students are not the same; everyone is unique and must be educated according to individual needs. Frequently parents and teachers become too involved in wanting students to be treated equally. Work toward a level playing field; not everyone should be handled exactly the same.

- Maintain a supportive and stress-reduced environment that is conducive to academic achievement. The amount of attention and cognitive energy that is applied to learning is often a reflection of how the student feels. A negative school and classroom environment significantly affects performance and behavior. If the student does not feel emotionally safe to take risks, make mistakes, and display a handicap, the student may experience frustration, anxiety, stress, and/or anger. These feelings decrease attention and concentration, exacerbate hyperactivity, negatively impact executive and memory skills, interfere with learning, increase tics, and impair self-esteem. (1)

- Establish a school-wide policy of no bullying.

    - *The Health Resources and Services Administration (HRSA) of the U.S. Department of Health and Human Services has formed a federally funded campaign based on research-validated information entitled "Take a Stand. Lend a Hand. Stop Bullying Now!". (3) 30%-40% of students report frequently being victims of bullying, participating in bullying, or both. Approximately 20% are victims, 10% are bullies, and 10% are both victims and bullies. (4, 5) Bullying is defined as "aggressive behavior that is persistent, intentional, and involves an imbalance of power or strength." It is often "repeated over time and can take many forms. Many young people who bully see their behavior as justified. Many are viewed by peers and teachers as popular at school… Bullying is wrong and no one deserves to be bullied." (3)*

    - Be aware that bullying occurs in many different forms.

        - Physical – pushing, pinching, hitting, tripping, kicking

        - Verbal – teasing, name-calling, gossiping, harassing, embarrassing, humiliating, intimidating, threatening

        - Nonverbal – gesturing; deliberately avoiding, ignoring, excluding, rejecting socially

- Cyber – emailing; blogging; spreading rumors or writing negative, derogatory, insulting remarks on websites to victims or peers
  - Bullying can have physical, psychological, and educational consequences.
    - Physical – fatigue, headaches, stomachaches
    - Psychological – fearfulness, anxiety, helplessness, loneliness, sleeplessness, nightmares, low self-esteem, depression, suicidal ideation
    - Educational – academic underachievement, absenteeism, school avoidance
  - Recognize that students with **ADHD** are vulnerable to peer bullying. They are also more likely to bully others. (6) A survey of parents of students with **TS** indicated that 39% of their children experienced teasing and 28% were rejected. (2)

> **One of the teachers of my son with TS made it clear to the other students that there would be zero tolerance for teasing him about his tics. That was his favorite teacher and best year in school!**
> **A Grateful Mother**

- Follow recommendations offered by the HRSA.
  - Set clear and specific rules and expectations regarding bullying and repeatedly stress that it is unacceptable behavior.
    - *The teacher sets the tone and standards of the school regarding the treatment of students with disabilities.*
  - Establish a positive relationship with the student. Give permission and encourage the student to report bullying. Emphasize that there will be no consequences for telling about the incidents.
  - Take all reports of bullying seriously.
  - Help the student feel a member of the class.
  - Hold class meetings to discuss bullying, the physical and emotional consequences it engenders, and solutions to the problem. Design lessons that teach victims and those who observe bullying how to appropriately request help.
  - Be alert for signs of bullying and victimization and immediately intervene. An episode of bullying takes only a few seconds.
    - *Teachers have been found to have difficulty identifying students who are bullied and underestimate the extent of the problem. (5, 7)*
  - Provide close supervision in less structured situations (hallways, recess, P.E., cafeteria, restroom, bus).
  - Hold peers who bully responsible for their behavior.
    - *Recognize that the impulsivity and impaired social functioning associated with **ADHD-H/I** and **ADHD-C** may cause the student to bully and try to control others. Use cognitive interventions, social skills training, and anger management to handle inappropriate behavior. However, these interventions will not be effective when bullying is intentional and planned.*

Section III

- Meet <u>individually</u> with the student who bullies and explicitly explain that bullying is against the school rules and unacceptable. Consistent consequences will be administered no matter what the provocation, and parents will be notified. "The message for children who bully should be, 'Your behavior is inappropriate and must be stopped.'" (3)

- Do <u>not</u> hold a meeting between the bully and student or use conflict resolution or negotiation strategies. These interventions are based on the assumption that both the bully and student are involved. "Bullying is a form of victimization, not conflict." (3) The victim has done nothing wrong and does not need to negotiate, compromise, or change behavior.

- Challenge excuses that minimize the bullying ("I only said he was ticcing like a weirdo.") or place the blame on the student ("He kept on making those annoying noises so I hit him.").

- Help the bully view the situation from the victim's perspective so that the effect of the bullying is understood and experienced. Offer positive reinforcement when the bully is being kind, helpful, and responsive to the needs of the victim.

○ Encourage parents to report all incidents of bullying.

○ Help the student try to personally stop the bullying.

Suggest that the student:

- <u>always</u> tell a trusted adult (e.g., teacher, parent, school counselor, coach, relative) what happened. Provide accurate details - who, what, when, where, and how of the situation. Avoid "why" because the student is not responsible for the bullying. Discuss the feelings generated.

  > *The student must understand that reporting bullying is not "tattling" but the most important action to take. (3)*

- realize that the problem belongs to the bully. Do not accept the blame and feel guilty for being victimized. The cruelty was unwanted and unprovoked. Bullying is an attempt to have power and to control.

- try to stand up to the bully, if possible. Use self-talk to remain calm; pretend not to see or hear the bully and continue with the ongoing activity; smile, do not respond, and then walk away; calmly tell the bully to stop; or make a joke out of the teasing. However, do not fight back or bully the student.

  > *Sometimes a bully will stop when there is no reaction and power and control over the student cannot be achieved.*

- never respond to cyberbullying. Print a copy of the message to show to an adult.

- avoid situations that are likely to present problems. Remain with a friend or group of students (e.g., play with others at recess, sit with peers in the cafeteria, change classes with another classmate, sit at the front of the bus).

- join extra curricular activities and make friends with peers who have similar interests.

○ Enlist assistance from classmates and friends to "Take a Stand and Lend a Hand" to stop the bullying. The support of teachers, school personnel, peers, and parents reduces the distress experienced by victims. (8)

  > *A study involving 15,185 students revealed that 70% of students reported witnessing bullying. When observing bullying, 35% indicated that they ignored it, only 25% tried to stop it, and 9% joined in the bullying. (5)*

Suggest that peers:

- report all incidents of bullying to an adult. Tell exactly what happened using who, what, when, where, and how. Only 10% of students report incidents to a teacher or parent. (5)

  🐾 *Peers are often reluctant to report bullying for fear of retaliation by the bully, that adults will not consider the problem serious, or that attempts to intercede will make the situation worse. (5)*

- report cyberbullying and provide printed evidence.
- confront the bully and say that it is wrong to be cruel to another student.
- ask the other classmates to help.
- be a "buddy" to the student who is being victimized (e.g., playground, cafeteria, hall, bus buddy).

• Encourage administrators to increase awareness of bullying and provide training for effective interventions. A bully program should include the teachers and all of the school staff who are likely to be present when bullying occurs (e.g., playground monitors, coaches, cafeteria employees, custodians, bus drivers). Recommend an anti-bullying program such as *Take a Stand. Lend a Hand. Stop Bullying Now!* (3) or *Olweus Bully Prevention Program*. (9)

  🐾 *A comprehensive review of intervention programs to prevent bullying found that multidisciplinary school-based programs were more effective. Curriculum interventions (videotapes, lessons, written programs) did not consistently decrease bullying. Social and behavioral skills training, mentoring, and social work support had less positive effects. (10)*

• Provide consistent <u>classroom rules</u>, <u>expectations</u>, and <u>limits</u>.

  🐾 *If the rules, expectations, and limits are not understood or if they change frequently, students often remain in a constant state of anxiety and hyper-vigilance that interferes with learning.*

  ○ Select only a few (four to seven) of the most important rules.

  ○ Always state the rules positively. If a rule is phrased negatively, the student with **TS** may have an uncontrollable urge to do the action stated in the rule. The student with **ADHD** may have a milder, but similar, suggestibility and response. The student with **OCD** may perseverate on the negative rule. (1)

  ○ <u>Teach</u> the rules.

  ○ Refer frequently to the rules, expectations, and limits.

• Create a consistent, predictable, and structured <u>classroom routine</u> for the student to follow. An anxiety reaction accompanied by withdrawal or aggression may be the result of an unexpected change in routine.

  ○ Post daily work, schedules, duties, and homework assignments.

  ○ Follow the same schedule every day.

  ○ Design visual and cognitive cues that show what is expected.

  ○ Provide teacher-prepared schedules to assist the student with planning and organization.

Section III

- Hold <u>class meetings</u> to discuss rules and to solve problems.
  - Schedule the first class meeting as soon as possible after the beginning of the year.
  - Plan regular class meetings rather than meeting only when crises arise.
  - Allow all students to offer suggestions when making important classroom decisions (e.g., establishing classroom procedures; setting rules, limits, consequences; solving problems). Involvement promotes compliance.
    - *Students may give input but need to understand that the final decision belongs to the teacher.*
  - Provide assistance by mediating and offering solutions to problems occurring in the class.
  - Use a cognitive strategy such as "**GET A CLUE**" or "**PLAN**" (p. 109) to resolve problems (e.g., determining how to handle teasing and fighting).

- <u>Arrange a classroom</u> that provides support and assistance.
  - Place the student's desk in a location where most teaching occurs. This will allow monitoring of classwork and behavior so that more frequent feedback can be provided.
    - *If tics are severe enough to cause embarrassment, the student with **TS** may need to be seated in the back of the classroom or in close proximity to the door so that an unobtrusive exit can be made.*
  - Maintain visibility to and from all students.
  - Be sure that the student can be observed while working so that interventions can be made, if necessary.
  - Surround the student with peers who model appropriate behaviors and who will not encourage or stimulate inappropriate behaviors.
  - Provide a carrel for the hyperactive and/or tic-disordered student to use as needed. Reward the student for going to the "office."

- <u>Organize a classroom</u> that stimulates learning and reduces behavior problems. Organization allows the student to gain confidence in the ability to function independently. The more competence a student exhibits, the more motivation the student brings to each task.
  - Set up specific activity areas such as learning centers or labs.
  - Create quiet reading and studying areas, listening centers with headsets that play white noise or subdued music during work periods, spaces for small and large group activities, large tables for working on classroom projects, etc.
    - *Studies suggest that listening to background noise improves the performance of students with **ADHD**. (11, 12)*
  - Have clearly defined rules for moving between and working in the activity and study areas.
  - Place desks for completing assignments away from other areas. Provide adequate space between desks.
  - Arrange, if needed, a study area (carrel) separated from the rest of the class.
  - Designate a private area to which a student who needs some time alone can withdraw.

- ○ Keep busy areas (door, pencil sharpener, waste basket, group projects) away from quiet areas and learning centers.
- ○ Take into consideration the students' learning preferences (proper spacing, lighting, temperature, type of furniture). (pp. 65–67)
- ○ Modify the environment when the room arrangement is causing learning and behavioral problems.

- Organize resources and materials in order to reduce the frustration which accompanies the disorganization associated with executive dysfunction (EDF). (pp. 107–130)

  - ○ Minimize disorder by removing everything from the room that is not needed.
  - ○ Keep all materials and equipment in designated and labeled storage areas (e.g., reading, science, art, computer). Select a specific area for personal possessions.
  - ○ Place frequently used supplies next to each study and activity area. This lessens unnecessary movement, eliminates disruptions and confusion while preparing for activities, decreases the stress and frustration associated with trying to locate materials, and increases work completion.
  - ○ Color code all materials. Color code textbooks, notebooks, and folders. For example, the blue science book cover corresponds with the blue science notebook and folder. Copy assignments and handouts on matching colored paper, if possible.
    - 🐾 *Use the same color for the same subject every year.*
  - ○ Create labeled and color coordinated assignment bins for students to turn in classwork and homework (e.g., science assignments are placed in the blue container). Teach students to use them.

- Provide frequent cooperative learning experiences and group activities (e.g., working on a project, performing an experiment, writing and printing a class newspaper, making a bulletin board, creating a mural, completing an art project). Assignments that require working together increase attention, promote learning and academic achievement, develop communication skills, enhance social interactions, and improve self-esteem.

  - ○ Establish learning centers or work stations that offer a variety of materials and methods of instruction. Such diversity helps maintain interest and attention and provides freedom of movement.
  - ○ Schedule group activities when the student is most likely to successfully interact with others (e.g., before rather than following recess, lunch, P.E..).
  - ○ Assign the student to a group that will be accepting and supportive.
  - ○ Keep the size of the group small so that the student can frequently participate. If the student is unable to function in a group, plan an activity with one peer and gradually increase the size of the group as success is achieved.
  - ○ Highlight and point out interests shared between students.
  - ○ Guide the group process (e.g., "Before starting, let's brainstorm and allow everyone to have a chance to express an idea. Be sure to listen to all ideas without interrupting or making critical comments.").
  - ○ Predetermine roles and tasks (e.g., secretary, group artist, computer expert, research specialist, oral presenter). Capitalizing on the student's talents and interests, assign a role in which the student can be successful.
    - 🐾 *Students with **ADHD**, **TS**, and/or **OCD** often have well-developed computer skills.*

Section III

- Review group rules and expectations before beginning any activity.

- Monitor group interactions. Allow the student to return to independent seatwork when group participation becomes difficult.

- Frequently rearrange the composition of the groups to provide opportunities for interacting with different classmates.

CHAPTER 9
STUDENT INTERVENTIONS

> <u>Children Learn What They Live</u>
>
> If a child lives with criticism, he learns to condemn
> If a child lives with hostility, he learns to fight
> If a child lives with fear, he learns to be apprehensive
> If a child lives with pity, he learns to feel sorry for himself
> If a child lives with ridicule, he learns to be shy
> If a child lives with jealousy, he learns to feel guilt
>
> BUT
>
> If a child lives with tolerance, he learns to be patient
> If a child lives with encouragement, he learns to be confident
> If a child lives with praise, he learns to be appreciative
> If a child lives with acceptance, he learns to love
> If a child lives with honesty, he learns what truth is
> If a child lives with fairness, he learns what justice is
> If a child lives with security, he learns to have faith in himself and those about him
> If a child lives with friendliness, he learns the world is a nice place in which to live
>
> WITH WHAT IS YOUR CHILD LIVING?
>
> Dorothy L. Law (1959). <u>Children Learn What They Live</u>. Torrence Schools Board of Education Newsletter. Torrence, CA: Unified School District

General Interventions

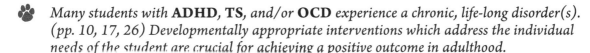 *Many students with **ADHD**, **TS**, and/or **OCD** experience a chronic, life-long disorder(s). (pp. 10, 17, 26) Developmentally appropriate interventions which address the individual needs of the student are crucial for achieving a positive outcome in adulthood.*

- Assign the student to classrooms with understanding and flexible teachers.

- Be <u>sensitive to the emotional needs</u> of the student.

  - Be patient. Be nurturing. Be supportive. Be positive.

  - Understand that teacher modeling has a powerful influence on how students with neurological problems are treated by their classmates. If the teacher is thoughtful in dealing with the symptoms, friendship and kindness will be exhibited by peers. If the teacher is not thoughtful, intolerance will act as a catalyst for insensitivity and rejection. This impacts the student's ability to experience academic and social success.

  - Separate the student from the disorder(s).

    - Think about and imagine the feelings experienced by the student.

Section III

- Instill the realization that the student is fundamentally a good person.
  - *Many students feel that they are "bad," "stupid," "lazy," or "crazy" because of their unusual behaviors.*
- Be aware of the internal distractions that the student is experiencing. Reported comments include:
  - **ADHD** student: "I feel like the ideas in my head are like popcorn and go in all directions. I can't hang on to them!"
  - **TS** student: "Oh, no! That great looking girl is sitting behind me and I have to try and hold in my tics. I can't concentrate on the teacher and do that at the same time. "
  - **OCD** student: "I worry that if I don't do everything 'just right' something bad will happen to my family!"
    - *Even if the symptoms of the disorders remit or are not observable in the classroom, do not assume that the associated problems (e.g., executive dysfunction, memory deficits, academic underachievement, impaired socialization) are not present.*
- Celebrate the uniqueness, special interests, and natural talents of the student (e.g., verbal, visual, artistic, musical, physical abilities). Incorporate them into classroom activities.
  - *All students possess different learning styles, strengths, interests, weaknesses, and needs.*
- Reduce competition between students. Emphasize cooperative learning. Many academic and behavioral problems are eliminated when students work together rather than competing.
- Be tolerant of mistakes. If the student repeatedly makes the same mistakes, do not focus on them. Instead, offer strategies for dealing with the problems.
- Reinforce the student frequently in front of peers both inside and outside the classroom. Emphasize what the student "can do" rather than "can't do." If the student can experience a sense of accomplishment, it will improve self-esteem and provide an incentive for appropriate behavior in the future.

- Maintain a respectful relationship with parents. Positive communication between home and school affects the student's ability to have a successful school year. Becoming angry interferes with finding solutions to problems.
  - *Teachers and parents must demonstrate mutual support and understanding and work together for the student's success.*
  - Express understanding and sensitivity to the student's unique needs.
  - Communicate appreciation for the student's positive characteristics (e.g., creativity, special interests and talents, academic strengths).

- Use cooperative problem solving with parents to generate appropriate strategies to help the student. For example, if the student with executive dysfunction has difficulty having the necessary supplies, ask the parents to provide a box of pencils and a ream of paper marked with the student's name.
    - 🐾 *Be aware that middle and high school students often resist using the interventions created by teachers and parents. The developmental task of this age group is to become less dependent on adults and to conform to the values and opinions of peers. Therefore, it is important to include students when designing interventions so that the motivation to use them is enhanced.*
- Establish daily communication with the parents by writing comments in the assignment notebook (pp. 116–117) or sending an email.
    - 🐾 *Some students have excessively large handwriting which does not allow room for the teachers' comments. It is often necessary to email, fax, or staple a separate sheet inside the front cover of the assignment book.*
    - Review <u>important</u> events (e.g., academic progress, behavior, activities, social interactions).
        - 🐾 *Avoid reporting only negative situations and areas of concern.*
    - Share information regarding special projects and long-term topics so parents can preview information and assist with their preparation.
    - Record homework assignments and provide suggestions for helping the student complete the tasks. This will negate the "I don't have any homework" statements.
    - Call the parents on the telephone or schedule a meeting if problems become too complex to discuss or solve with a note.
- Enhance a sense of mastery and control over academic and behavioral functioning. "<u>Learned helplessness</u>" is a concept introduced by Seligman which posits that some individuals learn that there is no relationship between what they do and their ability to master and control their environment. (2) The student who is confronted with frequent failure often learns that no response or behavior will impact a situation or alleviate a problem. The perceived inability to influence and control events causes the student to become discouraged, give up, place responsibility for learning and behavior on others, and respond passively as though "helpless." Learned helplessness often leads to a lack of persistence, impaired academic performance, social incompetence, low self esteem, and depression.
    - 🐾 *A positive school environment impacts beliefs about competence and self-control. A study investigating the relationship between a student's sense of mastery and control over school functioning and achievement indicated that self-perceptions develop around the age of 8-9 years. Researchers found that inattention negatively influences not only school adjustment but also self-perceptions. (3)*

Section III

- Structure learning experiences that reduce the chance of failure.
  - *Success improves motivation and self-esteem.*
  - Present teacher-directed and teacher-monitored lessons at the <u>instructional</u> level.
    - *Research suggests that when students are presented classroom activities at the proper instructional level (70%-85% of the information is understood), attention to task, work completion, and comprehension are enhanced. (4)*
  - Assign unmonitored seatwork and homework at the <u>independent</u> level.
    - *Understanding and task completion are adequate when learning materials are assigned at the independent level (90% of the material is familiar). (4)*
  - Assign no work at the <u>frustration</u> level.
    - *When students are provided work at the frustration level (less than 70% of the items are known), learning and on-task behaviors are negatively impacted. (4)*
- Grade work on <u>abilities</u> rather than disabilities. For example, grade the content of the science exam, not the handwriting, punctuation, or spelling.
- Allow mistakes made on assignments to be corrected. Permit tests to be retaken. Score the best effort.
- Use some <u>ungraded</u> assignments to evaluate knowledge and provide feedback.
- Emphasize what the student does right by marking the number of correct answers, rather than the number of incorrect answers.
- Provide acceptable choices to encourage success and active involvement in learning.
  - Offer a selection of assignments. Have the student choose the tasks to be completed, (e.g., present 8 academic tasks of which 5 must be completed before the end of the school day).
    - *If students with **OCD** insist on completing all assigned tasks, do not provide choices.*
  - Give positive reinforcement when the assignment is finished.
    - *For younger students or students who struggle to finish tasks, offer positive reinforcement for effort as well as completion. Use tangible rewards as appropriate for the individual student.*
- <u>Teach learning strategies</u> and how to use them to demonstrate mastery and control of academic skills and social interactions.
  - *Students with **ADHD** often cannot automatically generate strategies or solve problems.*
  - Suggest that the strategies be recorded in a list, on a chart, or in a <u>strategy ("trick") book</u>. (5) A strategy book is a collection of metacognitive strategies (thinking or learning "tricks") that the student accumulates from year to year. Strategies might be those used for reading narrative and expository texts, writing term papers, solving math problems, improving social relationships, and recognizing when to ask for help. Place examples of the student's work in the book to illustrate the correct use of the strategies.

    Advantages of the strategy book:

      The book itself is a physical reminder of the student's need to collect and use strategies to solve problems.

The teacher can cue the use of the "trick" book as an active, independent method for solving problems if the student is unsuccessful when attempting to solve problems, responds passively, or requires constant supervision.

Teachers and parents do not have to continually recreate strategies each time they help the student.

- Consult with the student periodically to review strategies and work samples.

○ Make sure the student is able to function independently. Doing too much for the student is as detrimental to self-concept as doing too little. The student needs to feel that success can be achieved without assistance.

- Encourage independent task completion, even if the work does not fully meet expectations.
- Offer praise, no matter how small the success. State clearly and enthusiastically comments regarding the student's ability to succeed. ("You organized your time well and worked on your report 15 minutes every day. Your report is ready on time!").

○ Help the student learn to accept responsibility for failure.

Ideally, <u>mistakes provide valuable learning experiences</u> and offer opportunities to correct errors. When mistakes are made, it is not time for students and others to get upset and angry. Prohibiting consequences prevents students from learning how to function successfully as adults.

- Use instructional methods that are congruent with the student's <u>learning style preferences</u> as proposed by Dunn and Dunn (6, 7). Learning styles are the ways in which students are best able to focus and sustain attention, apply executive skills, and acquire unfamiliar and complex academic and social information.

A large-scale analysis of research studies during the last 20 years which included over 7,000 individuals found that when students received educational instruction that was based on learning style preferences their attitude toward learning and academic achievement significantly improved. **"Students exposed to learning styles responsive instruction have an expected success rate of 70%. Students taught with traditional instructional methods have only a 30% expected success rate and, therefore, a 70% expected failure rate."** *(8)*

○ Assess at the beginning of each school year the student's learning style characteristics across a variety of learning situations.

Learning style preferences may change with age and differ for each academic area.

○ Determine the student's learning style by answering the following questions:

- Does the student prefer a quiet or noisy environment?
- Does the student prefer low, bright, incandescent, or fluorescent light?
- Does the student prefer a warm or cool environment?
- Does the student prefer sitting on hard (wood, metal, plastic) or soft classroom furniture (upholstered chairs, pillows, carpeting)?
- Does the student work best in a formal (chairs in rows) or informal study area?
- Is the student more alert in the early morning, late morning, afternoon, or evening?
- Does the student remain seated while studying or need to move?

Section III

- Is the student able to persist or need breaks?
- Does the student prefer learning and working alone, with a peer, in a group, or with an adult?
- Does the student internally structure tasks and activities or require external structure from adults?
- Is the student's motivation high or low? Is the student self-, peer-, or adult-motivated?
- In each academic area, through which sensory/perceptual modality does the student learn best (auditory, visual, tactile)?
- Does the student prefer to process information globally/holistically (understand the whole concept before focusing on details) or analytically (learn information presented sequentially and build upon existing knowledge)?

    🐾 *Teaching experience suggests that students with **ADHD, TS**, and/or **OCD** are often whole to part learners.*

• Design instructional methods based on Howard Gardner's theory of "Multiple Intelligences." (9, 10, 11, 12)

    🐾 *Teachers tend to provide instruction using their own learning style rather than adapting to the student's. That is often the reason why some students learn more easily with one teacher rather than with another.*

  ○ **Linguistic/Verbal Learner**

    Strengths: being responsive to spoken/written language – reading; writing; expressing one's self verbally; telling stories; joking, making puns; enjoying prose and poetry; having a large vocabulary; thinking/remembering with words

    Teaching Methods: provide a language enriched environment – use reading, listening, speaking, word games, computers, tape recorders, multi-media, lecturing

  ○ **Visual-Spatial Learner**

    Strengths: being visually-spatially aware - thinking in images/color; focusing on visual details; drawing, designing, building; solving jigsaw puzzles and mazes; reading maps

    Teaching Methods: design activities that use visualization – use drawing, art, designing/building models; look at videos, slides, television, pictures, diagrams, charts; use photography; furnish graphic organizers; give computer assignments

  ○ **Tactile/Kinesthetic Learner**

    Strengths: using whole body or parts of body to learn – moving; touching; handling, manipulating objects; participating in physical activities such as sports, exercise, games, dance, drama, role playing; communicating through body language

    Teaching Methods: present information physically and encourage interacting with space (moving; touching; manipulating; doing hands-on projects such as constructing, building, sewing, making crafts); use acting, role playing, miming

- **Logical/Mathematical Learner**

  Strengths: reasoning clearly, concisely, logically; being interested in patterns, relationships; questioning; experimenting; problem solving; making connections and drawing conclusions; using computers; learning math and science materials; using formulas; planning/utilizing time management skills

  Teaching Methods: use an organized, step-by-step approach to teaching; encourage categorization, classification; work with abstract numbers, patterns, relationships; provide logic/math games and mysteries; apply mathematical concepts to everyday activities

- **Musical Learner**

  Strengths: using rhythm, pitch, melody, and beat to learn - remembering through music and lyrics; singing, humming tunes, whistling; hearing rhymes, rhythms, repetitions in language; responding to music and sounds in the environment

  Teaching Methods: associate academic content with rhythm, melody, and music (e.g., listen to various songs from *Schoolhouse Rock*; use musical instruments, radio, stereo, CDs; tap out math facts rhythmically; permit studying with music; play music to calm/relax)

- **Interpersonal Learner**

  Strengths: socializing; empathizing; being diplomatic; understanding others/interactions; intuiting; leading/organizing; communicating; negotiating/mediating/problem solving; being "street smart"

  Teaching Methods: create cooperative learning experiences, seminars, class discussions, peer tutoring, study groups; assign interviewing and surveying activities; use audio/video/computer conferencing; provide personal attention

- **Intrapersonal Learner**

  Strengths: functioning independently; engaging in introspection; understanding self; being motivated to pursue personal interests, projects, hobbies; being intuitive/wise; having a strong will/confidence/opinion

  Teaching Methods: arrange independent study; provide self-paced instruction and learning; allow to set own goals, follow personal interests, projects; use books/diaries

• Incorporate more than one learning style into each lesson.

  > *Most students use each learning style to varying degrees. If students are unable to learn something through the preferred method, they may acquire the information through another modality.*

• Use technology to provide interactive teaching and learning.

  - Use computer-based software to help the student master academic skills and subject matter, remediate deficiencies, and provide enrichment (e.g., computer games and programs, interactive learning web sites). The best programs are appealing, present both auditory and visual input, and provide immediate feedback and rewards.

  - Suggest watching DVDs and listening to talking books.

  - Promote reading, writing, math, history, science, and problem solving with the use of an electronic interactive whiteboard. The board can be used to display Internet web sites, educational software, videos, Power Point presentations, and *Inspiration/Kidspiration* graphic organizers. (13)

Section III

- Use technology to bypass learning deficits (e.g., voice-recognition programs to accommodate written expression difficulties, typing programs for handwriting problems, visual mapping programs for disorganization).

- Recognize that research has consistently shown that students with **ADHD**, **TS**, and **OCD** have neurologically-based <u>graphomotor (handwriting) problems</u>. Handwriting difficulties in turn interfere with the ability to complete assignments quickly and effectively. (14, 15, 16, 17)

  - 🐾 *82% of students with **ADHD-C** and 57% of those with **ADHD-I** have been identified as having penmanship problems. (14)*

  - Provide remediation to the younger student in letter formation, automaticity, and fluency. Writing is a critical life skill that cannot be completely avoided (e.g., making lists, writing notes, taking telephone messages, filling out forms, taking the current SAT/ACT).

    - 🐾 *Pediatric occupational therapists teach handwriting skills.*

  - Recognize that handwriting is often slow and laborious. The need to finish the work within a specified time frame affects both legibility and content. Waive time limits on writing tasks.

    - 🐾 *Eliminating time constraints frequently reduces stress and anxiety enough to allow students to finish written tasks within the time limits.*

  - Understand that impulsivity associated with **ADHD** may result in rapid, unplanned handwriting that impacts legibility.

  - Maintain flexibility when **TS** hand/arm tics interfere with writing.

  - Be sensitive to **OCD** compulsions to write and rewrite words, count letters, or erase until the work is considered perfect.

  - Suggest using a pencil with soft lead or a mechanical pencil to relieve undue pencil pressure.

  - Provide a pencil with a gripper to help the student stabilize the pencil.

  - Allow either manuscript or cursive writing, depending on which is easier and produces better results.

  - Reduce copying aspects of assignments (e.g., provide a preprinted math worksheet rather than having the student copy the problems out of a book or off the board).

  - Modify writing expectations. For example, when the class is assigned the task of writing the definitions of words, provide the definitions and ask the student to highlight or underline the most important words or phrases. Alternatively, provide the definitions with important words omitted and have the student supply the missing information. If the class is required to answer questions in complete sentences, allow the student to select three or four and answer the rest in phrases.

  - Avoid requiring the recopying of illegible handwriting. Muscle soreness and fatigue can cause handwriting to deteriorate and produce stress and inappropriate behavior.

  - Grade handwriting separate from content.

  - Scan work sheets into the student's laptop so that the work can be completed on the computer.

  - Provide a partially completed outline instead of having the student write a complete set of notes.

  - Allow the student to dictate some assignments to a "scribe."

  - Suggest creating models, designing posters, making scrapbooks, giving demonstrations, or making oral presentations instead of writing reports.

- Allow <u>computer</u> use to offset handwriting deficits, to increase attention, and to assist with organization. (1)

  - Provide direct instruction in computer skills, word processing, and voice-activated software.

  - Modify and de-emphasize keyboarding instruction.

    - Do not require motor accuracy and mastery of home key position as prerequisites for the use of a word processor since impulsivity associated with **ADHD**, hand tics associated with **TS**, and the **OCD** urge to type and retype may interfere with accuracy and the ability to hold home key position.

    - Eliminate mandatory requirements for timed practice tests and long practice sessions. It is critical that the student view the computer with enthusiasm rather than another boring, difficult chore.

      - *The computer for the student with handwriting problems is like the electric wheelchair for students with mobility impairment.*

    - Assign short tasks or games that require accurate typing of responses.

    - Positively reinforce achievement.

    - Allow some responses to be dictated to an adult for transcribing on the computer until the student can manage longer sessions at the keyboard. If a "hunt and peck" approach is too slow and laborious, the student may become discouraged and not want to use the computer. As the student masters keyboarding, increase the amount of typing required.

- Teach, model, prompt, assist, and repeatedly practice the use of <u>self-talk strategies</u>. Self-talk helps increase attention to task, interrupt and control impulsive behaviors, generate and use problem solving strategies, modulate intense emotional reactions (anxiety, frustration, anger), monitor and adapt behavior, encode and retrieve information, self-evaluate, and self-correct.

- <u>Be flexible</u> and <u>adjust expectations</u> when the severity and intensity of the symptoms associated with the disorder(s) increase. (1)

  - *When symptoms are more noticeable, performance and behavior may deteriorate. The student may not be neurologically available to learn new information.*

  - Recognize that the student with **TS** and/or **OCD** may be so preoccupied with attempting to control tics and obsessions/compulsions that there is little cognitive energy available to sustain attention and perform with mental efficiency.

  - Understand that the student with **OCD** may be unable to stop a ritual such as checking, lining up, arranging, counting, erasing, rewriting, getting things "just right," and other perfectionistic behaviors.

  - Prepare and keep a packet of materials ready for use as a review for previously learned skills.

  - Allow use of the computer to reinforce previously learned skills. The student often is able to focus on the computer when focusing on other types of learning activities is impossible.

- Understand that a fluctuation in daily performance is a hallmark of many neurological disorders and is not due to a lack of caring or interest.

  - Do not penalize the student for uneven performance.

  - Have the student on "on days" complete enough work to reinforce concepts presented on "off days."

Section III

- Allow the student to choose as a mentor one of the school's personnel with whom problems can be shared.

- Utilize a peer "buddy" system to assist the student with tasks that are too difficult (e.g., a homework buddy to ensure that the homework was copied correctly and the bookbag packed with the necessary materials).

    - *Make sure that the student is comfortable having a buddy assigned and that the buddy wants the job.*

- Report all observations of medication side effects to the parents and doctor. Include both positive side effects (improved attention and concentration, reduction of tics and obsessions/compulsions, increase in work completion) and negative side effects (fatigue, sleepiness, thirst, nausea, irritability, increased anxiety and aggression, school phobia).

    - *Obtain written permission from parents before communicating with the doctor.*

- Allow the student to select, from a list of possible options, a safe place to go when symptoms become severe (e.g., nurse's or counselor's office). Use an agreed upon signal to communicate when it is necessary to leave.

- Refrain from retaining at grade level the student who experiences academic underachievement. Research findings fail to support the policy of using grade retention to improve learning and socio-emotional adjustment. Retained students have more impaired academic skills, are more aggressive during adolescence, tend to drop out of high school, and obtain poorer education/employment ratings when compared to groups of low-achieving promoted students. (18, 19, 20) Instead, design developmentally appropriate interventions based on the student's strengths to address academic needs.

CHAPTER 10
UNDERAROUSAL/SLOW COGNITIVE PROCESSING SPEED

Underarousal and slow, variable cognitive tempo impact the ability to sustain focused attention, to quickly and efficiently assimilate information, and to perform tasks fluently and automatically. Retrieval of information from long-term memory may be slow and require extra effort, thereby reducing the resources available to manipulate and integrate material. Slow processing speed may be experienced in one or more academic areas or be observed when the student is required to process information through the weakest modality (auditory, visual, tactile, motor).

The following behaviors serve as general indicators. The student will not exhibit every characteristic listed. These behaviors may also be indicative of other problems.

- Appearing fatigued/sleepy (yawning/putting head on desk)
- Looking bewildered/confused/absent-minded
- Seeming "lazy"/"unmotivated"
- Lacking persistence
- Moving slowly
- Appearing not to listen
- Avoiding tasks requiring focused and sustained attention
- Struggling to grasp/understand/follow instructions/explanations
- Being unable to pay close attention to details
- Becoming overwhelmed when confronted with complex information
- Processing slowly
- Hesitating to initiate assignments/tasks/activities
- Needing additional time to think/respond to questions/requests, even when knowing correct answers/behavior
- Answering questions with short, unclear answers
- Participating reluctantly in class discussions
- Having trouble quickly accessing information stored in long-term memory (vocabulary/math facts and procedures/history facts/science formulas)
- Possessing ability to do assignments, but being unable to complete them in the allotted time
- Having difficulty keeping up with lectures and taking notes
- Reading slowly despite having age appropriate reading skills
- Understanding math concepts, but being slow to recall math facts
- Expressing ideas in writing slowly
- Handwriting slowly despite ability to form letters properly
- Requiring extra time to finish timed tasks
- Completing homework/studying slowly
- Having difficulty finishing tests/proofreading/checking mistakes
- Exhibiting inconsistent academic performance
- Forgetting material learned yesterday

Research suggests that students with **ADHD** have processing speed deficits. (1, 2, 3) A "sluggish cognitive tempo" (SCT) or slow speed of processing characterizes one-fourth to one-half of students with **ADHD, Inattentive type.** (4, 5, 6, 7, 8) Cognitive slowing may also be associated with **TS** and **OCD.** (9, 10, 11)

Section III

Interventions for reduced cognitive speed that impacts academic and social skills can be located in Part IV and Part VII of this handbook.

Interventions

- Recognize that the student who lacks physical and mental energy is underaroused and insufficiently alert to perform adequately in the classroom.

- Determine if underarousal or a speed of processing deficit underlies the student's slowness in completing tasks and activities or if it is related to another problem (e.g., tic, obsession, compulsion, inattention, perfectionism, reflective cognitive style, graphomotor impairment, working memory deficit, sleep disorder). A neuropsychological evaluation may be required.

- Assess whether slow processing speed is format-specific (verbal, visual, tactile, motor) and/or content-specific (reading, writing, math, history, literature, science).

- Consult with the teacher(s) from the previous year to find out which interventions increased alertness.

- Teach strategies for recognizing and modifying arousal levels.

    Suggest that the student:

    - self-monitor alertness (e.g., feelings of tiredness, lethargy, or reduced attention in contrast to those of anticipation, excitement, energy, or full concentration).

    - compare task requirements to the level of arousal required (e.g., alertness needed to read a chapter in the textbook, write a term paper, listen to music).

    - adjust arousal if alertness is not congruent with task demands.

        - complete short segments of work with mobility breaks between tasks (read 10 pages, take a break).
        - utilize a computer when appropriate to increase interest and attention.
        - have a protein snack (e.g., cheese and crackers) before studying.

- Schedule, when possible, core subjects during the student's optimal arousal time.

    Fatigue and daytime drowsiness increase during the teenage years due to physiological changes in the body's circadian rhythms (internal clock that regulates the hormones and other chemical systems that physically affect functioning). Uncoordinated signals make it difficult to fall asleep early enough to get sufficient sleep and be alert the following day. (12)

    - Plan a subject of special interest to the student for first period.

- Provide many opportunities for <u>movement</u> to stimulate alertness. (13)

    - Use interactive teaching activities such as class discussions, group projects, and electronic whiteboards.

    - Permit changing work sites.

    - Give short movement breaks (e.g., stand up, reach for the sky, stretch arms and shoulders, touch toes, twist waist).

    - Ask the student to make a trip to the office, take a note to another teacher, sharpen pencils, hand out materials, collect papers, or get a drink.

- Suggest pressing hands together, doing push ups against the wall, kneading modeling clay, carrying heavy objects, or rearranging classroom furniture. (14, 15, 16)

  🐾 *For further information on these techniques consult with a pediatric occupational therapist.*

- Capitalize on the student's <u>learning preferences</u> when assigning academic tasks. (p. 65) Many students with **ADHD** are underaroused when confronted with dull, "boring," repetitive tasks, classwork, and homework. These students need the stimulation of new, different, and interesting assignments that offer immediate reward to maintain arousal.

  - Offer a variety of materials and methods of instruction through different modalities.
  - Alternate seatwork with other kinds of learning activities by creating learning centers, labs, or stations in the classroom.
  - Use games and hands-on projects.
  - Vary the pace and change tasks frequently.
  - Follow less interesting tasks with more interesting tasks. Have the student complete the first, less interesting, assignment before being allowed to perform the second, more interesting, work.
  - Allow the student to quietly recite the instructions or think aloud while following through on tasks. Using self-directed speech increases alertness. Arrange a place to work where subvocalization will not disturb the other students.

- Reduce the length and requirements of class assignments. (13)

  🐾 *Completing assignments is very tiring and frustrating for the student who processes information slowly.*

  - Provide work that can easily be completed.
  - Divide lengthy assignments into smaller, more manageable segments that appear as several independent tasks.
  - Assign shorter tasks requiring accuracy and quality of response.
  - Design cooperative learning activities to prevent the need to work on an entire assignment alone.
  - Permit use of a word processor, calculator, or tape recorder.

- Modify the manner in which directions are delivered.
- Present verbal information at a slower-than-normal rate.
- Pause frequently to allow time between statements for the material to be processed.
- Be alert for confusion and loss of focus. Repeat, rephrase, or summarize material periodically.
- Allow sufficient time to formulate verbal responses.

  - Pose a question to the class, call upon another classmate, then ask the student to respond.
  - Provide in advance a list of questions or topics that will be discussed during the lesson.

- Schedule frequent practice and rehearsal of cognitive and academic skills until mastered. When information is automatized, speed of processing increases.

Section III

Underarousal and slow processing speed may be secondary to a sleep disorder.

SLEEP DISORDERS

Sleep helps students learn and remember. During sleep, the brain reviews, reprocesses, and consolidates into long-term memory recently-acquired skills and concepts. These memories become more permanent and resistant to interference and, thus, enhance the ability to quickly recall information and efficiently perform tasks. (17, 18, 19)

Sleep-related problems are frequently associated with **ADHD** and **TS**. (20, 21, 22, 23, 24) Inadequate or fragmented sleep has been found to affect 48 percent of students with **ADHD only**, 26 percent of students with **TS only**, and 41 percent of students with **TS plus ADHD** as compared to 10 percent of typically developing students. (25) Students with **OCD** may stay up late because they feel compelled to complete all homework perfectly and perform compulsive routines before going to sleep. Furthermore, anxiety interferes with sleep.

A review of studies addressing the sleep disturbances associated with **ADHD** suggests that the most common problems include excessive motor movements and disturbed breathing during sleep. (26, 27) The severity of sleep disturbances may be impacted by comorbid oppositional, anxiety, and/or mood disorders. (28)

 Medication side effects often produce drowsiness or sleepiness shortly after being ingested and affect daytime arousal. Other side effects keep the student from falling asleep and make it difficult to wake up and become fully aroused.

Parent and student questionnaires indicate that students with **ADHD** have problems preparing for bed, falling asleep, waking up, getting ready, and remaining alert during the day. (29, 30) Sleep deprivation is cumulative and may lead to daytime feelings of fatigue, tiredness, or drowsiness; periods of sleepiness; irritability and emotional fluctuations; increased vulnerability to stress; and worsening of the symptoms associated with the disorders. (31)

General Interventions

- Be aware that normally developing 5- to 12-year-old students are usually optimally aroused and display little or no daytime sleepiness. Chronic sleepiness may be indicative of a sleep disorder. (12)

    Recommend that the <u>parents</u>:

    ○ complete the Sleep Survey. (32) (Appendix p. 404)

    ○ keep a sleep diary for several weeks. Record medication(s), early evening activities, foods consumed, bedtime routines, bedtime, bedroom environment (temperature, light, noise level), amount of time before falling asleep, behaviors during sleep, time of awakening, and ease of completing morning routines.

    ○ consult with a physician who is a sleep specialist if signs of sleep problems are present.

- Recognize that insufficient sleep affects focused and sustained attention (30); executive functions, especially working memory (33); academic performance (34); behavior (35); and socialization (35).

    The student with a sleep disorder should not be considered "lazy," "unmotivated," or "resistant."

Chapter 10

Difficulty Falling Asleep

The following behaviors serve as general indicators. The student will not exhibit every characteristic listed. These behaviors may also be indicative of other problems.

    Having too much energy to relax and settle down
    Resisting bedtime
    Becoming overstimulated by TV programs/video games/computer
    Getting upset at bedtime
    Tossing and turning
    Being unable to stop thinking/mind racing
    Overfocusing on events that occurred during the day
    Worrying/feeling anxious about unfinished homework/school incident/fight with family member or peer
    Fearing the dark/sleeping alone/weather/dangerous event
    Wanting parent in room to fall asleep/to sleep in parents'/sibling's bed

Interventions

- Offer suggestions for developing healthy sleep habits.

    Recommend that the <u>parents</u>:

    - encourage regular exercise in the morning or early afternoon rather than late in the day.

    - develop a <u>bedtime routine</u> that begins at dinner time and signals the body to calm down for sleep.

        - avoid having large meals just before going to sleep. Serve dinner two hours before bedtime to allow enough time for the food to be digested.

        - offer a light snack before going to bed. Dairy products such as a glass of warm milk or turkey contain tryptophan which induces sleep. Do not provide drinks or foods that contain caffeine (e.g., colas, chocolate) after 4:00 PM.

        - have the student take a warm bath 90 minutes before going to bed. While a bath may initially raise body temperature, the subsequent drop in body temperature may promote sleep.

        - refrain from overactive, overstimulating activities before bedtime. Instead, listen to music and/or read stories together.

        - limit all telephone calls, telephone text messaging, TV, computers, IM (instant messaging), and other electronic devices to one hour before bedtime.

            - *Television viewing, electronic game playing, Internet use, and mobile phone calling or text messaging after bedtime leads to sleep deprivation and impaired daytime functioning. (36, 37)*

        - avoid arguments and power struggles before bedtime.

            - *Clinical experience suggests that the best rule for avoiding power struggles at bedtime is to have no major questions answered, demands debated, or decisions made after 9PM (or before 9AM). Any discussion during that period is "off limits." The answer to all questions is "NO!"*

        - insist that all decisions about clothes for the following day be made at least one hour before going to bed. Organizing what to wear is as difficult as organizing term papers or cleaning rooms. (13)

            - *Organizing on Sunday a hanger of clothes for each day of the week will eliminate a great deal of stress on weekdays.*

- set a <u>regular time</u> for going to bed and getting up. Maintain the schedule seven days a week. Do not allow the student to "catch up" by sleeping late on weekends.

  > *Students require varying amounts of sleep to function effectively and efficiently. A 5-year-old student requires 11 hours of uninterrupted nighttime sleep, a 9-year-old needs 10 hours, a 13-year-old needs 9 hours, and a 16-year-old requires 8 hours. (12)*

- create a <u>bedroom environment</u> that is conducive to sleep. For example, maintain a comfortable temperature (neither too warm nor too cold), darken the room (use a nightlight if needed), or install blackout shades or curtains if early morning light interferes with sleep.

- suggest listening to calming music, white noise, or nature sounds to block out overstimulating household noises. Be sure the student listens to an audio tape, CD, or iPod and not to a radio or television program with distracting commentaries and commercials.

- consult with the student's physician if stimulant medication appears to affect the ability to fall asleep. The physician may adjust the dosage, change to a different stimulant, or try a nonstimulant medication. (38)

Difficulty Remaining Asleep

The following behaviors serve as general indicators. The student will not exhibit every characteristic listed. These behaviors may also be indicative of other problems.

Having excess energy/being restless/moving frequently
Feeling anxious/worried/fearful
Being easily awakened by noises/talking
Moving to someone else's bed
Having tics while sleeping (23, 39)
Jerking of the arms/legs/body (periodic limb movements) (23, 27)
Sleep-talking (somniloquy)/sleep-walking (somnambulism)
Snoring/difficult breathing (sleep disordered breathing) (27)
Experiencing nocturnal enuresis (bedwetting) (25)
Having unpleasant dreams/nightmares
Experiencing night terrors (waking up confused/crying/screaming/sweating/incapable of full arousal/inconsolable; being unaware of episode following morning)
Waking in middle of night (often at same hour – 3 or 4 AM)
Waking too early

Interventions

- Provide recommendations to maintain sleep.

  Suggest that the parents:

  - insist on a low noise level in the house.

  - use white noise such as a fan or provide earplugs.

  - limit fluids after dinner if the student is enuretic (bedwetting).

    > *7% of students with **TS-only**, 16% with **ADHD-only**, 25% with **TS plus ADHD** compared to 11% of unaffected students experience nocturnal enuresis. Bedwetting may be due to arousal problems, a developmental delay, or an immature physiological control system. It is <u>not</u> purposeful and should <u>not</u> be punished. (25)*

  - suggest screening for a mood or anxiety disorder if the student wakes at the same time each night.

Chapter 10

- consult a sleep specialist if sleep disordered breathing (snoring, difficult breathing, intermittent cessation of breathing) interferes with sleep.

Difficulty Awakening

The following behaviors serve as general indicators. The student will not exhibit every characteristic listed. These behaviors may also be indicative of other problems.

> Being unable to hear loud alarm
> Needing to be awakened by parent/sibling rather than waking spontaneously
> Being unresponsive to/unaware of person trying to awaken student
> Having a "storm" when unable to be awakened
> Needing frequent reminders to get out of bed
> Taking a long time to become alert
> Waking feeling tired
> Waking in irritable mood
> Dressing slowly
> Forgetting to groom self
> Oversleeping and missing breakfast
> Forgetting bookbag/homework/books
> Missing school transportation
> Being late to school

Interventions

- Recognize that failure to get enough sleep impacts the ability to awaken. Offer suggestions that help the student wake up independently.

- Recommend that the <u>parents</u> wake the student at the same time every day for thirty days and use the <u>Four Alarm Clock System</u>. (13)

  - purchase two dual alarm clock radios. Place one next to the student's bed and the other across the room.
    - set one of the alarms on the bedside clock radio to play music of the student's choice 45 minutes before it is time to get up. Allow the student to hit the snooze button several times.
    - set the other alarm on the bedside clock radio to sound an alarm 30 minutes before time to get up. Permit the student to hit the snooze button.
    - set one alarm on the clock radio across the room to play music on a different station of the student's choice 15 minutes before it is time to get up. Allow the student to return to bed.
    - set the final alarm on the clock radio across the room to sound when it is time to get up. Do <u>not</u> permit the student to return to bed. Have the student start getting ready for school.
  - insist that the student wake independently after thirty days of using the Four Alarm Clock System.

- Be aware that, once the student is out of the bed, underarousal may make completing morning routines very difficult and stressful. Students with **OCD** may feel pressured and become irritable because morning rituals must be performed "just so" before leaving for school (e.g., grooming, dressing). (13)

  Suggest that the parents:

  - encourage the student to shower after rising. Showering raises body temperature and increases arousal.

Section III

- do not allow the student to turn on an electronic device (e.g., TV, computer, hand-held game) as it interferes with getting dressed and eating breakfast. However, music of the student's own choice may reduce the stress produced by having to complete morning routines.

- do not criticize or lecture the student during <u>morning routines</u>. Waking, dressing, and leaving for school (a sometimes stressful destination) frequently produce overarousal. (pp. 81-95)

- have breakfast prepared and on the table.
    - encourage the younger student to eat breakfast to provide energy.
    - have available high energy health bars that can be consumed on the bus for the adolescent who refuses to eat. Low blood sugar levels, resulting from skipping meals, reduce energy levels and exacerbate fatigue, distractibility, and inattention.
        - 🐾 *The student with* **OCD** *may get "stuck" on a particular food or eating ritual. Drawing attention to the ritual increases the likelihood of the behavior continuing. The sensory defensive student may have an aversion to certain food textures. Trying to force the student to eat these foods is not worth a "storm" before leaving for school.*

- expose the underaroused student to a light therapy device or natural light (e.g., open curtains and blinds, use light therapy for about 30 minutes, suggest walking outside for 15 minutes).

- be sure that the bookbag that was packed the previous night is in front of the door through which the student leaves in the morning. Use this area to put anything that needs to be taken to school.
    - 🐾 *Refer to the area as the "loading dock" or "launch pad." The use of these terms allows an adult to address a problem in a way that is not interpreted as a critical remark.*

- apply natural consequences for missing the bus and having to be driven to school, (e.g., losing weekend privileges; not being allowed to stay up late, go to an arcade, play on the computer, drive the car, go out on Friday night; doing a chore for parent that takes the same amount of time that was spent driving to and from school).
    - 🐾 *Real sleep disorders are medical problems and do not deserve anger or judgment.*

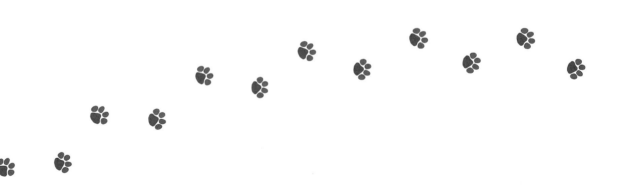

CHAPTER 11

ANXIETY/"STORMS"/OVERAROUSAL

Anxiety

Anxiety is a tendency to experience chronic and excessive fears or worries that significantly impact the student's ability to perform in the classroom and in social situations. The anxious student often feels "helpless" and is unable to effectively cope with stressful situations. About one-third of students with **ADHD** (p. 7) and more than one-half of those with **TS** (p. 16) and **OCD** (p. 24) have a variety of clinically diagnosed anxiety disorders. Many experience symptoms which accompany more than one of these disorders.

Symptoms associated with anxiety disorders are typically manifested in three areas: cognitive, behavioral, and physical (somatic). (1) The following behaviors serve as general indicators. The student will not exhibit every characteristic listed. These behaviors may also be indicative of other problems.

Cognitive Symptoms
- Having daily anxious/worrisome thoughts about both important and unimportant problems/situations/events/activities
- Fearing transitions or changes in routine/environment
- Worrying about being embarrassed/humiliated
- Fearing reading aloud/speaking up in class/performing in front of others
- Worrying about failing/school grades
- Fearing social situations (initiating/maintaining conversations/asking peers to get together)
- Fearing unstructured school activities (assemblies/cafeteria/P.E.)
- Engaging in persistent self-doubt/self-criticism/low self-esteem
- Fearing storms/burglary/danger to self or others

Behavioral Symptoms
- Avoiding eye contact/speaking very softly/mumbling
- Hesitating to engage in new experiences
- Avoiding academic tasks/refusing to even try
- Having difficulty focusing/sustaining attention
- Being hesitant to participate in discussions/oral presentations
- Being inflexible
- Isolating self from peers
- Feeling frustrated/restless/irritable/angry/aggressive
- Saying "NO!" as first response
- Having tantrums ("storms")
- Being reluctant/refusing to attend school
- Being overly dependent/constantly seeking reassurance and approval

Physical Symptoms (2)
- Being restless
- Having stomachaches
- Flushing/sweating
- Rapid beating of heart
- Tensing of muscles
- Trembling/shaking
- Being fatigued

Section III

Other symptoms
    Feeling dizzy
    Having headaches
    Experiencing chills/hot flashes
    Using loud, repetitive speech
    Exhibiting increased activity level
    Having exacerbation of ADHD/TS/OCD symptoms

Adolescents experience more physical symptoms than younger students. (2) Cognitive, behavioral, and physical symptoms interact with each other to increase the anxiety level. (1)

Research suggests that anxiety may moderate the impulsivity or inhibitory dysfunction associated with ADHD but significantly impact attention and working memory. (3, 4) Students with **ADHD-I** and Slow Cognitive Tempo exhibit higher levels of anxiety than the hyperactive and combined types. (5, 6) It is hypothesized that ADHD anxiety reflects worries about cognitive, academic, and social competency rather than the fears and phobias of several anxiety disorders. (7, 8)

Interventions

- Provide a cooperative rather than competitive environment. Fear of failure may cause the student to become anxious and refuse to complete assignments or try to succeed.
    - Design small group projects to develop competency.
    - Pair students to complete class assignments, take tests, and do homework.
    - De-emphasize grades and comparisons between classmates.
- Establish routines and schedules to build predictability. (p. 57)
- Organize the classroom to minimize anxiety. (p. 58)
- Remain calm and be sensitive to anxiety.
    - Listen empathetically to the problem and feelings being expressed. Rephrase the issue, clarify it, and then ask "How can you solve the problem?" Be solution-oriented and use "**GET A CLUE**" or "**PLAN**" as a strategy to resolve the problem. (p. 109) Using this strategy, the student learns competence in problem solving, gains self-confidence, and thereby reduces anxiety.
    - Identify with the student antecedent (preceding) events that precipitate anxiety.
    - Discuss how the student can gain control over those situations.
    - Help the student select a strategy to use in different anxiety-producing situations (e.g., When the reading book cannot be located, ask a friend to share. When a pencil breaks, resharpen it or get another one. When a homework assignment is forgotten, ask to turn it in the next day. When a play date is desired, practice a script for asking a friend to get together.).
    - Provide reassurance by noting that the student handled similar situations appropriately ("You were worried yesterday about not completing your assignment because there were so many difficult problems. However, you worked diligently despite the anxiety and finished every problem!").
    - Offer positive reinforcement for all efforts to conquer anxiety.

- Encourage the use of positive, coping self-talk.
  - Help identify and reframe negative cognitions.
  - Teach scripts to use when anxiety becomes overwhelming (e.g., "My brain is tricking me. I can do this!" "I've done this before so I know I can do it!" "If I get started, I will feel better.").
- Implement interventions to reduce anxiety (e.g., modify assignments, provide movement breaks, use distraction, change activities, suggest moving to a less stressful work area).
- Use relaxation techniques to help decrease both the worries and accompanying physical symptoms (e.g., breathing deeply, counting to 10, progressively relaxing, visualizing a calming scene, listening to soft music).
- Prepare the student for transitions which are accompanied by worry and anxiety. (pp. 123-124)
- Intervene if the student is frequently absent or refuses to come to school.
  - Determine the cause. The problem is not always separation anxiety (fear of leaving home and parents) but may be related to anxiety about school (bullying, overly critical teacher), or social anxiety.
  - Address the core problem.
  - Initiate a plan with the parents to have the student return to school as quickly as possible (e.g., attending for one hour or half day until symptoms improve).
  - Avoid overreacting to physical complaints.
    - 🐾 *Do not explain the criteria for determining when a student may be sent home (e.g., vomiting, fever).*
  - Positively reinforce the student for attending school.
- Prearrange a "safe" place to which the student can retreat when feeling overwhelmed and anxious. Establish guidelines for moving between and using the safe place (e.g., making a "graceful exit" (p. 90)).

"Storms"/Overarousal

Students with **ADHD** and/or **TS** may have deregulated arousal systems which fluctuate unpredictably between underarousal (pp. 71-78), optimum arousal (p. 27), and overarousal (pp. 81-95). Clinical experience indicates that other disorders such as **OCD** and sensory defensiveness have varying levels of arousal that can also lead to "storms." Arousal levels may change throughout the day and vary from minute to minute, hour to hour, day to day, and even week to week. Fluctuating arousal produces inconsistent learning, variable academic performance, erratic behavior, and impaired socialization. (9)

Teachers often report:

"He knew the information yesterday, but forgot it on the test today."

"His handwriting was neat this morning, but messy this afternoon."

"He was happy one minute, but something as insignificant as demanding eye contact produced an angry outburst."

"He was playing nicely with his friend, but the next thing I knew he was hitting him."

Section III

The following behaviors serve as general indicators of overarousal. The student will not exhibit every characteristic listed. These behaviors may also be indicative of other problems.

    Becoming overly nervous/anxious
    Crying over a minor occurrence
    Exhibiting increase in activity level/impulsivity/tics
    Having a low tolerance for frustration/reacting with irritation
    Being unable to self-regulate behavior/emotions
    Becoming angry and/or aggressive/experiencing temper outbursts
    Having difficulty thinking clearly
    Being unable to complete assignments/tasks/activities
    Performing inconsistently
    Experiencing anxiety attack (test/social anxiety)
    Responding negatively to sensory stimulation
    Running away

Students with **ADHD, TS,** and/or **OCD** are often overaroused by many situations that other students take in stride. They live day in and day out with symptoms that infrequently remit. Their bodies are rarely still and are constantly making unwanted movements. Persistent tics cause embarrassment and at times pain. Students with **OCD** may become highly anxious and frightened when obsessions and compulsions are present. It takes very little stimulation to arouse feelings of anxiety, frustration, heightened arousal, and anger. (9)

Situations That Produce Overarousal

    Becoming frustrated/irritated/angry
    Engaging in power struggles
    Feeling anxious/afraid
    Experiencing hopelessness/despair
    Being unable to concentrate in presence of background noises
    Trying to listen/speak when several people are talking at the same time
    Becoming overstimulated by visual input
    Insisting on eye-contact
    Having movement restricted
    Being assigned handwritten work/lessons at frustration level
    Needing assignments/order of things to be "perfect"
    Needing to do homework/take tests
    Receiving criticism/lectures by teacher/parent (especially before peers)
    Being told "NO!"/not getting one's way
    Believing "That's NOT FAIR!"
    Being told to stop/transition to new task/activity/game
    Being confronted with unpredictable rules/expectations
    Losing when playing games
    Being teased/ridiculed/left out/ignored/socially ostracized
    Going to school assemblies/on field trips
    Having substitutes teachers/bus drivers
    Being mainstreamed for unstructured activities (P.E./cafeteria/recess)
    Walking in crowded/noisy hallways
    Being lightly touched in class/hall/line/assembly/cafeteria/bus
    Being overly sensitive to texture of clothes/smells/food
    Fearing dark/weather/animals/insects/reptiles
    Participating in holidays/family occasions/birthdays

Loss of self-control or a "storm," is a common outcome of overarousal.

Chapter 11

STORMS

The following behaviors serve as general indicators. The student will not exhibit every characteristic listed. These behaviors may also be indicative of other problems.

> Becoming intense/rigid/inflexible/"stuck"
> Yelling/screaming/using abusive language/swearing
> Kicking/punching/pushing/hitting
> Being unable to carry on rational discussion
> Failing to understand/listen to another person's point of view
> Panicking
> Threatening harm to self/others
> Hurting self/others
> Throwing/damaging property (putting hole in wall/door, breaking objects)
> Running away

A "storm" (10) or rage attack is a sudden, dramatic, uncontrolled, and explosive outburst of anger and aggression that occurs at the height of sensory overload and overarousal. The storm may be associated with the situational stressors described above or may occur in the absence of external provocation. During overarousal, access to abstract reasoning and problem-solving skills is unavailable. The student's ability to stop and think through the consequences of abusive attitudes, actions, and verbalizations is impaired. Any sensory input, including verbalizations, increases the storm and leads to a more violent reaction. When the storm subsides, there is a release of tension, irritability, and anger. The student may feel guilty and remorseful for displaying behaviors that others interpret as "bad," "stupid," "lazy," or "crazy." At times, there is loss of memory for the events that occurred during the rage attack. A storm often interferes with academic achievement, interpersonal relationships, and psychosocial development and leads to demoralization and poor self-esteem. (9)

> *Some students have implosive storms during which overwhelming feelings such as anxiety, hurt, or a sense of injustice are internalized. These students experience "lockdown" and become rigid, "stuck," and unresponsive for a period of time.*

Research examining the types of irritability associated with **ADHD** indicated that three-fourths of the students were easily annoyed, lost their temper, and felt angry or resentful. More than one-third experienced "mad/cranky" irritability, and one-fifth suffered from "super-angry/grouchy/cranky" irritability. (11) Extreme irritability, anger, stubbornness, negativism, oppositional behavior, and temper outbursts were found in another study to be exhibited by more than two-thirds of clinic-referred students with **ADHD** (12).

Findings suggest that up to one-third of students with **TS** who are evaluated in clinical settings experience episodic behavioral outbursts. (13, 14, 15) 94% of the rage attacks occur at home and are directed toward parents and siblings and 35% happen at school and target peers. During the storms, 60% of the attacks result in the destruction of property. (15) However, the majority of students with **TS-only** do not have anger control problems. The likelihood of explosive storms is not related to the severity of the tics but to the comorbidity of **ADHD** and **OCD**. (14, 16)

One-half of clinic-referred students with **OCD** have out-of-control, angry episodes. (17) They often become excessively angry when others try to interfere with their obsessions or compulsions.

> *Clinical experience suggests that students with anxiety disorders and sensory issues frequently have storms.*

Section III

Storms are sometimes, but not always, preceded by signs or behaviors suggesting imminent loss of control. (9)

Pre-storm Warnings

The following behaviors serve as general indicators. The student will not exhibit every characteristic listed. These behaviors may also be indicative of other problems.

> Tensing of muscles in jaw/forehead
> Overreacting to sensory input (touch/noise)
> Raising voice/becoming loud/using hostile tone of voice/angry words
> Increasing activity level/movements/intensity
> Showing low frustration tolerance
> Demanding things "NOW!"
> Becoming stubborn/rigid/inflexible/"stuck"
> Becoming agitated/anxious

Classroom Modifications to Minimize or Avoid Storms

- Create a classroom climate that enhances the student's ability to maintain emotional control. The student who experiences overarousal is too stimulated to function effectively. (9)

  - Ensure that the classroom environment is accepting and safe. Insist on zero tolerance for teasing, humiliation, harassment, intimidation, scapegoating, or bullying. (pp. 54-57)

  - Create a positive relationship with the student. Before the student will accept help during difficult times, the student must sense the teacher's respect and concern.

  - Model controlled behavior by expressing anger without blame. Avoid lecturing and using the word "you." Instead, use "I" messages that address the problem not the student.

    🐾 *Teachers' attitudes and actions are modeled by students.*

    - Describe the situation. Say, for example, "When students ask for extra time after school to complete tests, I agree to provide them the time. However, when they do not keep the appointments, I feel angry because they are not considerate of my time and feelings."

    - Validate the feelings of the student (e.g., "I hear that you are angry because you have to stay after school.").

    - Clarify expectations ("If students are unable to keep appointments, I expect them to cancel.").

- Allow the student to choose a compatible "buddy." A buddy will help alleviate stress and diminish the impact of the student's neurological disorder. (p. 70)

  🐾 *Make sure the student is comfortable having a buddy assigned and that the buddy wants the job.*

- Hold class meetings to discuss rules and to solve problems. (p. 58)

- Modify classroom procedures to reduce stress and prevent the occurrence of frustrating, anger-producing situations. (9)

  - Seat the student near the teacher.

    🐾 *If the teacher's desk is at the front of the room, the student with **TS** and severe tics should be seated in a less conspicuous location.*

- Provide consistency. The predictability of consistent routines provides security, decreases stress, and allows the student to direct more energy to self-control and learning.

- Privately prearrange appropriate mobility options. (pp. 72, 105) Stress occurs naturally and waxes and wanes in the body. Frequent movement allows this natural build-up of energy to be modulated or alleviated. This not only decreases stress, but also increases attention, provides tic relief, reduces anxiety, and helps the student calm down.

- Notify the student of impending changes in routine to facilitate readjustment (e.g., 5 minutes prior to the end of an activity, several days before the teacher's absence and each day there after).

  > *Changes in routine increase stress and may produce anxiety, anger, overarousal, and the feeling of being "stuck." The student may not be able to adjust and respond in a rapid, integrated fashion.*

- Structure the environment to prevent aggressive behavior from happening rather than reacting to it after it has occurred. For example, if the student with **TS** has a touching or hitting tic, or if the tactilely reactive student becomes agitated or aggressive when touched, move the student's desk far enough away from neighboring desks to provide more space.

- Minimize academic failure. Always assign tasks at the appropriate instructional level. (p. 64)

- Assign short tasks that can be easily completed. The student tends to become frustrated, agitated, and overwhelmed when confronted with long assignments. Gradually increase the length and difficulty of the assignments as the student demonstrates success.

- Do not allow the student with **OCD** to start any activity that cannot be finished in the allotted time frame. The student may be unable to change tasks or sets without subsequent anxiety which can produce inappropriate behaviors. The student may experience a compulsive need to complete the task and be unable to be redirected. A lengthy assignment can be broken up to appear as several independent ones.

- Arrange social situations so that they do not stimulate overarousal.

  - Plan social activities in which the student can excel and be praised.

  - Be sensitive to the tactilely reactive student who responds negatively when touched. If an activity or game requires physical contact such as playing tag or touch football, make arrangements for the student to be a referee, coach's assistant, score keeper, or library/office helper.

    > *Some pediatric occupational therapists are trained to treat sensory overreactivity.*

- Modify classroom procedures if the student with **ADHD**, **TS**, and/or **OCD** is easily overaroused by extra sensory input.

  > *Some of the most difficult situations occur in the hallways, between classes, in the cafeteria, at recess and P.E., during assemblies and pep rallies, and on the school bus. These are not only noisy, less structured times which produce destabilizing anxiety and stress, but offer limited, if any, adult supervision. Students often complain about being teased, embarrassed, and touched by the other students in these unstructured situations.*

  - Allow the student to leave the classroom two to three minutes early if loud noises and/or movement in the hallway are overstimulating and stressful.

  - Have an adult remain in close proximity to the student in the hallways and cafeteria. This will help prevent a possible confrontation.

Section III

- ○ Intervene if the student has a <u>problem on the bus</u>. (9)
  - 🐾 *All interventions must have parental consent in writing.*
- Educate the bus driver about the student's needs.
- Assign a bus "buddy" (willing peer to model appropriate bus behavior). (p. 70)
- Require the student to sit at the front of the bus.
- If modifications in the regular bus situation do not alleviate the problem, assign the student to a special education bus. These buses are smaller and frequently have monitors in addition to the drivers.
  - 🐾 *Use this procedure as a last resort. The student is usually embarrassed by the special education bus.*
- If the symptoms appear to be temporary, suggest that the parents drive the student.

Individual Interventions to Minimize or Avoid Storms

IS IT NAUGHTY OR NEUROLOGICAL

IF THE BEHAVIOR IN REALITY IS:

	NAUGHTY	NEUROLOGICAL
If The Behavior Is Treated As NAUGHTY	"Bad" behavior decreases Child gains respect for authority Child is calmer, happier "I better clean up my act. Every time I try to get away with something, I get caught. Crime does not pay."	Child may become frustrated, discouraged, depressed, despondent, suicidal, scared, fearful, and anxious Child quits trying, caves in, stops caring, avoids school authorities "Why should I try when I know no one will see me trying. I'll just get punished no matter what I do. I will give up or get even!"
If The Behavior Is Treated As NEUROLOGICAL	"Bad" behavior increases Child loses respect for authority Child may feel: anxious ("Who's in charge?") entitled ("I will do what I want to do!") "I'm in charge. No one has authority over me. I am getting scared. That makes me angry to be in charge. I'm too young!"	Child is hopeful. Child feels understood and works with team to solve problems Child feels affection for authority "There is hope for me. I will keep trying because when I try, everyone knows and encourages me. They give me strategies that can help me succeed."

Figure 11.1. Is It Naughty or Neurological? – Approaches to treating behavior (16)

🐾 *If a symptom such as impulsivity or overactivity is treated as a voluntary behavior and consequated, the student becomes discouraged, feels helpless, and quits trying. If it is appropriately treated as neurological, the student calms down, feels more successful, and performs better.*

Chapter 11

- Always treat the behaviors associated with **ADHD**, **TS**, and **OCD** as neurological in origin and design interventions accordingly.

  🐾 *Overarousal and "storms" are not expressions of "bad" behavior or "emotional" problems; they are manifestations of a neurological disorder.*

- Recommend that the student who is experiencing storms be assessed for a mood disorder by a psychiatrist or other health care professional trained to diagnose mood disorders.

  🐾 *Clinically, many professionals have observed that storms frequently occur with an accompanying bipolar disorder. For a more indepth discussion of mood disorders consult <u>Challenging Kids, Challenged Teachers!</u> by Leslie E. Packer, Ph. D. and Sheryl K. Pruitt, M. Ed., ET/P (working title, manuscript in press. Bethesda, MD: Woodbine House)*

- Overlook minor, unimportant behaviors. Teach the other students to do the same.

- Teach the student how to use "I" statements and verbalize <u>feelings</u> before losing control ("This is too much work for me to do." "I do not understand this assignment." "Please let me have some time alone. I am frustrated and beginning to feel angry.").

- Acknowledge the student's feelings. Do not confuse the student's behavior with the feelings being expressed.

  🐾 *Feelings are always valid even if the behavior is inappropriate. Be sure to provide consequences for the <u>behavior</u>, not the feeling.*

- Develop the student's understanding of personal <u>feelings of frustration and anger</u>. (9)

  🐾 *Negative emotions and deficient regulatory skills affect the ability to assess and interpret situations, generate solutions to problems, analyze proposed responses, and self-monitor and self-correct behavior. The ability to self-regulate the expression of feelings is related to an understanding of the emotions.*

  ○ Indicate that anger is a response to experiences and one's reactions to those experiences.

  ○ Explain that there is nothing wrong with feeling angry. Everyone experiences anger. What is important is how the individual reacts to those feelings. Although it is difficult to control aggressive impulses caused by neurological problems, aggression is unacceptable and appropriate strategies for releasing anger and aggression must be learned.

  ○ Teach the student how to identify <u>signs</u> indicating imminent loss of control (e.g., feeling anxious, out of control, fearful/panicked, tightening of the stomach, flushing of the face, breathlessness, sweaty, shaky/tremulous, rapid heart palpitations).

  ○ Help determine what happened just before the feeling occurred.

  ○ Emphasize the importance of learning self-control strategies to remain calm when confronted with stressful situations. Responding aggressively is <u>not</u> an acceptable way to solve problems.

  ○ Point out that angry feelings often produce negative thoughts ("I can never do anything right." "I quit." "I'm no good." "I hate him." "I'm going to get even with him.") and that those thoughts often affect the ability to remain in control.

  ○ Discuss the negative consequences of angry, aggressive acts (e.g., social ostracism, bodily harm to self and others, school expulsion, juvenile detention, jail).

Section III

- Act out different negative feelings and use the appropriate expressions and body language. Describe the feelings engendered.

- Encourage the sharing of past situations in which angry feelings were experienced.

• Recognize <u>signs of impending loss of control</u> and immediately use <u>de-escalation strategies</u>. (9)

- Respond in a nonthreatening, matter-of-fact, and caring manner.

- <u>Never enter into a power struggle</u> or try to add input to the student's sensory system. Once the "storm" begins to build, further input increases the overstimulation already occurring in the body and leads to an automatic escalation of the event. Sensory input includes requiring eye contact, saying "NO!," arguing, insisting on an immediate response, and touching the student (even when one is trying to be supportive).

  🐾 ***Power struggles during a storm can never be won!***

- Reflect the feelings being expressed (e.g., "You are really angry at ____. You feel like you never want to play with him again.").

  🐾 *Recognize the feelings before dealing with the situation.*

- Help the student verbalize frustration and anger appropriately before losing control ("I feel ____ because ____.").

- Encourage the student to make positive self-statements to lessen intense feelings and control angry reactions ("Relax." "Calm down." "He's not going to bother me.").

- Use a problem solving strategy such as "**GET A CLUE**" or "**PLAN**" that includes the following executive skills: defining the problem, generating a goal, identifying possible solutions, analyzing the positive and negative consequences of each proposed solution, making a decision, using the best solution, and evaluating the outcome. (p. 109)

- Use a <u>cognitive self-talk technique</u> to help the student identify and reframe angry, aggressive behavior and regain control. (19)

  🐾 *Traditional management techniques, except for positive reinforcement and time-out, are usually ineffective in modifying the behavior of students with neurological disorders. These methods rely on their ability to attend, concentrate, and neurologically remain in control. Cognitive interventions are sometimes more effective.*

Teach the student how to:

- <u>identify the problem</u> and state it orally.

  Teacher: "What is the problem?"
  Student: "I keep hitting my classmates."

- recognize the <u>controlling factors</u> in the situation that caused the problem.

  Teacher: "Do you know why you hit them?"
  Student: "They keep teasing me and calling me names."

- think about the <u>consequences</u> of an inappropriate response.

  Teacher: "What happens when you hit other children?"
  Student: "I'm the one who gets in trouble, is sent to the principal's office, or has detention."

- identify an appropriate <u>goal</u>.

    Teacher: "What will you gain by solving the problem?"
    Student: "I won't get into trouble and I'll get along with my classmates better."

- <u>generate alternative responses</u> or solutions to the problem.

    Teacher: "Can you think of something you could do instead of hitting?"
    Student: "I don't know anything."
    Teacher: "What about fighting back with words instead of fists?"
    Student: "My mother and father get upset when I say certain words!"
    Teacher: "What if you and your parents look at our list of acceptable words and add some of your own. Then you can use words they approve."

- <u>analyze alternative solutions</u> generated.

    Teacher: "Will it work?"
    "Will you be able to do it?"
    "Have you ever tried that before?"
    "Will you break any rules?"
    "What will be the effect on you and others?"
    "How will others feel?"

- <u>evaluate the results</u> of changes in behavior.

    Teacher: "Did it work? Are you satisfied? Are there any new problems?"
    Student: "It worked! The kid was so surprised he left me alone!"

- make <u>self-directed, positive, reinforcing statements</u> about the results of changes in behavior.

    Student: "I did very well at not getting into a fight when I was teased. How do I feel? Great! Proud!"

🐾 ***Once a behavioral intervention proves successful, do not assume it is no longer useful. It may be needed indefinitely.***

- Use <u>humor</u> to defuse tension. Humor often introduces novelty into the situation, distracts the student, deflects an impending impasse, and restores calm.

    🐾 *Sarcasm <u>intensifies</u> storms and is not considered humorous to the student who is frustrated or angry.*

- Use the student's need for <u>diversity</u> to redirect behavior. For example, assign lessons on the computer or at learning centers to break up seatwork.

- Take a break and check the appropriateness of the task if signs of frustration become apparent while the student is working on an assignment. If the task is consistent with the student's ability level, change activities until calm is restored. The student's own distractibility possibly can be used to redirect attention to another task.

- Change the student's focus of attention by suggesting a resistive physical activity (e.g., push against the wall with hands, do push ups on the floor, jog in place, lift something heavy, hit a pillow, use stretchy exercise bands). (20)

- Recommend a calming activity (e.g., listening to music, playing an electronic game, drawing, writing thoughts and feelings in a journal, using relaxation or breathing techniques, talking with a trusted friend or adult).

Section III

- Intervene <u>when anger and aggression cannot be redirected</u>. (9)
    - Arrange for a trusted adult to be available when a crisis occurs to help restore calm and defuse the situation.
    - Provide a quiet, safe place to which the student may go to spend some time alone, release stress, and regain control. This area might be supplied with a plastic bat with which to beat a pillow, a heavy cylinder-shaped punching bag, or other nonbreakable items. The student should be reinforced for using the objects to release anger.
        - 🐾 *Do not use a light, pear-shaped punching bag. It fights back and sometimes makes the student even angrier.*
    - Teach the student how to make a "<u>graceful exit</u>." (21) A graceful exit occurs when the student, anticipating or experiencing a "storm," leaves the room according to a previously agreed-upon procedure.
        - Plan in advance with the student a set of options which delineate how to exit and where to go because the student may not be able to ask to leave the room during a "storm."
        - Privately prearrange cues for saving face. These cues may be auditory, visual, motor, tactile, or represent a cognitive frame. For example, the student agrees that when the teacher notices that loss of control is imminent, the elementary student is given a color pass to leave the room and perform an errand. (Allow the student to choose the color of the pass. Color choice may promote a positive feeling about using the pass which enhances the ability to leave gracefully.) The older student is handed a pass that is typically used in the middle and high school setting.
            - 🐾 *A student often saves face by muttering and grumbling while exiting. Understand that this is in fact a <u>compliant</u> response. A better or more graceful exit might be a future expectation and goal.*
        - Reinforce the student for exiting rather than allowing the situation to escalate, even if the exit is less than graceful.

- Explore <u>alternative solutions to resolve conflicts</u>.
    - Hold a class meeting. Have the group generate nonaggressive alternatives to hypothetical or real problems that occur within the social context of the class. For example, if the student is being teased or ridiculed, the group might propose telling the teacher, walking away, or fighting with words rather than fists.
    - Discuss and generate with the student effective strategies to use in problem situations.
    - Teach and practice <u>negotiation and compromise</u>. (22)

    Suggest that the student:
    - determine whether there is a problem that needs to be solved.
    - arrange a meeting with the peer or adult with whom there is a problem.
    - state the problem clearly and use "I" messages. Use feeling words rather than angry words. Be assertive rather than aggressive.
    - discuss what went wrong without placing the blame on the other person. Analyze the who, what, when, where, how, and why of the situation.
    - listen to and try to understand different perspectives. (p. 328)
    - paraphrase the various perspectives.

- think about similarities and differences in the points of view.
- propose and consider various solutions.
- offer a personally acceptable solution to solve the problem.
- listen to an alternate solution.
- negotiate and try to reach a compromise.

○ Frequently review and practice these strategies so they are available for use in stressful situations. The student under stress is unable to easily or spontaneously generate ideas.

○ Use a previously agreed-upon cue to remind the student to think about an alternative solution when a real problem occurs.

> *The student who has learned maladaptive responses to frustration and anger will impulsively use those responses even after learning more appropriate strategies. Therefore, it will be necessary to frequently remind the student of more acceptable ways of expressing frustration and anger.*

- Use <u>nonjudgmental correction procedures</u>. Correction procedures should leave the dignity of both the student and teacher intact. (9)

○ Remain calm, speak quietly, and avoid giving long sermons and logical reasons. Do not debate or argue with the student.

○ Suggest rating the intensity of feelings (anxiety, frustration, anger) experienced during the episode on a "feeling thermometer." (23, 24)

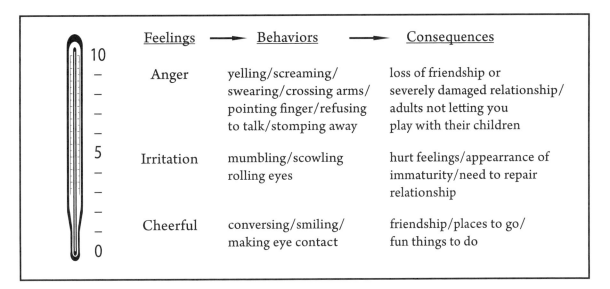

Figure 11.2. Feeling Thermometer

> *The "feeling thermometer" helps the student analyze feelings through both the verbal and visual modalities.*

- Talk about the intensity of the feelings and the reaction to them. Be sure to separate the self-worth of the student from the misbehavior.
- Deliver the feedback as clearly and dispassionately as possible, rather than in a passive-aggressive manner (e.g., angry tone of voice, angry facial expression, sarcasm).

Section III

- Discuss the consequences associated with the behavioral reactions to the emotions.
- Use the problem–solving strategy "**GET A CLUE**" or "**PLAN**" to determine what to do the next time that might prove successful. (p. 109)

• Eliminate public hangings. (25)

**Children may forget what you say,
but they will never forget how you make them feel.**

Ross Greene, Ph.D. (2001). Southeastern Tourette Syndrome Conference. Atlanta, GA.

  ○ Do not discipline and embarrass the student in front of peers. This focuses the other students' attention on the misbehavior and wounds self-esteem. Deliver reprimands privately and in a calm, unemotional manner. Pain and embarrassment are not appropriate management tools.

  🐾 *Everyone can remember being the victim of a public hanging at the hands of a teacher and most can remember the name of the teacher many, many years later.*

• Use contingency management known as "Grandma's Rule." (source unknown)

Student:	"I do NOT want to do all these math problems. I want to use the computer."
Teacher:	(without anger) "As soon as you finish your assignment, you can have 30 minutes of computer time."
Student:	"But I want the computer NOW!"
Teacher:	(calmly and sympathetically) "Of course you do, and, as soon as you finish your work, you can use the computer."

  🐾 *Avoid the temptation to be sarcastic when responding.*

• Try to discern the underlying reason for the student's behavior. (9)

  🐾 *At times responsibility is incorrectly placed on the student.*

  ○ Ask who, what, when, where, how, and why questions about behavior.
    - Was the behavior caused by the neurological condition?
    - Was the problem the result of an ADHD need for movement?
    - Was the problem caused by tics (e.g., hitting, kicking, spitting tic)?
    - Was the problem related to an OCD compulsive need to produce a perfect handwritten report?
    - Was the behavior a side effect of medication?
      🐾 *Some medications increase anger and aggression.*
    - Was the problem caused by the teacher(s), parent(s), or peer(s)?

- Was the behavior elicited by the need for:

    more structure?
    more strategies?
    more emotional support?
    obsessive reassurance?
    more movement?
    more personal space?
    more stimulating and interesting work?
    not wanting to fail?
    less stimulation?
    avoiding embarrassment?
    relieving anxiety?
    leaving the situation to calm down?
    cleanliness?
    perfectionism?

- Was the behavior caused by:

    insisting on eye-contact?
    being lightly touched?
    listening to loud noises in the hallway/cafeteria/assembly/pep rally?
    needing to wait when lining up/speaking/getting on or off bus?
    being required to undress in P.E.?
    mentioning student's handicap in front of class without permission?
    criticizing student in front of other students?
    insisting on response before being able to access needed information?
    sitting near inappropriate models?
    teasing and ridicule by peers?
    being penalized for inherent disorganization (loss of books, pencils, papers, homework, materials)?
    assigning a boring task (too easy, too short)?
    giving work at the frustration level (too hard, too long)? (p. 64)
    assigning too much handwritten work?
    giving an unclear direction?
    giving multi-step directions?
    handing out illegible worksheets?
    assigning too many problems, poorly spaced on the page?
    being punished for behaviors associated with neurological disorder(s) (inattention, impulsivity, tics, obsessions, compulsions)?
    having another neurological disorder that is undiagnosed?

○ Evaluate the efficacy of reinforcement. Ask the following:

- Was the behavior the result of ineffective reinforcement?
- Was the reinforcer considered positive and meaningful to the student?
- Was there a stronger reinforcer in the environment that was stimulating inappropriate behavior?
- Was the delay too long between the behavior and the reinforcement?
- Had the student become satiated with the reinforcer?

Section III

- Follow the general <u>principles of behavior management</u> when dealing with angry, aggressive, and oppositional behaviors. (9)

  - 🐾 *Always determine the event that happened just **before** the behavior occurred.*

  ○ Develop a set of explicit limits and rules. The rules should be clearly defined so the student knows exactly what is expected.

    - 🐾 *All students need boundaries and limits established. Limits make students feel cared for and safe.*

    · Avoid setting so many rules that it is impossible for the student to remember all of them.

      - 🐾 *Four rules are generally adequate. One rule needs to be "respect" for self and others.*

    · Post the rules at eye level in the front of the classroom.

    · Always state the rules positively. If the rule is phrased negatively, the student with **TS** may have an uncontrollable urge to do the action stated in the rule. The student with **ADHD** may have a milder, but similar, suggestibility and impulsive response. The student with **OCD** may perseverate on the negative rule.

    · Restate the rules frequently.

    · Reinforce positive, rule-governed behavior frequently and emphatically.

  ○ Prearrange natural, logical <u>consequences</u> for misbehaviors and communicate those consequences to the class and/or the student during a time when no emotional problems are occurring. Establishing consequences in advance allows the student to make choices ("If I _____, the consequence will be _____.").

    · Choose an appropriate consequence.

    · Do not impose a major consequence for a minor offense. Be fair and consistent. If the consequences are fair, the student will learn to be accountable for misbehavior and learn correct behavior.

    · Do not punish the student for behavior caused by the neurological disorder (e.g., impulsivity, impersistence, hyperactivity, inattention, tics, obsessions, compulsions, being "stuck").

    · The consequence should be imposed <u>immediately</u> after the inappropriate behavior occurs. Similarly, when rewards are promised, give them immediately after the appropriate response is exhibited.

      - 🐾 *Implement the consequence privately to lessen embarrassment.*

    · Do not spend excessive time punishing inappropriate behavior at the expense of rewarding appropriate behavior. Positively reinforce behavior as soon as it occurs. Rewarding good behavior builds self-esteem.

    · Do not threaten consequences that are not intended to be carried out.

    · Always respond the same way to the same specific misbehavior.

      - 🐾 *Remain calm and in control so that the student is able to focus on the behavior itself rather than the reaction to the behavior.*

    · Reward the student for remaining in control. Allow the student to earn chips/points that can be used for extra free-time, computer use, being excused from a homework assignment, etc.

- Hold the student responsible for cleaning up or correcting any problems that may have resulted from the incident after a "storm" has passed and self-control has been regained (e.g., If the student marks on the walls, have the student stay after school or come early to clean the walls. If the student must be removed from the room because others are being disturbed by a behavior within the student's control, have the student complete unfinished assignments during free-time or after school.

    🐾 *Do not give the student additional consequences for a "storm."*

- Help the student recognize that everyone makes mistakes, but it is important to learn from one's mistakes.

- Explain, without blaming, the specific behavior that was inappropriate and why. Listen to and reflect back the student's point of view. Encourage the student to problem solve and plan a strategy for avoiding the behavior in the future.

    🐾 *For a more indepth discussion of punishment consult <u>Challenging Kids, Challenged Teachers!</u> by Leslie E. Packer, Ph. D. and Sheryl K. Pruitt, M. Ed., ET/P (working title, manuscript in press. Bethesda, MD: Woodbine House)*

• Help the student learn to <u>apologize</u> for inappropriate behavior and repair relationships.

    🐾 *The student who is in a state of overarousal will be unable to accept responsibility for the disruptive incident. However, when calm has been restored, the student must assume accountability and apologize.*

Suggest that the student:

○ stop and consider whether teachers and other students might feel hurt, resentful, or fearful following an out-of-control episode.

○ decide the best way, time, and place to apologize.

○ learn and follow a script for apologizing. (22)

- admit the mistake.

- explain why it happened.

- acknowledge the peer's or adult's hurt, angry, or resentful feelings.

- apologize.

    🐾 *Initially, apologies may be more forthcoming and appropriate when done by email or IM (instant messaging). This eliminates the overstimulation of a direct apology.*

- ask how the relationship can be mended so that the friendship can be maintained.

- correct the mistake.

CHAPTER 12
INATTENTION/IMPULSIVITY/HYPERACTIVITY

INATTENTION

Inattention significantly impacts academic achievement, behavior, and socialization. Students with **ADHD** do not intentionally fail to "pay attention," and may in fact be exerting more effort to attend than other classmates. Students with **TS** may be distracted by or struggling to suppress tics. Research indicates that students with **TS plus ADHD** have more trouble focusing and sustaining attention than those with **TS-only**. (1) Students with **OCD** may be so preoccupied with obsessive thoughts or trying to resist expressing compulsions that they are unable to pay attention to the material being taught. Failure to focus and sustain attention to task, resist distractions, and prolong concentration is due to the student's neurological disorder.

The following behaviors serve as general indicators. The student will not exhibit every characteristic listed. These behaviors may also be indicative of other problems.

Impact on Behavior
- Appearing underaroused (tired)
- Exhibiting attentional inconsistencies ("tuned in"/"tuned out")
- Being off-task after initially starting work
- Experiencing auditory/visual/tactile/other sensory distractions
- Daydreaming/looking around/staring into space
- Being distracted by/preoccupied with one's own thoughts/worries
- Free-associating (mentally/verbally)
- Interjecting irrelevant comments
- Fiddling/doodling
- Getting out of seat frequently
- Seeking stimulating activities rather than focusing on assigned tasks
- Requiring high interest materials to remain on-task
- Seeming "lazy"/"unmotivated" when confronted with goal-oriented tasks
- Becoming overwhelmed when given too many choices
- Needing immediate reinforcement

Impact on Academics
- Overlooking important details
- Misunderstanding directions for assignments/homework
- Struggling to follow complex instructions/explanations
- Needing reminders to remain on task/complete classwork
- Lacking the ability to do assignments/homework independently
- Performing handwritten and cognitive tasks slowly
- Becoming quickly bored with/losing interest in schoolwork and homework
- Being unable to finish tasks/assignments/homework
- Having difficulty completing long-term reports/projects
- Attending to social activities during academic tasks
- Displaying inconsistent academic performance
- Switching from one uncompleted activity to another
- Forgetting materials needed for tasks

Section III

Interventions

- Assess auditory and visual attention.
- Determine <u>where</u>, <u>when</u>, <u>how</u>, and <u>why</u> the student is inattentive.
    - Is the student easily distracted by noises and movements in the classroom?
    - Is the student seated near classmates who interfere with the ability to attend?
    - Is the student more inattentive in the morning or afternoon, before or after lunch, before or after recess?
    - Does the student need to move before a task is completed?
    - Is inattention <u>modality-specific</u> (verbal or visual)?
        - 🐾 *Most students today are audio-visual learners.*
    - Does the student struggle to listen to or follow verbal or written instructions?
    - Is inattention <u>content-specific</u> (e.g., reading, writing, math, literature, science, history)?
    - Does the student become overwhelmed when given too many choices?
    - Does the student seem preoccupied with inner thoughts?
    - Are interesting learning materials needed to attract and maintain attention?
- Consult with teacher(s) from the previous year to determine which interventions proved successful.
- Modify requirements and length of assignments when the student is unable to maintain focused attention. (2)
    - Schedule, if possible, more demanding tasks middle to late morning when the student is most alert. Attention and concentration tend to wane in the afternoon.
    - Plan less demanding, more active learning activities when the student has difficulty paying attention.
    - Assign work that can easily be completed. The student may become frustrated and agitated when confronted with long assignments that require sustained attention.
    - Break a lengthy assignment into small segments to appear as several independent tasks.
    - Assign shorter tasks requiring accuracy and quality of response.
    - Divide study periods into several short sessions with breaks between tasks.
- Arrange the classroom environment to <u>minimize distractions</u>. (2) Students with **ADHD** are susceptible to being distracted in the presence of background noises. (3)
    - Place the student's desk away from doors, windows, heating and air conditioning ducts, pencil sharpener, work stations, and other high traffic areas.
    - Seat the student near peers who will remain on-task and not encourage or stimulate inappropriate behaviors.
    - Limit the size of groups so that the student's attention is not interrupted by other students.

- Assign a peer with good on-task behaviors to act as a work "buddy." (p. 70)

- Reduce the noise level in the classroom.

- Permit the student easily disturbed by noises to use earplugs or a headset with white noise or music. White noise has been found to enhance the cognitive performance of students with **ADHD**. (4)

    - *If the use of music interferes with learning, the privilege is lost and earphones with white noise or no sound must be used.*

- Provide a carrel for the student who is easily distracted by objects, movements, and events. Reward the student for going to the "office" when necessary.

• <u>Gain attention</u> before beginning lessons. (2)

- Stand near the student, say the student's name, or use a hand gesture.

- Do not require eye contact. Requiring eye contact is often overstimulating to the visually sensitive student and produces academic and behavioral problems. Look for cues other than eye contact to determine if the student is attending. A student looking out the window or at another student may in fact be paying attention. Check the student's comprehension before giving a consequence for not listening.

    - *Just because the student is not looking at the instructor does not mean that the student is not listening. Sometimes the student avoids looking at the person talking to concentrate on the words.*

- Use introductory words to direct focus such as "Ready," "Listen," or "Let's begin."

- Provide novelty or do something unusual (e.g., show illustrations, pictures, and objects; make sudden noises or movements; add color; interject humor or music).

• Modify the manner in which <u>directions</u> are delivered. (2)

    - *Understanding the directions is a prerequisite for completing an assignment correctly.*

- Present directions and explanations facing the student. Focusing is more difficult when the teacher does not speak directly to the student (e.g., giving instructions while writing on the board).

- Avoid giving multi-step directions. If necessary, deliver one instruction at a time and be specific (e.g., "Get out your math book." Pause. "Turn to page 45." Pause. "Work problems 1-10.").

    - *Pausing allows time for the direction to be processed and followed before the next one is delivered.*

- Repeat and/or paraphrase instructions. Use a calm, reassuring voice when repeating.

- Incorporate a variety of modalities (e.g., verbal and written instructions, cognitive cues with laminated visual cue cards, demonstrations).

- Suggest marking written directions with a highlighter or underlining with a mechanical pencil with a grooved grip and dark, strong lead.

- Have the younger student add visual cues to specific words in directions by putting a circle around the word "circle," underlining the word "underline," or drawing two dots (eyes) over the word "read."

- Check understanding of the instructions. Ask the student to restate the directions, do the first step of the task, or work one example and have it checked before continuing.

    - *Avoid using this approach in front of classmates.*

Section III

- Provide more assistance and structure than usual if the student is having difficulty maintaining focused attention.

- Remind the student during the lesson as to which information attention should be directed (e.g., answers to questions, main ideas, relevant facts).
  - Stress what is most important about the information.
  - Cue attention to who, what, when, where, how, and why of material.

- Alter the <u>presentation of information</u>.
  - Offer a variety of materials and methods of instruction using different learning styles. (pp. 65-67)
    - Verbal – reading, discussing, writing, listening, playing word games
    - Visual – drawing; building; making charts, maps, graphs; watching DVDs
    - Tactile – manipulating/building objects, experimenting, role playing, board games, hands-on projects
    - Logical/Mathematical – solving logic/math puzzles, discovering patterns/relationships
    - Musical – writing lyrics for songs, playing musical instruments
    - Interpersonal – working on group projects, interviewing others
    - Intrapersonal – completing individualized projects, writing in diary
  - Use interactive teaching methods such as class discussions and group projects.
  - Establish learning centers, labs, or stations which offer a variety of materials and methods of instruction. Such diversity helps maintain the student's interest and attention to task and also allows freedom of movement.
  - Adjust the pace and change topics and tasks frequently.
    - *The student with **ADHD** often becomes inattentive when confronted with dull, boring, repetitive subjects and activities. The student needs the stimulation of new, different, and interesting schoolwork that offers more satisfaction, provides immediate reward, and maintains arousal and attention.*
  - Follow less interesting tasks with more interesting tasks. Have the preferred task contingent upon adequate completion of the first task (e.g., writing assignment/math problems must be completed before free-reading/computer time).

- Be alert for confusion and loss of focus.

- Repeat information frequently to allow for lapses in attention.

- <u>Always</u> assign seatwork at the appropriate <u>instructional</u> level. (p. 64)

- Encourage the student to use <u>cognitive strategies to enhance on-task behavior</u>.
  - Tape a visual cue card of the selected cognitive strategy to the desk or place it inside the notebook as a reminder to pay attention and finish the assignments. Stand near the student and touch the cue to prompt attention to task.

- Teach a think aloud or <u>self-talk strategy</u> that helps the student maintain focused attention when confronted with unfamiliar, demanding tasks and activities or when mastering new skills. Suggest quietly reciting while following through on tasks. Arrange a workplace where subvocalization will not disturb the other students.

- Circulate around the classroom during independent study. Discreetly point to the assignment to which the student should be attending.

- Privately prearrange with the student a nonpunitive hand gesture or signal to be used during listening and work periods as a reminder from the teacher to refocus attention.

- Set a <u>timer</u> or clock for the amount of time needed to focus on and complete a task. (2)

    - Initially set the amount of time required to perform a task commensurate with the student's attention span. Gradually reduce the amount of time when tasks begin to be consistently finished in the allotted time frame.

    - Allow the student to set own time estimates for work periods.

    - Assess the appropriateness of the task and adjust the time requirements if the work is not completed.

    - Encourage the student to work more slowly and accurately if the assignment is finished too quickly and inaccurately.

- <u>Reinforce on-task behavior</u> and <u>work completion</u>. (2)

    - Provide positive feedback to classmates who demonstrate the appropriate behavior. Always define on-task behavior during reinforcement ("I like the way John is sitting quietly at his desk and concentrating on his work.").

        - *Check to see that the student knows appropriate on-task behavior. Sometimes the student has not learned the behavior.*

- Use the following progression of <u>interventions when off-task</u> behaviors interfere with the rest of the class: (2)

    - <u>Cueing</u> – give the student a previously agreed upon signal to jump-start attention and increase persistence.

    - <u>Redirection</u> – use the student's own distractibility to switch from off-task to on-task behavior. Refocus the student's attention with a change of physical location or a change of activity.

    - <u>Time-out (opportunity to regain self-control)</u> – prearrange with the student a safe place to go to regain control. When determining the location of time-out, initially provide a place within the classroom (e.g., chair or desk in back of the classroom, behind a bookcase or carrel, in the reading center for quietly reading a book of the student's choice). If the student is unsuccessful, select a more restrictive environment.

    Time-out procedures include:
    - Student voluntarily goes to time-out without being prompted.
        - *Reward initiation of time-out.*

Section III

- Teacher signals the student to go to time-out.

  - 🐾 *Never act as if time-out is a punishment. Time-out should be a tool that is viewed as positive. For many students, this will become a "lifelong" coping strategy to be used in school, social, and family settings. One minute for each year of age is usually sufficient.*

  - 🐾 *For a more indepth discussion of time-out procedures consult <u>Challenging Kids, Challenged Teachers</u>! by Leslie E. Packer, Ph.D. and Sheryl K. Pruitt, M.Ed., ET/P. (working title, manuscript in press. Bethesda, MD: Woodbine House).*

  - <u>Apply natural consequences</u> – a student learns best from consequences related to the behavior. Be sure that the consequences are <u>reasonable</u> and <u>fair</u>. Administer consequences consistently.

- Never use punishment (loss of recess or social activities, additional homework) for situations and behaviors over which the student has no control (e.g., not attending to lectures, being off-task, making careless errors). Being punished for these types of behaviors creates stress which increases the likelihood of inappropriate behaviors. (2)

  - Be aware that inconsistent performance from one day to the next may be due to the student's neurological disorder and not due to disinterest, lack of motivation, or laziness.

    - Do not penalize the student for uneven performance.
    - Have the student on "good days" complete enough work to reinforce concepts presented on "off days."

- Avoid sending <u>unfinished class assignments</u> home. It is not productive and is frequently psychologically harmful to the student. Finishing school work at home creates astonishing and traumatic power struggles between the student and the parents. (2)

  - 🐾 *The student who is unable to finish classwork at school will <u>not</u> be able to complete it at home due to a decrease in physical and cognitive energy.*

  - Evaluate the appropriateness of the assignments and modify expectations until the student can be successful. Gradually increase expectations for work completion.

  - If the teacher is certain the workload has been reduced to a level at which the student can be successful, have the student stay after school to complete the unfinished classwork. It usually takes only a few episodes of remaining after school to ensure work completion. However, this consequence must occur consistently, even when inconvenient for the parents or teacher.

    - 🐾 *This recommendation is not appropriate if the severity of the disorder(s) makes the student unable to comply.*

Chapter 12

IMPULSIVITY

(ACTING BEFORE THINKING)

The following behaviors serve as general indicators. The student will not exhibit every characteristic listed. These behaviors may also be indicative of other problems.

Impact on Behavioral/Emotional Responsiveness

Being distracted by auditory/visual/tactile/olfactory (smell) stimuli
Having difficulty waiting in line and taking turns
Being unable to inhibit inappropriate behavior
Neglecting to ask "What if?"
Having difficulty learning from consequences of behavior
Demonstrating inability to use internalized speech to follow rules/control behavior/solve problems
Having difficulty feeling satisfied
Needing instant gratification ("I have to have it NOW!")
Engaging in risk-taking behaviors
Being unable to regulate emotions (too high/too low)
Having difficulty separating thoughts from feelings
Being easily irritated
Having low tolerance for frustration/stress/disappointment
Reacting with anger to unanticipated situations (e.g., reacting negatively when unable to be first)
Responding too quickly and strongly to criticism
Experiencing emotional outbursts
Giving up/quitting when confronted with stressful tasks and activities

Impact on Academic Functioning

Doing things without planning/organizing before starting
Doing the first thing that comes to mind
Failing to delay/inhibit before acting/speaking (blurting out/interrupting)
Talking during group activities/while working on assignments
Starting tasks/activities without fully understanding instructions
Having difficulty following directions
Answering question before entire question has been posed
Impulsively interrupting lesson with inappropriate humor
Rushing through tasks/activities without stopping to think about them
Making careless errors

ADHD involves deficits in self-regulation and inhibition of behavior. The prevalence of impulsivity has been identified in approximately three-fourths of clinic-referred students with **ADHD-only**, one-third of students with **TS plus ADHD**, and one-tenth of the students with **TS-only**. (1) The presence of more severe ADHD and OCD symptoms puts the student with **TS** at risk for inhibitory dysfunction. (5) The student with **OCD** is often unable to inhibit irrelevant and unwanted thoughts and responses.

Interventions

- Ignore impulsive behavior as much as possible. (2)

    - *Do not expect perfection. An expectation for perfect behavior makes the student more frustrated and exacerbates impulsivity.*

Section III

- Implement interventions that <u>reduce impulsive behaviors</u>. (2)
    - Address only those behaviors that disrupt and annoy other students (e.g., interrupting or intruding into ongoing games, grabbing objects from others).
    - Suggest using a <u>self-talk strategy</u>. Self-directed speech reduces impulsivity, slows down responding, and provides time for objectively evaluating tasks and situations before reacting.
    - Place a simple visual cue, such as a picture of a reward on top of the desk or inside the notebook to remind the student to stop and think before acting.
    - Positively reinforce behaviors that reflect appropriate impulse control.
    - Compliment other students for self-regulating their behavior rather than continuously correcting the student.
- Assign shorter tasks with a criterion for accuracy if the student rushes through classwork.
- Eliminate incentives for completing assignments quickly (e.g., free-time, computer use).
- Teach <u>turn-taking</u> routines. (2)
    - Be aware that the neurology associated with **ADHD** may make the student feel that time is moving excessively and unbearably slowly. When the student becomes impatient, bored, and frustrated with a seeming delay, interruptions become difficult to inhibit.
    - Practice turn-taking in structured, teacher-directed lessons.
    - Minimize problems with interrupting and waiting one's turn by assigning the student to a small group in which there are frequent opportunities to interact.
    - Explain to the student who tries to dominate conversations or control games that others often become angry.
    - Discuss the nonverbal cues classmates exhibit when they are annoyed (e.g., frowning, wanting to stop playing a game, not wanting to interact socially).
    - Positively reinforce other students who demonstrate the appropriate turn-taking behavior. Always define the behavior ("I like the way John waited before taking his turn to speak.")
    - Determine the interests of the quiet, withdrawn student and arrange topic-centered activities so the student has a chance to contribute. Pose questions or ask for opinions.
        - *Notify the student in advance of the topic.*
    - Supervise group activities and be sure the reticent student has opportunities to take turns.

Chapter 12

HYPERACTIVITY

The following behaviors serve as general indicators. The student will not exhibit every characteristic listed. These behaviors may also be indicative of other problems.

Continually moving (shifting position in seat/moving desk)
Fidgeting (shaking leg/tapping foot/drumming fingers/tapping pencil)
Moving around room when required to be seated
Shifting from one uncompleted activity to another
Talking excessively
Playing with objects during lessons
Throwing things
Requesting frequent restroom breaks as movement tactic
Excessive running and climbing
Disrupting class/family life

Interventions

- Ignore minor motor movements that allow the student to release hyperactivity. (2)

    - 🐾 *Students with **ADHD** and/or **TS** have difficulty following rules that restrict movement.*

    - Permit doodling during listening activities. Doodling allows fine motor movement which decreases the restlessness and overactivity experienced by the student with **ADHD**.

    - Offer a small, noiseless squeeze toy that does not roll or an eraser with which to fidget during times of needed concentration.

- Allow standing, shaking legs, kneeling, or repositioning self in chair during the completion of class assignments.

- Permit standing during groups lessons or small group activities.

- Privately prearrange appropriate mobility options. (2)

    - Assign the student two seats in different locations in the room and allow movement from one seat to the other when needed. Place a table with three or four chairs at the back of the room. Permit the student to change chairs as needed.

    - Demonstrate how to move from one desk to another (e.g., take the required materials, go directly to desk, refrain from talking to other students).

        - 🐾 *Do not use these procedures if they embarrass the student.*

- Periodically give the class a movement break. For example, have the class stand up, reach for the sky, stretch or shake arms and shoulders, press hands together, touch toes, or twist waist.

- Ask the restless student to press the hands together, do push ups against the wall, knead modeling clay, carry heavy objects, or help rearrange classroom furniture. (6, 7, 8)

- Suggest making a trip to the office, taking a note to another teacher, sharpening a pencil, collecting papers, handing out materials, or getting a drink.

- Schedule opportunities throughout the day for physical activity. This should be in addition to regularly scheduled P.E. and recess (e.g., running around track, throwing ball in gym). (2)

- Never punish the student for uncompleted class assignments or inappropriate behavior with loss of recess. Movement stimulates the neurochemicals and decreases hyperactivity.

CHAPTER 13
EXECUTIVE DYSFUNCTION (EDF)

> EDF plays a critical role in the educational, behavioral, and social problems that many students with ADHD, TS, and/or OCD experience. However, it is often misunderstood by school personnel, parents, family members, and peers.

Executive Dysfunction (**EDF**) may first be observed during childhood. However, it becomes more apparent as students progress through middle school, high school, and college and are confronted with increasingly complex tasks and situations that demand independence, sustained effort, and executive functions. Executive functions, which include problem solving (goal setting, planning, prioritization, organization, sequencing, time management), flexibility, initiation, self-monitoring, use of feedback, and self-correction, are neurologically-based skills. (pp. 29-33)

Attention Deficit Hyperactivity Disorder (ADHD) and EDF

Research suggests that students with **ADHD** have difficulty performing executive tasks requiring planning, problem-solving, organization, generation and use of strategies, flexibility, initiation, and self-monitoring. (1, 2, 3) **EDF** is more commonly exhibited by students with ADHD-C and ADHD-I than ADHD-H/I. (4)

EDF often persists into adolescence (5, 6, 7) and adulthood. (8, 9)

Tourette Syndrome (TS) and EDF

Students with **TS-only** generally perform normally on performance-based tests of executive functions. (10, 11)

Students with **TS plus ADHD** have more difficulty than students with **TS-only**. (1, 10, 12)
Students with **TS plus ADHD** and **OCD** are the most impaired. (11, 13)

Obsessive-Compulsive Disorder (OCD) and EDF

Few research studies have been conducted to assess the executive functioning of students with OCD. Some studies suggest that these students tend to have difficulty with response inhibition (14) and nonverbal organization. (15)

Interventions for ameliorating the impact of executive dysfunction on academic and social skills can be located in Part IV and Part VII of this handbook.

Section III

General Recommendations

- Be aware that there is considerable variation in executive deficits among students. This limits the specificity of **EDF** in **ADHD**, **TS**, and **OCD**. A weakness may be present in one or more of the executive skills. Impairments may range from mild to severe.

- Recommend neuropsychological evaluations to determine the exact nature of the executive deficits.

  🐾 *One of the best indicators of **EDF** is disorganization.*

- Modify the classroom environment to adapt to the student's executive deficits.

- Recognize that the student who is experiencing difficulty with an executive skill cannot be expected to perform it without adequate instruction and practice.

- Teach one skill at a time until it has been mastered before requiring the use of several different skills.

IMPAIRED PROBLEM SOLVING
(TASKS/ACTIVITIES/SITUATIONS)

- Teach a <u>cognitive, problem-solving strategy</u> that compensates for impaired executive skills and facilitates learning.

  🐾 *Many students with executive dysfunction do not spontaneously acquire, generate, and/or use strategies to enhance learning and problem solving. However, EDF can be offset by learning and using cognitive strategies.*

  Use the following progression of instruction when teaching a strategy:

  ○ Explicitly and clearly describe the strategy. Explain <u>why</u> the strategy should be learned, <u>what</u> it will achieve, and <u>when</u> and <u>where</u> it should be used.

  ○ Model or demonstrate <u>how</u> to use the strategy in a meaningful context.
    - Use an electronic whiteboard, LCD projector with Power Point, or other multi-media aid.
    - <u>Verbalize</u> each step of the process.

  ○ Supply a <u>visual cue card</u> that indicates how to apply the strategy. The cue card might be taped to the student's desk or placed in the notebook as a reminder to use the strategy.

    🐾 *A visual reminder lessens the demands placed on the capacity of working memory. (p. 36)*

  ○ Provide <u>guided practice</u> by giving prompts and assistance. Monitor the student's ability to follow the steps of the strategy. Offer positive, corrective feedback as the student completes the process.

  ○ Have the student add the strategy to the "trick" book. (p. 64)

    🐾 *Many students will not master the strategy and will need to frequently consult the "trick" book.*

  ○ Provide <u>independent practice</u>. After determining that the student understands the strategy, gradually withdraw modeling, prompts, and assistance. Encourage working without the visual cue.

  ○ Review and reteach the strategy, if needed.

- Select as few cognitive strategies as possible when teaching academic, behavior and social skills to reduce the need to remember a different strategy for each one.
  - *The strategy used throughout this handbook is "**GET A CLUE**" (16) or "**PLAN**" (17) and is based on cognitive principles. Webster's Dictionary defines "clue" as "anything that guides or directs in the solution of a problem."*

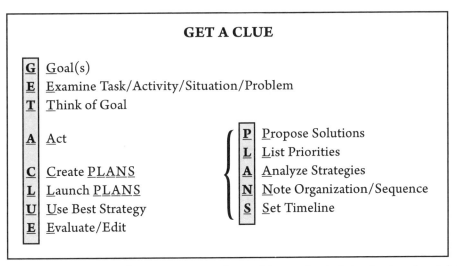

Figure 13.1. GET A CLUE – Cognitive strategy for teaching academic, behavioral, and social skills

Some students may not be able to follow the complexity of this strategy unless taught in incremental steps that must be mastered before continuing to the next step. Other students may need to learn a more simplified version "PLAN." If so, use "GET A CLUE" as a structure for discussing and teaching ways to solve tasks, activities, and problem situations.

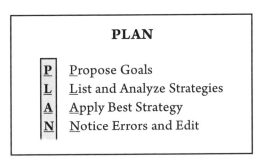

Figure 13.2. PLAN – Cognitive strategy for teaching academic, behavioral, and social skills

- *Examples of the use of these strategies are provided in the academic, behavioral, and social skills sections of this handbook.*

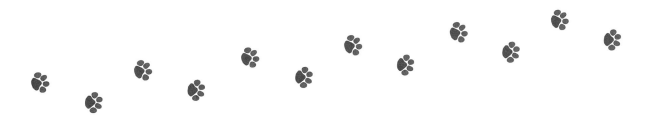

Section III

Difficulty Setting Goals

The following behaviors serve as general indicators. The student will not exhibit every characteristic listed. These behaviors may also be indicative of other problems.

- Being unaware that there is a problem that needs to be solved
- Failing to recognize need/usefulness of looking forward in time/setting goals/planning
- Having trouble identifying who, what, where, when, how, and why of a problem before setting goal
- Having difficulty stepping out of present to look at possible outcomes of tasks/activities/situations
- Being unable to generate goals when faced with an inquiry as to what to do (frequently responding, "I don't know.")
- Setting immature/unrealistic goals
- Confusing "wants" and "needs"
- Lacking understanding of need to do well in school
- Missing value of practicing toward mastery

Interventions

- Conference with the student in a location that does not allow others to overhear the discussion.

- Provide a template of "**GET A CLUE**," "**PLAN**," or another strategy for setting goals. (Appendix pp. 374–375)

- State and cue the first step – setting **GOAL(S)**.

    🐾 *Student involvement in goal selection may ensure motivation to achieve it.*

    Suggest that the student with teacher guidance:

    ○ define the skill/task/activity/situation in concrete, concise terms.

    Examples:

    <u>Academic skill</u>

    • self-evaluate mastery of an academic skill.

    • identify prerequisites to the skill that have not been learned.

    • discuss <u>what</u> the skill is, <u>when</u>, <u>where</u>, and <u>how</u> it might be used, and <u>why</u> learning it is important.

    <u>Problem situation</u>

    • think about <u>who</u> and <u>what</u> were responsible for the problem situation.

    • determine <u>when</u> and <u>where</u> the problem happened.

    • discuss possible reasons <u>how</u> and <u>why</u> the problem occurred.

    ○ break the skill, task, activity, or problem situation into its various parts and identify what needs to be accomplished.

    ○ establish long-term goals (e.g., improving reading comprehension grade, scoring well on the SAT, making and maintaining friendships).

- set <u>realistic</u> short-term goals as explicitly and clearly as possible. Be sure they are achievable (e.g., read a book about the American Indians, write a three page book report, turn it in two weeks from today; take a SAT preparatory course; apologize for making inappropriate comments to a peer).

  🐾 *When goals are unrealistic and success is rarely experienced, effort and motivation to achieve is diminished.*

  - determine whether the goals are practical (e.g., ask trusted adult).
- Help the student revise goals by asking open-ended questions.
- Offer alternatives to the student's suggestions, if necessary.
- Gradually decrease assistance until the student is able to establish goals independently.

Difficulty Planning

Interventions

- Meet with the student and devise **PLANS** for accomplishing goals.

  Suggest that the student:
  - <u>p</u>ropose ideas, solutions, or strategies for solving a task, activity, or situation.
  - <u>l</u>ist priorities to determine the most important issues to address.
  - <u>a</u>nalyze both the positive and negative outcomes or consequences of each idea.
  - <u>n</u>ote the <u>organization</u> and <u>sequence</u> of the idea, solution, or strategy so the goal can be solved efficiently and effectively.
  - <u>s</u>et a timeline for accomplishing the goal.
- Provide sufficient time for considering ideas and solutions to problems.
- Recommend <u>thinking aloud</u> during the planning activity.
- Aid, cue, and repeat each step until plans can be made independently.

Difficulty Proposing or Generating Ideas/Strategies/Solutions

The following behaviors serve as general indicators. The student will not exhibit every characteristic listed. These behaviors may also be indicative of other problems.

Lacking skills to generate/brainstorm ideas/solutions to tasks/activities/problem situations
Being unable to think of strategies to use to bypass weaknesses
Having difficulty analyzing steps needed to carry out a goal
Doing the first thing that comes to mind
Using a haphazard approach to problem solving

Section III

Interventions

- Provide assistance with the proposal of ideas, solutions, strategies to solve problems.

    🐾 *Avoid discussing and criticizing ideas as they are offered. Criticism suppresses creativity and idea generation.*

    Suggest that the student:

    ○ activate existing knowledge and personal experiences about the task, activity, or situation.

    ○ brainstorm as many practical and unusual ideas, solutions, or strategies as possible.

    ○ use a mind mapping strategy to stimulate ideas. Place a key concept in the middle circle. Record every idea that comes to mind, circle that word, and connect it to the closest related idea.

    ○ tape record proposed ideas, solutions, or strategies.

    ○ generate ideas on a computer (e.g., use a mind mapping program such as *Inspiration/Kidspiration*). (18)

    ○ brainstorm with a classmate who excels in generating original ideas.

Difficulty Prioritizing

The following behaviors serve as general indicators. The student will not exhibit every characteristic listed. These behaviors may also be indicative of other problems.

Having difficulty understanding reason to do tasks/learn facts and skills considered "BORING!"
Proclaiming, "I don't need to know that when I grow up!"
Overlooking importance of effort/value of practice toward mastery
Thinking practice work is boring and refusing to do it
Spending too much time on activities of personal interest (TV/video games/computers/sports/friends)
Spending less time on important tasks (completing homework/studying)
Having trouble determining most relevant information
Focusing on minor details and overlooking main ideas

Interventions

- Discuss the importance of setting goals, planning, and applying effort that results in achievement.

    ○ Explain how neurological disorders, especially **ADHD** and **EDF** contribute to a sense of boredom and tedium for normal everyday tasks (e.g., doing repetitive work even when the material has been mastered).

    ○ Stress that throughout life people are confronted with tasks and situations that are disagreeable. However, in order to succeed, one has to do things that are not considered interesting or entertaining (e.g., completing homework, taking tests, doing chores, cleaning).

    ○ Define the meaning of the saying "No pain, no gain." In order to succeed, one has to do things that are frustrating and "BORING."

    ○ Read and discuss stories of goal setting, persistence, and positive outcomes.

- - Point out examples of effort and accomplishments of individuals with **ADHD**, **TS**, and **OCD**. For example, Wolfgang Amadeus Mozart (famous composer) was considered to have ADHD, Jim Eisenreich (World Series baseball player) has TS, and Howard Hughes (Hollywood director and aviator) had OCD.
  - Ask the student to share personal results of persistence.
  - Talk about the importance of demonstrating responsible behavior in school and its relationship to a good job ("If you were an employer, would you hire someone with good working skills or someone whose record shows a dislike for working?").
  - Analyze how others use academic skills in their lives. For example, stress the advantages of learning math and its relationship to a good job (e.g., "The owner of a car dealership wants to hire employees who are able to calculate the cost of a car, order parts, write bills, and receive payments.").
  - Discuss the long-term results of having a good job (e.g., cars, electronics, house, vacations, happy family).
- Encourage the student to take an active role in learning.
  - Provide advance notice of classwork that might be repetitive and frustrating.
  - Point out the student's strengths and demonstrate how to use them when completing difficult tasks.
  - Emphasize that learning is a sequential process that builds on mastery of previous skills.
  - Explain how automatic skills require no effort and make academic tasks easier.
  - Offer words of encouragement while the student is completing tedious assignments and tasks (e.g., "I know this work is very hard, but persistence results in mastery." "I'm glad you decided to try. You're doing an excellent job on your assignment.").
  - Evaluate the student's work on the amount learned rather than comparing it to the achievement of others.
    - Have the student use a graph to record effort and its connection with achievement (e.g., mastery of vocabulary and spelling words, multiplication facts).
    - Reward effortful work and progress.
- Limit the number of tasks, choices, or options that the student is required to prioritize.
- Reinforce the prioritization of problem solving and conceptual understanding instead of the ability to quickly complete an assignment or be the first to answer a question.
- Stress the most essential concepts prior to starting the lesson.
  - Indicate what will be important about the information to be presented (answers to questions, main ideas, related facts).
  - Cue listening for who, what, when, where, how, and why.
- Identify and state the importance and purpose of each skill, strategy, and piece of information as it is presented.
- When speaking, use cue words or phrases to emphasize importance (e.g., "Listen carefully, _____." "It's important to know that _____." "In conclusion, _____.").
- Repeat, rephrase, or summarize key ideas frequently.

Section III

- Have the student paraphrase or summarize information.
- Provide a lettered or numbered outline that lists essential concepts and facts.
- Supply lettered or numbered graphic organizers to indicate main ideas and related details. (Appendix pp. 379–388)
- Prepare a list of questions assessing key concepts that will be asked after the lesson. Review the questions before teaching the lesson.
- Teach the student how to prepare a "To Do List" to prioritize, consolidate, and organize all of the essential tasks that need to be carried out during the day, week, and month.

  🐾 *A "To Do List" will help reduce the demands placed on working memory to remember several different tasks over an extended period.*

Ask the student to:

- list all the activities that must be accomplished during the day, week, and month.
- separate important tasks from time-consuming unimportant ones.

  🐾 *Check with an adult to see if priorities are correct.*

- divide difficult tasks and assignments into several smaller ones and add them to the list.
- include the steps needed to complete long-term reports and projects.
- add important dates such as deadlines, due dates, and tests.
- incorporate recreational activities.
- number the tasks in the order of importance.
- rewrite the list in priority order.

  🐾 *Be aware that when a student responds "yes" to completing tasks and activities, "when" it is to be accomplished often is not specified. The student needs to always define "when." (19)*

Difficulty Organizing

The following behaviors serve as general indicators. The student will not exhibit every characteristic listed. These behaviors may also be indicative of other problems.

Appearing bewildered/confused/overwhelmed when confronted with large tasks/activities
Having difficulty organizing ideas
Being unable to break down tasks into manageable subtasks
Having trouble generating/using organizational strategies when working on tasks/assignments
Finding it difficult to use assignment book
Lacking the skills to organize time
Becoming disorganized when changing from one activity to another
Having problems organizing materials/belongings/backpack/locker
Being unable to locate items in desk/backpack/locker
Losing personal possessions/materials needed for tasks/activities
Having difficulty remembering to take home needed books/study materials, returning books/materials/homework to school
Lacking/not understanding organizational strategy for cleaning (notebook/bookbag/locker/closet)
Relying on teachers'/parents' organizational skills

Students with **ADHD** and **OCD** have been found to be impaired on organizational tasks. Organizational deficits are in part considered to be a function of impulsivity, a lack of planning, and/or overlooking the need to use strategies. (20, 21)

 Clinical and teaching experience suggests that these students often experience anxiety, feel overwhelmed, and do not know how to proceed when confronted with disorganization both at school and at home.

Interventions

- Be aware that organizational skills tend to be better developed in a classroom that provides structure and routine.

- Teach organizational strategies to enhance learning.

     Strategies are important learning tools that help the student acquire, process, consolidate, store, and retrieve information. Teaching the strategies should be an essential component of the classroom curriculum.

    ○ Introduce a single strategy that can be used with various tasks such as "**GET A CLUE**" or "**PLAN**." Students are more likely to use a single strategy rather than multiple procedures.

    ○ Teach each step until mastered before introducing the next.

    ○ Cue use of the strategy until it can be applied independently.

- Encourage the use of graphic organizers to visually organize ideas and concepts. (Appendix pp. 379–388)

    ○ Use who, what, when, where, how, and why outlines to represent problems, attempted solutions, and outcomes.

       • Who were the main individuals involved?

       • Who were the others?

       • What happened during the event?

       • When did it occur?

       • Where did it take place?

       • Why was there a problem?

       • How was the problem solved?

    ○ Create mind maps to depict main ideas, subtopics, and details.

    ○ Use timelines to describe sequences of events, steps in a process, stages of something, or historical events and dates.

    ○ Use Venn diagrams to express the similarities and differences between ideas, people, places, events, or concepts.

    ○ Use circles with arrows to show how a sequence of events leads to results that are continuous and self-reinforcing.

    ○ Draw tables, bar graphs, pie graphs, or flow charts.

    ○ Use computer-generated graphic organizers.

Section III

- Require the use of a <u>notebook</u>. (22)

    - Recommend purchasing a three-ring notebook of business quality (metal rings) that is deep enough to hold materials for all classes and has pockets inside both covers.

    - Suggest using a notebook with Velcro fasteners on the outside to prevent papers and materials from falling out.

    - Obtain agreement from all of the student's teachers to allow the use of only <u>one</u> notebook.

    - Suggest placing a three-ring school supply pouch in the front of the notebook. The pouch should contain:

        - several mechanical pencils.
        - erasable pens (not for the left-handed student because the left hand and arm will smear the ink).
        - extra erasers (students erase frequently).
        - different colored markers/highlighters with visible ink.
        - small calculator (large enough for accurate key strokes).
        - scissors.
        - ruler.
        - small hole punch or a 3-hole punch designed to fit on the binder rings behind the pouch.
        - self-adhesive hole reinforcements for notebook paper (holes are often torn in notebook paper).

    - Recommend placing an <u>assignment sheet or book</u> in the front of the notebook. Make sure it is securely attached to the notebook.

        - 🐾 *If teachers insist on a separate notebook for each class, attach the assignment book to the school bag with a shoelace or other long cord so that it will not be lost.*

        - Allow the student to choose the type of assignment book. The student is less likely to use it if it feels awkward.

        - Suggest designing assignment sheets on a computer. List the subjects in the order in which they occur during the day.

    - Teach the student how to <u>organize the notebook</u>.

    Suggest that the student:

    - label subject dividers in the order of the student's schedule.
    - place a tabbed divider for each class.
    - color code tabbed dividers and book covers with the same color.
    - put a photocopy of the teacher's daily notes or notebook paper for taking notes behind each divider. Date all notes and place them in chronological order.
    - insert a color coordinated, manila folder with horizontal pockets at the end of each section. Use one side for class handouts and the other side for homework papers. Label accordingly.

- Use the assignment sheet in the notebook as a <u>communication log</u> with the parents.
    - 🐾 *Email or fax comments to the parents if the student's handwriting on the assignment sheet is too large or illegible.*
  - Initial that the homework assignments have been recorded correctly and that the homework was returned to school.
  - Have the parents initial that the assignment was completed to prevent unfair accusations if the work itself is misplaced between the home and school.
  - Use the log as a means of providing an accurate record if weekend privileges are being awarded for work completion. A Friday report can determine what rewards the student can earn (e.g., watching television, playing arcade games, using the computer, receiving an allowance, staying up late, going out socially, driving).
    - 🐾 *Do not use loss of social contact as a consequence if the student has difficulty establishing and maintaining friendships.*

- Recommend that parents purchase a heavy-duty <u>rolling bag</u> to help organize and keep track of belongings, assignments, and materials.

- Circumvent the student's <u>disorganization and forgetfulness</u>. (22)
  - Schedule extra time during the school day for organization.
    - Plan a study hall at the beginning or end of the school day so that the student can review and organize assignments, materials, and activities.
    - Assign an assistant or mentor to meet with the student at the beginning and end of the day to check the schedule and assignment sheet for the required books and materials.
  - Provide extra workspace to spread out materials (larger desk/table).
  - List necessary materials for each assignment/activity.
    - 🐾 *Minimize the number of items needed.*
  - Have an extra supply of materials, such as pencils and paper, available. Ask the parents to provide a large supply of materials at the beginning of each quarter.
  - Color code textbooks, notebooks, and folders so that each subject is color coordinated (e.g., red history book cover corresponds with the red history notebook and red folder). Color coding helps the student select the correct materials from the locker for the following class or homework. Teacher assignments might be written on matching colored paper.
  - Designate times during the day to organize materials.
  - Establish a weekly routine for cleaning out and reorganizing notebooks, folders, desks, lockers, and other possessions.
  - Provide extra transition time between classes.
  - Arrange for the student to go to the <u>locker</u> with an aide two to three minutes before the end of the day. Fine motor impairment, sequencing problems, and/or the need to repeat or do an act "just so" make opening the lock a very difficult task in a noisy, crowded hallway. The extra time also enables the student to calmly pack the school bag without the distraction of the other students. This helps ensure that the needed items go home.

Section III

- Ask the parents to purchase a <u>lock</u> with a key or a combination lock that requires no reverse sequencing to open. If the lock is built into the locker, provide the student with an alternative place to store books and materials.
- Tape a colorful list of needed homework materials at eye level inside the student's locker. ("Remember to take home _____.")
  - 🐾 *Change the list frequently to prompt attention.*
- Have an aide or resource teacher check the student's school bag to make sure the necessary items are included.

- Ask the parents to complete the Organizational Skills Survey to determine how disorganization is impacting functioning in the home. (23) (Appendix p. 405) Offer interventions as needed.

Suggest that the parents:

- purchase a heavy-duty rolling bag to help the student organize and keep track of belongings, assignments, and materials.
- label all belongings with the student's name.
- obtain from the school an extra set of books. This will alleviate worry and failure due to forgetting to take the books home.
- purchase, if necessary, the textbooks so that information can be underlined or written in the margins during lessons or reading assignments.
- do not allow any papers or tests to be thrown out until the courses have ended. Rather, put them in color coded, hanging files in the desk drawers at home.
  - 🐾 *Many students throw away homework or papers that were never turned in to the teacher.*

Difficulty Sequencing

The following behaviors serve as general indicators. The student will not exhibit every characteristic listed. These behaviors may also be indicative of other problems.

Lacking skills to break down and order steps for completing tasks/reports/long-term projects
Being unable to follow steps needed to accomplish tasks/assignments/problems
Having difficulty expressing oral/written ideas logically/sequentially
Experiencing problems interpreting/following multi-step explanations/instructions/oral directions
Completing only the first or last step of multi-step directions
Being unable to determine cause/effect and predict outcomes
Having difficulty logically/sequentially summarizing information

Interventions

- Teach sequencing words such as "before," "after," "first," "second," "next," "then," and "finally." Ask the student to relate personal stories using these words. (22)
- Practice sequencing by assigning a multi-step task (e.g., build a model airplane, bake cookies, make a pizza, perform an experiment). Use cue words to indicate the steps involved in planning and carrying out the task.
- Play classroom games in which the student practices sequencing to a logical outcome.

- Cut up a comic strip and arrange the sections in a mixed-up order. Have the student resequence the story.

- Use computer games involving sequencing (construction, planning an adventure).

- Write on the board or on an overhead transparency the order in which an assignment should be completed.

- Provide a list or outline of the steps required to complete an assignment, research paper, or long-term project. Insist that the list be placed in the strategy ("trick") book. (p. 64)

- Recommend using cognitive sequencing cues for abstract academic sequences (e.g., "**GET A CLUE**" or "**PLAN**" for problem solving (p. 109), "**D**irty **M**arvin **S**mells **B**ad" for the computation of a division problem. (p. 233))

- Provide templates of graphic organizers. (Appendix pp. 379–388)

- Monitor the completion of the first one or two problems to ensure that the correct sequence is being followed before allowing class assignments or homework to proceed.

  🐾 *The student with **OCD** and/or **EDF** may have great difficulty relearning a sequence that has been practiced incorrectly.*

Difficulty Managing Time

The following behaviors serve as general indicators. The student will not exhibit every characteristic listed. These behaviors may also be indicative of other problems.

> Having difficulty organizing schedule/using calendar
> Being unable to create timeline for completing long-term assignments/projects
> Lacking time estimation skills
> Misjudging available time/not allocating enough time to complete assignments/homework/reports/projects/studying for tests
> Being unaware of the passage of time (early/on time/late)
> Lacking a sense of time urgency (needing reminders to "hurry up")
> Failing to complete work within time limits/needing extra time
> Having difficulty organizing study time
> Procrastinating/starting assignments/homework/projects/studying for tests at last minute
> Losing track of the passage of time while engaged in absorbing activities (playing electronic games/socializing)
> Having trouble pacing self when studying for tests/taking tests
> Missing deadlines/due dates
> Arriving late for school/classes/activities/appointments

Students with **ADHD** may have an impaired sense of time that compromises their ability to complete tasks in an efficient and timely manner. Research suggests that they often have difficulty <u>estimating</u> time, reserving or <u>allocating</u> enough time to complete tasks within a given time frame, and being cognizant of the <u>passage</u> of time. (24, 25, 26, 27, 28). Time perception is considered to be dependent on attention, behavioral inhibition, and/or working memory. (27, 29, 30, 31)

Section III

Interventions

- Be aware that the "internal clock" of the impulsive student may be faster than that of the nonimpulsive student. The student is more likely to overestimate the passage of time (perceive time as moving slowly) and hurry to finish assignments, often making careless errors and becoming irritated with having to wait. Conversely, the student with a slower cognitive pace may underestimate time (think there is ample time) and fail to complete tasks and activities within the time limits.

- Develop an <u>awareness</u> of the amount of time spent on daily activities.
  - Furnish a day planner and list activities such as sleeping, eating, grooming, going to and from school, attending individual classes, studying, participating in sports, watching TV, playing video games, talking on the telephone, and socializing with friends.
  - Ask the student to record the time spent engaged in each activity.
  - Summarize at the end of one or two weeks.
  - Analyze and discuss the time spent.

- Provide instruction in time <u>estimation</u>.

  Suggest that the student:
  - estimate the amount of time that will be needed to finish an assignment (e.g., read a passage, answer questions at the end of a chapter, write a composition, solve a predetermined number of math problems).
  - record the estimate.
  - document the actual amount of time required.
  - discuss the difference between the estimate and time spent.

- Help the student monitor the <u>passage of time</u>.
  - Set time limits and provide reminders regarding the amount of time remaining.
  - Use a timer or stopwatch. After the designated amount of time, ask the student to estimate whether the work completion is early, on time, or late.
  - Indicate the remaining time 15 minutes, 10 minutes, and 5 minutes before the end of an activity.

- Require the student to use <u>daily and weekly schedules</u> and <u>monthly calendars</u>.
  - Explicitly and clearly describe the advantages of schedules. Explain <u>why</u> the schedules should be used, <u>what</u> they will achieve, and <u>when</u> and <u>how</u> they should be used. Emphasize that all successful students and adults use calendars/schedules.
  - Use an electronic interactive whiteboard, overhead projector, or a multi-media aid to demonstrate how to structure schedules and calendars.
  - Think aloud as the schedules are being organized.
  - Allow the student to design the type of schedule and calendar.

Suggest that the student:

- select the color, style, and size of the schedule and calendar. While there are many commercial styles available, a student often prefers to personalize schedules and calendars.

  🐾 *The student is less likely to use the schedule if the system feels awkward. If the student is allowed to select the type of schedule, motivation to use it may be enhanced.*

- create the schedules and calendars on the computer. List the activities in the order in which they occur throughout the day. Include free-time activities.

- add visual or pictorial cues to illustrate schedules for younger students.

- purchase an electronic or auditory style organizer. The student with visual strengths might choose a pocket-size electronic model that displays the daily and weekly schedules and the calendar on a screen. The verbally oriented student may prefer a voice-activated model. Select an organizer that has enough capacity for storage of daily, weekly, and monthly information.

- choose an organizer that provides external, time-based prompts (beeps, vibrations) to cue important activities (e.g., leaving for school, turning in homework, packing the bookbag, starting homework, going to bed, taking medication).

  🐾 *Monitor use of the calendar to be sure that the student is not distracted by games and the Internet.*

- Assist transferring the "To Do List" (p. 114) to the daily and weekly schedules and monthly calendar, estimating and allocating time required to complete tasks. Schedule accordingly.

Using the list, ask the student to:

- fill in during the weekend a week-at-a-glance schedule and large monthly calendar.

  - note due dates and steps for completing long-term assignments and studying for tests.
  - include special events such as field trips, athletic games, club meetings, holidays, birthdays, doctor's appointments, family events, and vacations.
  - schedule breaks between tasks.

    🐾 *More difficult tasks require more frequent breaks.*

  - highlight steps for completing a book report in one color, test dates in another color, etc. Always use the same colors (e.g., yellow for tests, light blue for term papers).

- Post the daily and weekly schedules and the monthly calendar for the class at eye level in the front of the room. (22)

  - Tape a smaller schedule to the student's desk, if appropriate.
  - Consult the daily schedule throughout the day to demonstrate and emphasize its usefulness.
  - Refer each day to the weekly and monthly schedules and point out due dates, field trips, and other important activities.
  - Cross off tasks as they are completed to provide a sense of accomplishment.

- Require placement of the daily and weekly schedules and monthly calendar in the front of the student's notebook.

- Recommend consulting with an academic assistant/tutor on a daily basis regarding schedules and time management. (p. 48)

Section III

INFLEXIBILITY

(COGNITIONS/BEHAVIORS/EMOTIONS)

Difficulty Being Flexible

The following behaviors serve as general indicators. The student will not exhibit every characteristic listed. These behaviors may also be indicative of other problems.

- Exhibiting rigid, concrete thinking
- Having difficulty using executive skills (analyzing tasks/activities/situations/problems; setting goals; making plans; initiating plans; self-monitoring/self-correcting)
- Perseverating (becoming "stuck" on one idea/detail/action)
- Being capable of doing only one thing at a time
- Being unable to think about a task/problem/situation one way and then think about it in a different way
- Being unable to change plans when confronted with obstacles/new information/mistakes
- Having difficulty modifying behavior in response to changing tasks/situational demands
- Using same approach to a problem even when it repeatedly has not worked/when told strategy was incorrect
- Becoming frustrated/overaroused by an unexpected change in plans/routine/activity
- Insisting on following rules/routines/plans
- Having trouble stopping/changing to new task/activity
- Finding transitions from one setting to another difficult (P.E./recess/lunch/bus)
- Overfocusing on electronic screens (TV/computer/video games) and not being able to stop when asked
- Being unable to adjust to multiple courses/different teaching styles/new expectations and rules
- Responding poorly to substitute teachers/bus drivers
- Being unable to shift from one emotion to another ("stuck" on hurt/angry feelings)
- Failing to generalize (carry over) learning to other situations

Cognitive inflexibility is at times a characteristic associated with **OCD** (32), but infrequently associated with **ADHD**. (33)

Interventions

- Teach the student who thinks concretely how to form concepts, use categories, generalize from one instance to another, apply rules, be aware of subtle aspects of a problem situation, and determine what is relevant, essential, or appropriate.

- Intervene when the student perseverates on just one thought or emotion.

    - Help the student identify and analyze the problem.

    - Demonstrate examples of being "stuck" on an idea.

    - Discuss situations that precipitate inflexibility.

    - Change the activity.

    - Provide movement breaks. Physical activity often can clear thinking.

    - Introduce a set of breathing exercises or relaxation techniques.

- Encourage the use of self-talk strategies to rephrase thinking ("My brain is tricking me. I <u>can</u> think about something else.").
  - 🐾 *Some students may <u>not</u> be able to alter thoughts regardless of the strategy used.*
- Assist the student who becomes overfocused on an emotion.
  - Speak calmly and slowly and provide reassurance.
  - Label what is happening (e.g., "It looks like you are "stuck" and having a hard time letting go of your angry feelings.").
  - Permit a "graceful exit" if the emotion is overwhelming. (p. 90)

- Provide a structured routine for the student to follow.
  - 🐾 *Changes in routine increase stress and can produce overarousal, anxiety, anger, withdrawal, and/or the feeling of being "stuck." The student may not be able to adjust and respond in a rapid, integrated fashion.*
  - Be consistent. The predictability of consistent routines provides security, decreases stress, and allows the student to direct more energy to learning.
  - Provide individualized schedules. Use pictures and/or words.
  - Distribute lesson plans in advance so that the student knows when lessons will change.

- Preview plans for future activities and events (e.g., fire drills, assemblies, field trips).
  - Clarify and discuss appropriate and expected behaviors.
  - Role play and rehearse how the student might respond.

- Inform the student several days before a teacher's absence and each day thereafter when possible. (22)
  - Prepare in advance a stimulating lesson plan to be used by the substitute teacher.
  - Video tape supplemental lessons to be shown to the class.
  - Prearrange with the student a strategy for avoiding trouble if a problem arises working while with the substitute (e.g., go to the resource room; nurse's, counselor's, school psychologist's, principal's office). This ensures the presence of a familiar adult

- Notify the student several times in advance of impending <u>transitions</u> to facilitate adjustment (e.g., recess, lunch, P.E., assemblies). (22)
  - Give several warnings, a few minutes apart (30 minutes, 15 minutes, 5 minutes) prior to the transition.
  - Use a timer as a reminder of the approaching need to change.
  - Hand the student a note indicating an imminent change in routine.

- Assist with <u>transitions between academic tasks and activities</u>. (22)
  - Provide additional time to shift from one academic task or classroom activity to another.
  - Make sure the student has put away all materials from the previous activity, located the appropriate items, and has everything necessary on the desk before beginning a new lesson. If not, discreetly help the student.

Section III

- Do not allow the student with **OCD** to start any activity that cannot be finished in the allotted time frame. The student may not be able to flexibly change tasks or sets. If the student cannot be redirected, the activity must be completed. A subsequent anxiety attack may produce inappropriate behaviors.
    - Provide work that can easily be completed.
    - Divide a lengthy assignment into several independent tasks.
    - Assign shorter tasks requiring accuracy and quality of response.

- Allow <u>no unstructured time</u>. For example, when the student finishes an assignment before the allotted time has expired, have a practice lesson available. When the student is returning to the classroom from an unstructured activity such as recess, have an assignment ready. (22)

- Provide extra structure and supervision during transitions. (22)

    > *The student with **ADHD** and/or **TS** may become overaroused by unstructured situations. Some of the most difficult ones may occur in the hallways between classes, in the cafeteria, at recess, during P.E., and on the school bus. They are not only noisy, less structured times, but also offer limited, if any, adult supervision. Students often complain about being teased, embarrassed, and touched by the other students. The amount of noise and jostling may overstimulate the student's sensory system and produce an explosive "storm" or implosive "lockdown."*

    - Have an adult remain near the student.
    - Stand at the end of the line in order to observe what is occurring and intervene if necessary.
    - Allow the student to leave the classroom two or three minutes early to avoid crowded hallways.

- Provide positive reinforcement for transitioning successfully.

- Prepare the student for a <u>change of schools</u> – elementary to middle school, middle to high school, high school to post-secondary facilities. (34)

    > *Many students experience considerable anxiety about transitions to new school environments. Worries include: finding the locker and using a combination lock; following a schedule; changing classes; finding classrooms in a large and unfamiliar building; getting to classes on time; adjusting to multiple courses and teachers; adapting to new and different teaching styles, expectations, and rules; meeting new classmates and making friends; avoiding teasing and embarrassment; being bullied; changing clothes in the locker room; and riding the bus.*

    - Provide activities in the late elementary grades that will facilitate the transition.
        - Teach the student how to use daily, weekly, and monthly schedules. (p. 120)
        - Teach organizational strategies that promote independent functioning.
        - Practice changing classes.
    - Role play situations that might occur in the new school.
    - Select a small group of students from the new school to provide information about the school and to answer questions.
    - Organize visits to the school.

Chapter 13

- Arrange for the student to accompany a middle or high school student to classes and activities for one day.
- Encourage students to write letters or send emails to new students.
- Suggest setting up a website that presents information about the school (e.g., yearly schedule, rules, routines, teachers and various courses taught, extra curricular activities, transportation).
- Meet with the middle or high school teachers to discuss problems that the student may encounter and strategies that have proven successful.
- Recommend that the new school establish peer mentoring and tutoring programs.

INITIATION/EXECUTION DIFFICULTIES
(TASKS/ACTIVITIES)

Difficulty Initiating/Executing

The following behaviors serve as general indicators. The student will not exhibit every characteristic listed. These behaviors may also be indicative of other problems.

Appearing hypoactive/lacking energy/uninterested when required to generate and carry out ideas/responses or solve problems
Seeming "lazy"/"unmotivated" when confronted with tasks/activities/problems
Not knowing where to start an assignment
Being slow to get started and finish tasks considered uninteresting/tedious/"BORING" (assignments/homework/chores)
Procrastinating (starting assignments/long-term projects/activities at the last minute)
Avoiding beginning and completing activities, even when knowing failure to do so will result in negative consequences
Needing frequent reminders to begin/continue working
Being reluctant to ask for help when needed

Interventions

- *Failure to initiate or complete tasks and activities is a behavior associated with the student's neurological disorder rather than purposeful behavior. It does not reflect noncompliance, irresponsibility, disinterest, or a problem performing the task.*

- Recognize that the student's arousal level fluctuates throughout the school day and from one day to the next. Deregulated arousal influences the ability to initiate problem solving or begin and carry out new tasks. (22)

  - Assign more demanding tasks when the student is optimally aroused (p. 27) and hands-on or less demanding activities when underaroused. (pp. 71-78)

    - *Many students are not fully aroused at the beginning of the day and experience a decline in energy and attention in the afternoon.*

  - Increase arousal or energy levels by including short movement breaks during the lesson.

Section III

- Always provide learning activities with which the student can experience success. A student learns to initiate and finish a task with repeated success.
    - Assign work at the appropriate instructional level. (p. 64)
    - Determine whether the student feels capable of performing the assigned task. Often the teacher is unaware that the student is unwilling to admit that simple tasks are sometimes too difficult to perform.
    - Divide assignments into short, manageable segments. The student may become discouraged and frustrated when confronted with a long assignment and then be unable to overcome the inertia caused by feeling overwhelmed. Gradually increase the length and difficulty of the assignments as the student demonstrates success.
- Design tasks and activities that are inherently interesting and motivating to the student.
- Provide reminders and cues regarding materials needed for starting and completing assignments ("You need to have your reading book and yellow and light blue highlighters to underline main ideas and important details.").
- Make sure the student understands the directions needed to initiate the task. Use a comprehension check before allowing the student to begin working.
- Pair the student with a "buddy" or place in a small group that will initiate and complete assignments without teacher intervention.
- Assist completion of the first one or two items to make sure the student knows how to do the assignment (e.g., read the first paragraph of the reading assignment to the student, complete one or two math problems with the student, provide the first sentence of a writing assignment).
- Give additional time for the student to self-start rather than expecting immediate initiation.
- Provide a prompt for task initiation. A hand signal or previously agreed-upon verbal cue might be used.
- Teach the student how to appropriately ask for help.

> **Children often misbehave when they have difficulty with an assignment. They are afraid to ask for assistance. Their experience has taught them that to request help is to risk rebuke. They would rather be punished for acting up than ridiculed for ignorance.**
>
> Dr. Haim G. Ginott. (1993). Teacher and Child: A Book for Parents and Teachers. New York, NY: Collier Books. (p. 60)

- *Asking for help is an important skill that students need to learn so that they can be successful at school, in the home, and with peers. Make the student feel comfortable asking for assistance. Many students will not ask for help because they are too embarrassed.*

Suggest that the student:

- share and discuss situations in the past when help was needed (e.g., not understanding an explanation of a math concept, not knowing how to complete a homework assignment, being unsure how to solve a social problem).
- identify the steps needed for seeking help.
    - determine if there is a problem that cannot be solved independently.
    - decide if help is wanted.
    - analyze the positive and negative consequences of not asking for help.
    - decide on the best person to help (teacher, aide, parent, peer).
    - ask that person to help.
    - use the suggestions offered to solve the problem.
- role play various situations in which help might be required. Follow the recommended steps and evaluate the outcome.

• Positively reinforce task initiation and completion.

　Praise the student no matter how small the success.

• Initiate a meeting with the student to schedule make-up work after an absence. Direct teacher intervention and monitoring may be required. The student may feel overwhelmed by the amount of work missed and be unable to initiate getting and completing make-up assignments. (22)

　The neurologically challenged student works harder than usual just to keep up and feels that it is an impossible challenge to complete all the unfinished assignments.

- Break the work into manageable units.
- Check with and support the student at regular intervals until the work is completed.

IMPAIRED SELF-MONITORING/USE OF FEEDBACK/SELF-CORRECTION

Difficulty Self-Monitoring

The following behaviors serve as general indicators. The student will not exhibit every characteristic listed. These behaviors may also be indicative of other problems.

Being unaware of personal strengths and weaknesses
Lacking insight into one's own vocal/motor/emotional/sensory behavior
Having difficulty understanding effect inappropriate behavior has on self/others
Failing to recognize behaviors that are disrupting class
Neglecting to use strategies to monitor academic/social behavior
Making careless errors (not attending to details)
Overlooking errors while completing assignments

Students with **ADHD** are often unaware of their own performance and behavior. They may deny or have difficulty accepting that there is a problem. Other students may recognize the problem but are unable to consistently use monitoring strategies. (35, 36)

Section III

Interventions

- Develop the student's <u>self-awareness</u>.

    Suggest that the student:

    - identify and list personal strengths.
    - analyze challenges or weaknesses that interfere with performance.
    - predict performance prior to initiating a task.
    - grade an assignment and explain how the grade was derived.
    - record the number of <u>correct</u> answers and compare results over time.
    - praise or reward self if the prediction was accurate.

- Recommend the use of <u>self-questioning</u> to monitor academic, behavioral, and social functioning. (37)

    - Explain the purpose of self-questioning and how it will help identify and evaluate performance and behavior.
    - Model or demonstrate how to use self-questioning.
    - Help generate questions such as:
        - "What did the teacher ask me to do?"
        - "Do I know how to do it?"
        - "What does this word/phrase/sentence/problem/direction mean?"
        - "Does this make sense to me?"
        - "Which strategy should I use?"
        - "Do I understand? I don't understand. What should I do?"
        - "Have I finished what I was supposed to do?"
        - "Is there something different that I should do next time?"
    - Suggest asking the questions aloud.
    - Prepare a checklist of the student's self-generated questions to serve as a visual guide.
    - Practice self-questioning with the student. Give positive, corrective feedback.
    - Encourage independent self-questioning without a visual cue when the technique has been mastered.
    - Recommend that the list of questions be placed in the students "trick" book. (p. 64)

- Teach the importance of making self-directed, positive, reinforcing statements and <u>rewarding one's self</u> for academic, behavioral, and social accomplishments.

    - *Self-rewards foster self-esteem and motivation.*

Suggest that the student:

- decide on a goal or achievement to be rewarded.

    - *Initially choose a readily attainable goal (improve history grade, make one new friend) before selecting a more difficult goal (making the honor roll, belonging to the "in crowd").*

- set criteria to earn rewards (verbal and/or material rewards).

- strive to meet goal.

- reward self when goal is reached. Verbally praise self and specifically relate reinforcement to achievements.

- accept "self-rewards" and acknowledge the positive feelings engendered.

Difficulty Using Feedback

The following behaviors serve as general indicators. The student will not exhibit every characteristic listed. These behaviors may also be indicative of other problems.

Being unable to learn from past mistakes/consequences and apply new strategies
Committing same mistakes over and over again
Failing to modify performance/behavior based on positive/negative feedback
Demonstrating inability to generalize from one situation to next
Appearing to not care when actually "clueless" about feedback

Interventions

- Be aware that prompt, specific, and corrective feedback often encourages the student to continue working, make corrections, and to persist until the assignment is completed.

- Prompt the use of a strategy that previously proved successful before beginning a similar task (e.g., "Be sure to take time to highlight the important words in the instructions before starting." "Remember to work more slowly and use the cue card to follow the steps of the problem.").

- Teach the student how to generate solutions to problems based on feedback.

    - Emphasize strategies or behaviors that produced <u>correct</u> responses. Stress success to build self-esteem.

    - Ask for incorrect answers and responses to be corrected.

        - *Finding correct answers to missed problems provides excellent feedback.*

    - Review assignments and tests and help the student analyze why responses or solutions were correct or incorrect (e.g., "I didn't read the directions carefully." "I was working too fast and forgot to use the cue card to solve the problem.").

- Provide suggestions that indicate what to do the next time in order to be successful. Eliminate consequences.

Section III

- Offer options when the student is confronted with a difficult problem. Analyze the outcome of the choice selected.

- Teach the concept of generalization. Discuss the similarities between situations and how an appropriate response in one situation applies to another.
  - Practice using same solutions in different settings.

Difficulty Self-Correcting

The following behaviors serve as general indicators. The student will not exhibit every characteristic listed. These behaviors may also be indicative of other problems.

Showing frustration when asked to correct assignments
Using same approach to a problem even when it repeatedly has not worked or when told strategy was incorrect
Having difficulty changing response/behavior even when it will help
Lacking solutions to problems when faced with inquiry as what to do (frequently responding, "I don't know.")
Turning in work with numerous errors despite knowing answers

Interventions

- Discuss benefits of self-correction (e.g., effect on mastery/grades).

- Cue the use of strategies that have proven successful.

- Encourage subvocalization (repeating aloud) as tasks and activities are being completed.

- Suggest using self-generated questions to implement corrections.

- Provide strategies such as editing strips, spelling lists, and grammar checkers to assist self-corrections.

  > *Help the student make editing strips or checklists to increase awareness and motivation to use them.*

- Positively reinforce use of self-correction.

CHAPTER 14

MEMORY PROBLEMS

School success, behavioral management, and social competence require efficient and effective short-term (immediate and working memory) as well as long-term (encoding and retrieval) memory skills. Insufficient arousal, inattention, slow processing speed, and inefficient working memory impact the encoding, storage, and retrieval of information. Executive dysfunction influences the ability to plan, organize, and use cognitive strategies to enhance learning.

Clinical and teaching experience suggests that the immediate, semantic, and episodic/autobiographical memories of students with **ADHD**, **TS**, and/or **OCD** are unimpaired while working memory; procedural, prospective, and strategic memory; metamemory; and information retrieval pose many problems. (p. 39)

Interventions for ameliorating the memory problems that impact academic and social skills can be located in Part IV and Part VII of this handbook.

General Interventions

- Recognize that students have difficulty with memory tasks for a variety of reasons. Students with **ADHD** may be restless and distractible and have difficulty paying attention. Those with **TS** often struggle to suppress tics while those with **OCD** are preoccupied with obsessive thoughts or trying to resist compulsions.

- Recommend a comprehensive neuropsychological evaluation to determine the source of the student's memory problems.

SHORT-TERM MEMORY PROBLEMS

Difficulty with Immediate Memory (Sensory Register)

The following behaviors serve as general indicators. The student will not exhibit every characteristic listed. These behaviors may also be indicative of other problems.

> Failing to recognize verbal/visual/tactile information
> Forgetting information immediately after presentation
> Having trouble listening to teachers/parents/peers
> Displaying academic inconsistencies/unevenness
> Misunderstanding instructions/assignments/homework
> Being unable to follow fast paced lessons
> Becoming overwhelmed by lengthy sentences/long explanations
> Missing important details
> Being unable to paraphrase/summarize information

Interventions

- Be aware that immediate short-term memory is dependent on a sufficient level of arousal and focused attention. Make the appropriate interventions as needed.

    > *Any sensory information that does not capture attention disappears from immediate memory within milliseconds.*

- Determine whether difficulty registering information is <u>modality-specific</u> (verbal, visual, tactile).
  - Introduce material through the student's strongest modality.
  - Combine different sensory modalities (e.g., verbal and nonverbal presentation of same material).
  - Provide additional assistance in difficult areas.
- Stress important information before beginning a lesson.
- Reduce the amount of material presented.
- Omit nonessential, irrelevant details.
- Link the material to what is already known.
- Repeat explanations and instructions.
- Pause frequently and ask for the information to be paraphrased or summarized.

Difficulty with Working Memory

Working memory (WM) plays a crucial role in the acquisition of complex cognitive and academic skills. (1, 2, 3, 4) Arousal, speed of processing, attention, and executive functions act as important mediators of WM. Working memory, on the other hand, is a significant factor in the successful performance of executive skills (self-regulation of cognitions, behavior, and emotions; flexibility; problem solving; self-monitoring/self-control).

The following behaviors serve as general indicators. The student will not exhibit every characteristic listed. These behaviors may also be indicative of other problems.

Impact on Executive Functions
Lacking skills to hold a goal in mind while planning/analyzing demands of future tasks/situations/activities
Being unable to determine cause-and-effect/foresee/predict the outcome of tasks/situations/activities
Having difficulty generating/evaluating different alternatives to achieve a goal
Thinking concretely rather than flexibly
Having difficulty drawing conclusions/making decisions
Using random approaches rather than strategies
Being unaware of the passage of time
Being unable to think about and respond to positive and negative feedback and adjust responses/behavior
Lacking ability to generalize (carry over) to other situations

Impact on Classroom Activities
Forgetting what one is doing while working
Rushing through assignments in order to limit forgetting what one is in the process of doing
Becoming overwhelmed when task has several parts or steps
Having trouble remembering the steps of task while executing it
Being unable to retrieve information from long-term memory during processing
Forgetting material and skills learned yesterday
Forgetting information when copying from the board/book
Forgetting instructions for assignments
Forgetting to turn in completed work

Impact on Behavior
- Interrupting during class discussions before forgetting ideas
- Becoming frustrated when assigned too many tasks
- Having problem thinking through responses before acting/speaking
- Being unable to consider consequences of behavior
- Acting out when forgetting or being unable to recall information
- Forgetting appropriate responses and becoming rude as anxiety/anger increase
- Lacking skills to generate alternatives to problem situations

Attention Deficit Hyperactivity Disorder and Working Memory

Research suggests that working memory problems are often associated with ADHD. Impairment is most often identified in the central executive (processing) and phonological and visual storage and rehearsal components of WM. Difficulty becomes more evident as the amount of information to be processed increases. (p. 36) (4, 5, 6)

- Disinhibition and difficulty suppressing or resisting distractions interfere with working memory. (7, 8, 9)
- Impaired verbal working memory has been found to compromise understanding of complex, unfamiliar information such as that presented in textbooks or during classroom instruction. (10, 11)

Tourette Syndrome and Working Memory

A behavior rating scale of executive functions, completed by both teachers and parents, indicated that TS students with and without **ADHD** tend to have working memory problems. (12)

Obsessive-Compulsive Disorder and Working Memory

Little research is available regarding the working memory of students with **OCD**. Numerous research studies examining working memory in adults have failed to find working memory impairment. (13) However, the student who is focused on obsessions and compulsions will be unable to successfully process demanding tasks.

Interventions

- Ensure a sufficient level of arousal to maintain attention. (pp. 71–78) (14)

    Adequate levels of arousal and attention are prerequisites for working memory.

    ○ Be alert for fluctuating arousal levels.
    ○ Assign complex cognitive tasks requiring working memory when the student is optimally aroused and less demanding activities when underaroused.

      Many students are not fully aroused at the beginning of the day and experience a decline in energy and attention in the afternoon.

    ○ Schedule frequent movement breaks.
    ○ Use high interest, multi-media presentations.

Section III

- Recognize that working memory is limited in <u>capacity</u>. (p. 36) The amount of information that can be maintained and processed is affected by the <u>amount</u>, <u>type</u>, and <u>complexity</u> of the activity. (15)

  - 🐾 *If a complex task requires effortful processing, less space is accessible for storage. Conversely, as more storage space is needed to temporarily hold information, less workspace is available for processing.*

  ○ Design well-organized lessons that are easy to understand and follow.

  ○ Pace the presentation of information so the student who is underaroused or processes slowly will not be penalized.

- Reduce the <u>amount</u> of material to be processed, particularly if the information is detailed and complex or requires sustained attention.

  - 🐾 *A normally developing 7-8 year-old student can hold in working memory approximately 3 pieces of information, an 11 year-old 4-5 items, and a 15 year-old 7 pieces or chunks. (3, 16) If the student has working memory problems, the deficit will impact the amount of information that can be processed. Be sure to determine the student's auditory and visual working memory span.*

  ○ Omit extraneous information.

  ○ Stress important information.

- Analyze the impact of different <u>types</u> of learning material on working memory.

  - 🐾 *The amount of space available may differ for each content area (e.g., the capacity to process reading comprehension materials may be different from the capacity to solve math problems; the capacity to follow a discussion of a novel may differ from the capacity to follow a science lecture). If the student has a strength in an area, enough storage and workspace will be available to efficiently and effectively maintain and process information presented in that modality. (p. 36)*

  ○ Create lessons that capitalize on the student's learning preferences (cognitive style). (pp. 65-67)

  ○ Compare the student's ability to remember nonmeaningful information (math facts, history dates) and material presented in a meaningful context (stories, relationship to own experiences, current events). If the student is able to recall meaningful information more readily, provide learning activities in a meaningful context.

  ○ Translate abstract concepts into concrete, <u>meaningful</u> examples.

- Minimize the <u>complexity</u> of the material to be introduced.

  ○ <u>Link unfamiliar, abstract concepts with the student's existing knowledge and personal experiences.</u>

    • Initially make associations for the student. Then teach the student how to attach new learning to previous learning. For example, plan a field trip to a battlefield before studying the history of the war.

    • Brainstorm what information is already known that relates to the topic.

  ○ Use the "**K**-**W**-**L**" method to generate what is **K**nown about a topic, what the student **W**ants to know, and what has been **L**earned. (17)

- Present unfamiliar or complex information with the use of visual aids (e.g., diagrams, illustrations, graphic organizers).
  - Include examples such as pictures and objects to provide the visual-cognitive association (e.g., "Mother Vowel's" house for positioning letters in space when handwriting). (18)

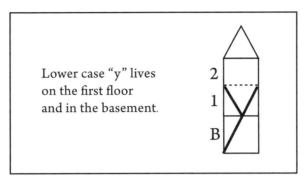

Figure 14.1. Mother Vowel's House – Visual cognitive cue for positioning letters in space

- Avoid introducing several concepts simultaneously. Wait for the first skill to be mastered before introducing the next skill.
  - *Some students can perform well when completing tasks individually but do not have enough workspace available to perform the same tasks simultaneously.*

- Design activities that keep information prolonged or <u>maintained</u> in working memory.
  - Pause and write information on an interactive whiteboard or overhead transparency.
  - Encourage the student with <u>verbal strengths</u> to subvocalize or <u>rehearse</u> the information several times. Information in working memory is subject to rapid loss unless the material is rehearsed.
    - *The spontaneous use of subvocal rehearsal emerges after 7 years. (19)*
    - Allocate rehearsal time during the lesson.
    - Repeat and paraphrase material.
    - Pose open-ended questions that prompt the student to think about, cognitively rehearse, and state information.
    - Ask for the information to be summarized.
    - Organize small groups of students to discuss the topic.
  - Have the student with <u>nonverbal strengths</u> use visualization (e.g., create in the mind mental illustrations or series of absurd or unusual images, picture a whiteboard and draw on it, sketch pictures on paper, use graphic organizers). Then suggest summarizing the information while looking at the images.
  - Combine as many different sensory modalities as possible (verbal, visual, motor, tactile). For example, supplement verbal material with visual aids, highlight or underline main ideas on electronic whiteboards, give demonstrations, and perform experiments.
  - Create cooperative experiences (e.g., experiments, projects, games, role play, field trips).

Section III

- Increase <u>automaticity</u> through repetition and frequent practice. A skill is considered automatic if it can be performed quickly, accurately, and outside conscious control. Automatic skills require minimal, if any, working memory capacity and free resources for processing.

  > *If skills have not been mastered at an automatic level (e.g., correct spelling, knowledge of math facts and formulas, regulation of emotional responses, understanding another person's point of view) and demand more effortful processing, the capacity of working memory will be limited. Less workspace will be available for performing complex tasks (e.g., written expression, math computation, anxiety and stress management, friendship development and maintenance).*

- Be aware that working memory problems result not only from trouble maintaining several pieces of information in mind during processing (e.g., understanding reading materials, steps of a math operation, ongoing social interaction), but also from difficulty <u>retrieving information from long-term memory</u> to use during processing (e.g., meaning of words, math facts, consequences of past behavior during a negative social exchange).

LONG-TERM MEMORY PROBLEMS

Difficulty Encoding or Consolidating (Learning)

The following behaviors serve as general indicators. The student will not exhibit every characteristic listed. These behaviors may also be indicative of other problems.

   Relying only on rote memory to learn
   Requiring meaning in order to learn
   Lacking skills to associate new information with what is already known
   Being unable to paraphrase/summarize information just presented
   Possessing partial knowledge of topic but not integrated whole
   Having difficulty selecting/learning/using efficient strategies
   Learning new skill one day and forgetting it the next
   Requiring additional practice to master information at automatic levels

Most students with **ADHD**, **TS**, and/or **OCD** have no difficulty encoding information. Research suggests that students with **ADHD** are able to learn information that is meaningfully structured for them. Deficits become apparent when efficient strategies are required to encode information that is presented with less structure (e.g., in expository texts, in situations that require extended study periods, with delays between studying and recall). Overlooking the need to use strategies makes it difficult to logically and systematically file and store material so it can be easily retrieved. Furthermore, these students tend to spend less time studying and apply less effort when needed. (20)

Most students with **OCD** have intact verbal memory but experience problems learning new, nonverbal material. Nonverbal memory deficits are considered to be secondary to deficient organizational skills. (21)

Interventions

- Recommend that the student get an adequate amount of sleep. (pp. 74-78) Research has found that sleep plays an important role in learning and is needed to consolidate and reconsolidate (organize and reorganize) information in long-term memory. (22)

   Suggest that the parents:

   - encourage review of study materials just before going to sleep. (15)

   - prohibit watching television, playing computer games, using the telephone, and communicating via the Internet between studying and going to sleep. (15)

- Gain attention prior to introducing a lesson. The longer the student is able to sustain attention, the greater the depth of processing and the more relevant the material becomes.

- Systematically introduce and repeat new concepts so that errors are minimized. "Errorless learning" has been found to improve encoding more than "trial-and-error" learning. (23, 24) Preventing errors during the initial learning phase will keep the student from practicing and, thereby, storing incorrect information.

   *Students with **ADHD** may not benefit from a trial-and-error teaching approach as they often do not learn from their mistakes due to inattention and inefficient working memory. Students with **OCD** may have difficulty unlearning errors that have become "stuck" in their minds.*

   - Limit the amount of new information that is presented.

   - Teach concepts at a concrete level before requiring abstract learning.

   - Introduce only one skill or concept at a time.

   - Do not allow the student to guess.

     - Immediately provide the correct answer.

     - Use prompts or cues to ensure correct responding.

     - Provide correct answers until the material is mastered.

       Mastery is defined as knowing the information 90 percent of the time over an extended period.

   - Do not expect mastery immediately after introducing new skills. Practice until skills become permanent and automatic.

- Recognize that the student may need to be explicitly and directly taught information that other students learn implicitly or automatically (e.g., reading skills, math facts and procedures, organization and preparation of projects and reports, establishment and maintenance of friendships).

Section III

- Use teaching methods that enhance encoding.

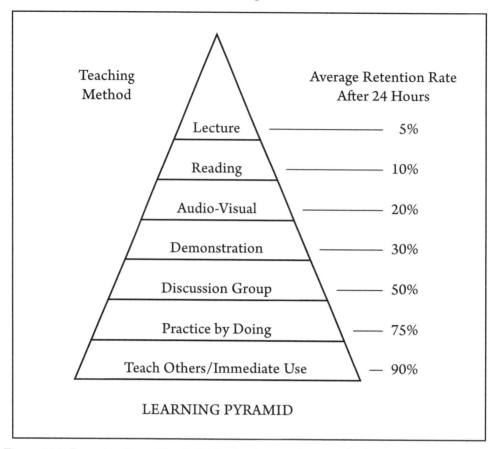

Figure 14.2. Learning Pyramid – Activities that increase learning (25)

- Share stories from personal life experiences.
- Show pictures, illustrations, and objects related to the topic.
- Assign group projects.
- Draw pictures to illustrate oral information.
- Use graphic organizers to visually consolidate information.
- Use Power Point presentations, interactive whiteboards, or other multi-media aids.
- Utilize manipulatives.
- Design hands-on activities.
- Conduct experiments.
- Plan academically relevant field trips.

- Be aware that information introduced at the beginning and end of a lesson is more easily and accurately recalled than that presented in the middle. (26)

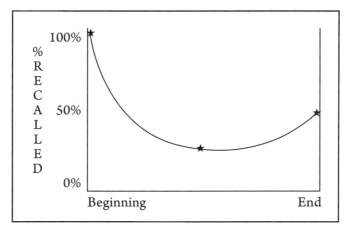

Figure 14.3. Recall During Lesson – Information recalled at beginning, middle, and end of lesson

- Divide lessons into segments with breaks in between. A lesson that is separated into several smaller units provides more opportunities to learn. (27)
  - Present the most <u>important and difficult information</u> at the <u>beginning</u> of each segment. Initial information is more effectively encoded due to a greater amount of attention, processing, and rehearsal that is applied to it.
    - *If the information is presented at a fast pace, the opportunity to process and rehearse is eliminated.*
    - *New concepts and skills presented at the <u>end</u> of each segment need to be briefly reviewed at the start of the following session.*
  - Emphasize material in the <u>middle</u> of the lesson to facilitate recall by introducing <u>novelty</u> or doing something unusual or unique (e.g., introduce humor, use audio-visual aids, show pictures and objects, add color, give demonstrations, conduct experiments). (28)
- Plan the <u>length of the segment</u> based on the age of the student and the complexity of the material.
  - *Teaching experience suggests that, during the early elementary grades, instructional periods should last for approximately 10 minutes. In adolescence, breaks should be given after 20 minutes. If the student is inattentive or has working memory problems, the length of the session should be shorter. More complex information requires more frequent breaks.*
- Breaks should last about 5 minutes. During the break, have the student do something <u>unrelated</u> to the topic being presented.

- Discourage <u>rote memorization</u>. Simply memorizing something does not ensure understanding and learning.
  - *Students who use rote memory to learn abstract, inherently uninteresting facts (e.g., math facts and procedures, rules of grammar, capitalization and punctuation rules, science formulas, history dates and facts, foreign languages) will not have enough cues available to efficiently retrieve the information.*

- Avoid expecting the student to memorize an excessive number of facts and details. Indicate which material should be learned.

Section III

- Stimulate learning during the encoding phase.

  - 🐾 *Passive review such as reading materials over and over is an ineffective and inefficient means of transferring information into long-term memory.*

  ○ Stress the similarities, differences, and associations between past and current information.

  - 🐾 *One of the most important factors in long-term memory is its associative links.*

  ○ Provide numerous, cooperative, hands-on learning activities (e.g., projects, experiments, role play, debates).

  ○ Ask open-ended questions that activate and structure the student's thinking about the material.

  ○ Apply concepts in different, real-life situations.

  ○ Suggest using self-talk with inflection during encoding.

  ○ Have the student explain the lesson to a classmate who needs assistance.

  ○ Encourage the use of flash cards.

  Suggest that the student:

  - use 3 x 5 or 4 x 6 index cards.
  - write vocabulary words, key concepts and facts, dates, questions, chemistry and physic elements, formulas, or foreign language words and phrases on one side and definitions, events, explanations, and answers on the other side.
  - respond orally to the cards.
  - review the cards in random order.
  - concentrate on the ones that are difficult to remember.
  - study the cards with parents or friends.
  - carry the cards in a pocket or notebook, and study them at various times throughout the day.

- Teach metacognitive encoding strategies overtly and directly. Emphasize the importance of learning and using strategies. Material that is encoded with the use of strategies and filed in a logical, organized manner is more readily accessed and recalled. Organization is an essential component of long-term memory.

  - 🐾 *Students with **ADHD** often use less efficient strategies when consolidating information into memory. While many of these students are able to identify and describe strategies that should be used, they frequently do not use previously learned strategies when confronted with difficult and complex memory tasks requiring more in-depth processing. (20)*

  ○ Assess the student's learning style preferences. (pp. 65-67) Select strategies that capitalize on the strongest modality.

  ○ Teach strategies recommended in the different academic areas in this handbook to help the student consolidate information.

  - 🐾 *The student may not be able to generate strategies and will need assistance.*

- Include explicit instruction about <u>when</u>, <u>where</u>, and <u>why</u> strategies are important and <u>how</u> they will increase learning.

    Ask the student to:
    - analyze task demands/problems.
    - consider various strategies.
    - select a strategy that has previously been useful when memorizing similar information.
    - subvocalize the steps of the strategy as they are applied.
    - evaluate and monitor the effectiveness of the chosen strategy.
    - try a different strategy if the one being used proves ineffective.

- Prompt the use of strategies, if necessary.
- Suggest consulting the "trick" book when a strategy cannot be recalled. (p. 64)
- Help the student learn how to generalize (transfer) the use of a strategy from one learning situation to another once a strategy is mastered.

- Encourage the <u>association</u> and <u>integration</u> of new information with existing knowledge and personal life experiences. Material is not stored as a single item but recorded throughout the brain in multiple interconnecting locations. Therefore, the more connections that are made, the more likely the information will be remembered and retrieved.

    - Link an abstract concept with a previously learned meaningful experience. For example, relating the Shakespeare's play *Romeo and Juliet* with Stephen Sondheim's musical *West Side Story* places the play in the vernacular, both culturally and linguistically. Watching *Glory* before studying that era of history provides more meaning to the Civil War.
    - Plan academically relevant field trips to associate topics with real-life experiences.

- Teach <u>verbal strategies</u> to maximize learning. (14)

    Suggest that the student:
    - compose humorous or absurd <u>stories</u> incorporating the material to be learned. The more ridiculous or silly the stories the more likely they will be remembered (e.g., story relating how Pierre from South Dakota fell in love with Helena from Montana as a means to learn the capitals of those two states).
    - combine the first letters of each word to be learned to form <u>acronyms</u>. For example, an acronym for the names of the Great Lakes would be HOMES – Huron, Ontario, Michigan, Erie, Superior. (source unknown)
    - create <u>acrostics</u> by using the first letter of each word to be learned to make a sentence. For example, an acrostic for E, G, B, D, F, the lines in the treble clef music staff, would be "Every Good Boy Does Fine." (source unknown)
    - form <u>abbreviations</u> to enhance recall. Write the key words to be remembered, arrange them in order if they must be remembered sequentially, and underline the first letter of each word (e.g., ADHD, <u>a</u>ttention <u>d</u>eficit <u>h</u>yperactivity <u>d</u>isorder).
    - make up <u>rhymes</u> when words in the information sound alike (e.g., "In 1492, Columbus sailed the ocean blue." or "Thirty days hath September, April, June, and November.").

Section III

- put new information to <u>music</u>. For example, it is a daunting task for a four-year-old child to learn the sequence of the twenty-six abstract letters of the alphabet. However, singing the "ABC" song makes encoding of the alphabet much easier. The songs from *Schoolhouse Rock!* make educational topics easier to learn (e.g., "Lucky Seven Sampson," "Figure Eight," "Naughty Number Nine" from *Multiplication Rock*; "Lolly, Lolly, Lolly Get Your Adverbs Here," "Conjunction Junction," "Busy Prepositions" from *Grammar Rock*; "The Body Machine," "The Energy Blues," "A Victim of Gravity" from *Science Rock*"). (29)

- Teach <u>categorization</u> skills (placing new information into existing categories). (14) Grouping or chunking strategies improve the encoding and subsequent recall of information. (30)

  Suggest that the student:

  - reduce information to be learned into categories or chunks (memory units). For example, names, dates, places, and spelling words are easier to remember if they are grouped together into small categories that are related to each other rather than one long list (e.g., all spelling words with the same prefix or root word).

  - ensure that the size of the chunk matches the length of the verbal and nonverbal memory spans. The ability to learn information decreases significantly when an effort is made to encode more than the memory span can retain.

- Encourage the use of <u>visualization</u>.

  Suggest that the student:

  - create <u>images</u> or series of pictures about the events in a story. The pictures should be nonsensical, humorous, or unusual to enhance learning.

    🐾 *Check to make sure the student can visualize (make a mental picture). This skill can be taught.*

  - <u>draw</u> pictures that illustrate important concepts.

  - use <u>graphic organizers</u> to visually structure information. Most of the information is encoded by the time the organizer is completed. (Appendix pp. 379–388)

    - use who, what, when, where, how, and why outlines to represent problems, attempted solutions, and outcomes.

    - create <u>mind maps</u> to depict main ideas, subtopics, and details.

    - draw <u>timelines</u> to describe a sequence of events, steps in a process, stages of something, or historical events and dates.

    - fill in <u>Venn diagrams</u> to express the similarities and differences between ideas, people, places, events, or concepts.

    - use <u>circles</u> with arrows to show how a sequence of related events produce results that are continuous and self-reinforcing.

    - draw <u>tables</u>, bar graphs, pie graphs, or flow charts.

    - emphasize various concepts and related facts by highlighting with different colors.

  - encode information using the <u>Method of Loci</u> (Ancient Rome).

    - visualize a familiar location such as the home and choose specific places (e.g., living room, dining room, family room, kitchen).

    - place the information to be remembered in the various rooms.

- remember the information by walking through the rooms and recalling the items associated with each room.
- use the same sequence each time that the method is used.

• Provide adequate review by using repetition and rehearsal strategies to ensure overlearning and mastery.

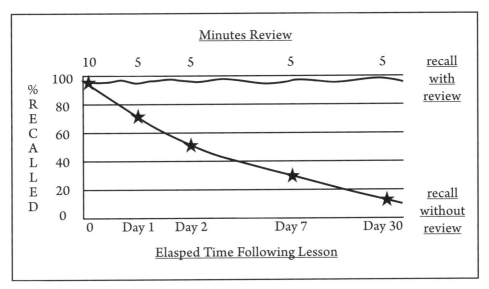

Figure 14.4. Elapsed Time and Review Following Lesson – Passage of time on retention of information, with and without review.

> 🐾 *Most forgetting occurs in the first few minutes after the information is processed. A quick review helps ensure that learning is permanent. (27, 31, 32)*

Suggest that the student:

○ review information 5-10 minutes after the lesson is completed and while recall is at its strongest.

> 🐾 *Studying the material at a later time requires relearning, not just reviewing.*

- subvocalize (whisper under breath) during the review.
- recite while covering or looking away from the material.
- paraphrase or summarize information.
- spend extra time studying the middle sections of learning materials. Beginning and ending sections are more easily remembered. Middle sections need extra review and emphasis.

○ do something different each time the material is studied.

- color code the material.
- reorganize or outline notes.
- transcribe the information on a word processing program.
- use voice-activated software on a computer.
- put visually presented information into words.
- review the most important facts just before going to sleep.

Section III

- review 24 hours after material has been consolidated during sleep.
- review materials and class notes as part of daily study sessions.
- review at regular but increasingly longer intervals (one week, one month, throughout the school year).

> 🐾 *Reinforcing learning at intervals negates the 80% decrease in memory over time.*

Difficulty Retrieving (Recalling)

The ability to recall information and skills accurately and at a rapid rate becomes increasingly important during the late elementary and junior high school years. The student in the upper grades is expected to have acquired basic information and mastered reading, writing, and math skills at automatic levels so that the demands of more complex learning can be met.

The following behaviors serve as general indicators. The student will not exhibit every characteristic listed. These behaviors may also be indicative of other problems.

- Having trouble recalling on demand correct spellings/math facts and procedures/history facts and dates/rules of grammar
- Lacking knowledge of or not using strategies to aid retrieval
- Pausing often when speaking/responding slowly to questioning
- Using simple, concrete vocabulary when speaking/repeating words
- Producing vague rather than specific answers
- Using filler words ("thing," "stuff," "um")
- Inventing stories/facts to substitute for forgotten information
- Having difficulty maintaining topic/talking in circles
- Forgetting information learned yesterday
- Being unable to answer test questions even when material is known
- Having more difficulty retrieving information on free-recall tests (fill-in-the-blank/essay) than on recognition tests (multiple-choice/matching/tests accompanied by word banks)
- Having trouble completing tests in allotted time

Research studies suggest that students with **ADHD** initially learn new, unfamiliar material but have difficulty quickly and efficiently retrieving and articulating previously memorized information. (33, 34) They often "know" more than they can recall. Ineffective use of strategies during the encoding phase frequently interferes with the ability to remember information.

Interventions

- Determine whether the inability to remember represents a true retrieval problem or is related to failure to attend to material, to efficiently process tasks in working memory, to apply strategies to encode and systematically store information, to rehearse and practice skills, and/or to use retrieval cues to assist recall.

- Postpone recall tasks if the student is underaroused (pp. 71-78) or overaroused. (pp. 81-95)

    > 🐾 *Arousal levels have a significant impact on ease of retrieval.*

- Allow extra time if the student is slow to retrieve information.

- Stimulate recall by providing retrieval cues for the younger student.
  - Supply phonetic cues.
    - Say the beginning consonant sound of the intended word.
    - Provide a word fragment containing the beginning syllable.
  - Present an associated word which belongs to the same semantic (conceptual) class.
  - Offer multiple-choice cues.
  - Provide sentence completion cues.
- Supply a word bank from which to choose the answers, especially for fill-in-the-blank assignments and tests.
- Furnish in advance specific questions to be answered in class or on tests.
- Place more emphasis on assessing <u>understanding</u> of concepts rather than recall of specific facts.
- Permit demonstration of what has been learned in an alternative form (e.g., poster, diagram, timeline, newspaper article, video or Power Point presentation, 3-dimensional project).
- Be aware that <u>free recall</u> tasks that require the student to remember information without the assistance of <u>cues</u> (bits of information that stimulate recall) are considerably more difficult than <u>recognition</u> tasks.
  - Use a multiple-choice or matching test format rather than a short-answer format.
    - *Fill-in-the-blank questions are difficult for the student with retrieval problems.*

There are several forms of long-term memory that affect academic, behavioral, and social performance. Review the definitions of these memory disorders in Chapter 6.

Difficulty with Procedural Memory

The following behaviors serve as general indicators. The student will not exhibit every characteristic listed. These behaviors may also be indicative of other problems.

Having trouble remembering multi-step explanations/instructions
Having problems recalling the sequence for accomplishing tasks/assignments/problems
Omitting steps/carrying out tasks in the wrong order

Interventions

- Write on the board or an overhead transparency the order in which assignments should be completed.
- Provide a list or outline of the steps required to complete an assignment, research paper, or long-term project.
- Provide models of graphic organizers. (Appendix pp. 379–388) Have the student place examples of the organizers in the strategy ("trick") book and consult them as needed. (p. 64)

Section III

- Monitor the student to ensure that the correct procedure is being followed before allowing classwork or homework to proceed.

    🐾 *The student with **OCD** or **EDF** may have difficulty relearning procedures that have been practiced incorrectly.*

- Recommend using cognitive sequencing cues for abstract academic sequences (e.g., "**GET A CLUE**" and/or "**PLAN**" for problem solving (p. 109), "**D**irty **M**arvin **S**mells **B**ad" to maintain the order of computation in a division problem. (p. 233))

Difficulty with Prospective Memory

Prospective memory becomes increasingly important as the student progresses through school. The elementary student is frequently reminded of future activities and due dates by teachers and parents. However, the middle or high school student is expected to "remember to remember" responsibilities and deadlines independently.

The following behaviors serve as general indicators. The student will not exhibit every characteristic listed. These behaviors may also be indicative of other problems.

> Having difficulty looking to the future
> Forgetting to carry out assigned/planned tasks
> Forgetting to check assignments/homework in assignment book/electronic organizer/calendar
> Forgetting to take books home to study/return materials to school/turn in homework assignment
> Forgetting to take make-up tests
> Forgetting to keep appointments/social commitments

Effective prospective memory requires planning a task or activity, retaining the plan in working memory, monitoring the passage of time, and/or flexibly switching from an ongoing activity to initiate the action. Students with ADHD often have deficient prospective memory skills resulting in failure to carry out a planned task, achieve a goal, or finish a task or activity at a specified time in the future. (35, 36, 37, 38)

🐾 *Impaired prospective memory is more evident in unfamiliar, complex situations rather than routine ones.*

Interventions

- Consult recommendations offered in the Prioritization and Time Management sections regarding "To Do" lists, daily and weekly schedules, and monthly calendars. (pp. 114, 120-121)

- Promote the use of external memory systems such as assignment notebooks and electronic organizers. (p. 116)

- Review interventions for Homework in Chapter 23.

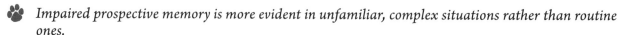

Difficulty with Strategic Memory

The following behaviors serve as general indicators. The student will not exhibit every characteristic listed. These behaviors may also be indicative of other problems.

> Overlooking need to use strategies to increase understanding/complete assignments/solve problems
> Forgetting to use strategies to encode information
> Forgetting to use strategies to facilitate retrieval
> Being unable to recall strategies from one year to the next

Students with **ADHD** at times present with strategic memory deficits. They tend to use less efficient strategies during encoding. Although they are able to identify and describe strategies that should be used, they overlook the need to use them when confronted with difficult and complex tasks. The deficit is not related to an inability to use the strategies as they are able to use them when prompted to do so. Executive deficits in self-regulation, planning, organization, and monitoring impact strategic memory. (18, 38)

Interventions

- Offer direct assistance in use of the appropriate cognitive strategies to efficiently encode and recall information. (pp. 136-145)

- Provide verbal/visual cues to elicit known strategies.

- Prompt the use of strategies as necessary.

- Remind the student to consult the strategies and work samples that were placed in the strategy ("trick") book. (p. 64)

- Pair the student when studying for a test with a classmate who uses successful memory strategies.

Difficulty with Metamemory

The following behaviors serve as general indicators. The student will not exhibit every characteristic listed. These behaviors may also be indicative of other problems.

> Lacking awareness of one's own memory strengths and weaknesses
> Being unaware that there are strategies available to aid memory
> Lacking knowledge of effective/efficient strategies
> Not knowing when/where certain types of strategies should be used
> Being unaware that a strategy was applied inappropriately
> Having difficulty deciding what information needs to be memorized
> Failing to determine if the material has been sufficiently mastered
> Overlooking need to self-monitor while performing memory tasks

Early elementary students are less cognizant of their memory problems and less aware of the need to use strategies to enhance memory. Metamemory is normally developed by 12 years of age. (19)

Section III

Interventions

- Assess the student's awareness of personal memory capabilities and the strategies that have been most effective for different types of memory tasks.

    Suggest that the student:
    - identify and list individual memory strengths.
    - analyze challenges or weaknesses that interfere with performance.
    - predict performance prior to initiating a recall task.
    - select and use a strategy.
    - grade the assignment/test and explain how the grade was derived.
    - record the number of <u>correct</u> answers and compare results over time.
    - discuss the effectiveness of the chosen strategy.
    - praise and reward self if prediction and strategy were accurate.

- Demonstrate and discuss procedures normally used to memorize learning materials.

- Use memory strategies that are congruent with the student's learning style preferences. (pp. 65-67)

    🐾 *Insight into how the student best learns will have a direct impact on the motivation to select and use strategies.*

SECTION IV
ACADEMIC INTERVENTIONS

CHAPTER 15

ORAL EXPRESSION

Students with **ADHD, TS,** and/or **OCD** generally do not have expressive language disorders involving deficits in articulation (pronunciation and clarity of speech), phonology (awareness of speech sounds), semantics (knowledge and use of vocabulary), or syntax (understanding and use of grammar). In fact, when expressing themselves spontaneously they often pronounce words correctly, possess age adequate vocabularies, are verbally fluent, and produce sentences with correct grammar.

Verbal expressive difficulties occur when the students are expected to interact and communicate with peers and adults, participate in classroom discussions, and work in groups with other students. These on-demand and pragmatic language deficits (difficulty using language in social situations) are often secondary to inattention, impulsivity, executive dysfunction (difficulty planning, prioritizing, organizing, sequencing, self-monitoring, self-correcting), inefficient working memory, and/or retrieval problems. (1, 2, 3, 4, 5)

> *Interventions for expressive language deficits are beyond the the scope of this handbook. If the student with **ADHD, TS,** and/or **OCD** has expressive language problems, recommend a comprehensive evaluation by a speech and language pathologist. The language assessment should also include hearing and auditory processing tests as these processes often contribute to language disorders.*

General Recommendations

- Understand that stammering and <u>stuttering</u>, behaviors that interfere with fluent speech and cause repetition of syllables and blockage or hesitation when trying to speak, may be involuntary vocalizations associated with **TS**. Speech abnormalities such as echolalia (repeating the other person's words), palilalia (repeating one's own words), and coprolalia (uttering inappropriate or obscene words) are not language disorders.

    > *Vocal tics are not amenable to speech or language therapy.*

- Be aware that speech dysfluencies of the student with **TS** and/or **OCD** may reflect a need to complete a sequence of actions (count to ten, tap ten times) or think about a response until it sounds "just right" before speaking.

Recommendations for pragmatic language deficits or difficulty communicating effectively and appropriately with others are included in Chapter 27 - Social Skills Interventions. Suggestions for retrieval problems are located in the individual chapters.

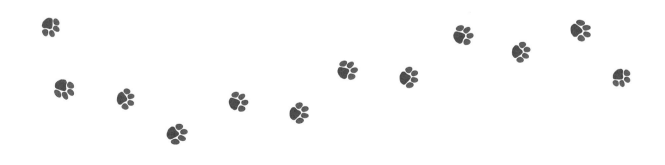

CHAPTER 16

LISTENING COMPREHENSION

A significant portion of the elementary school day is spent listening to teachers give instructions, introduce academic materials, and explain ideas. As the student progresses through the middle and high school years, listening skills are increasingly required. To be a good listener, the student must be able to attend and use executive skills and working memory for enhancing comprehension and remembering information presented in lessons.

General Recommendations

Review Classroom and Individual Student Interventions in Chapters 8 and 9.

- Distribute listening activities throughout the day. Several short periods with frequent breaks will improve comprehension.

- Evaluate the student's learning style preferences for listening activities and design lessons accordingly. (pp. 65-67)

    - Ask the student with auditory strengths to paraphrase or summarize materials or to put graphically presented information into words.

    - Have the student with a visual-spatial learning style watch movies, DVDs, or Internet websites related to the topics; complete graphic organizers during the lessons; or draw pictures of the material.

    - Suggest that the kinesthetic (tactile) learner act out or role play, participate in hands-on activities (e.g., demonstrations, experiments, model building), or play educational games related to the topic.

    - Have the logical thinker categorize, connect ideas and draw conclusions ("if _____, then _____."), make predictions, use Venn diagrams to demonstrate similarities and differences, or create time lines to show the series of events.

    - Recommend that student who prefers to learn interpersonally discuss lessons with a partner.

    - Permit the intrapersonal learner to read independently about the topics and choose the formats for demonstrating comprehension of the lessons.

    - Maximize learning by incorporating auditory, visual, and kinesthetic materials into each lesson.

- Recommend that the student be assessed for a receptive language disorder (difficulty processing and understanding spoken language) by a speech and language pathologist when interventions do not alleviate listening comprehension problems.

- Suggest a comprehensive audiological examination to rule out a hearing or auditory processing disorder (difficulty correctly distinguishing sounds in words).

    🐾 *Incorporate the teaching techniques and ideas used by the speech and language pathologist and/or audiologist into the daily curriculum.*

- Recommend a neuropsychological evaluation to determine whether underarousal/slow processing speed, inattention/impulsivity/hyperactivity, executive dysfunction, and/or memory problems are impacting listening comprehension.

Section IV

Before Oral Lesson:

- Provide the parents, resource teacher, and/or tutor with the class syllabus so that they can offer assistance previewing the concepts and facts to be covered in class.
- Assign as homework, reading material about the topic to be discussed the following day.
- Suggest reviewing the notes from the previous lesson during the homework study session.
- Provide an organized overview of the concepts to be discussed (e.g., teacher-prepared outline that lists main ideas and relevant facts, graphic organizer or mind map that highlights important information).
- Furnish a partial outline or mind map to be completed during the lesson.
- Prepare and hand out a list of questions to be answered.
- Review previous lesson.
- Preview the topic to be introduced.
  - Plan an academically relevant field trip (e.g., outing to a battlefield before studying the history of a particular war, visit to an aquarium before learning about sharks, trip to an interactive science museum before studying magnetism).
    - Provide advance information about the topic.
    - Create activities to be completed during the field trip (e.g., scavenger hunt, questions to be answered, objects to be drawn or photographed).
    - Discuss the field trip before initiating the lesson.
  - Link unfamiliar, abstract concepts with the student's existing knowledge and personal experiences.
    - Initially make the associations for the student. Then teach the student how to attach new learning to previous learning.
    - Brainstorm what information is already known that relates to the topic.
    - Include examples such as pictures and objects to provide a visual association.
  - Use the "**K**-**W**-**L**" method to generate what is **K**nown about a topic, what the student **W**ants to know, and, at the end of the lesson, what has been **L**earned. (1)
- Define vocabulary.
  - Associate definitions with something meaningful to the student.
  - Hand out a prepared sheet with proper spellings and acceptable definitions. Allow the student to use it while listening.
- Use a pre-listening activity to introduce the learning material (e.g., perform a science experiment, watch a video from the Nova series such as the January, 2004 program *Mars Dead or Alive* before discussing the planet).
- Have the student who is able to take notes independently organize the pages before the following day's lesson.

During Oral Lesson:

- Always review vocabulary and concepts from the previous lesson.
- Circulate around the classroom while talking.
- Be aware that listening comprehension is impacted by the <u>amount</u>, <u>rate</u>, and <u>complexity</u> of the information presented.
    - Use short, concise sentences when speaking.
    - Use vocabulary words that the student understands.
    - Provide clear explanations and instructions.
    - Omit extraneous details.
    - Present material at a slower-than-normal rate.
    - Increase vocal volume and use more expressive intonation to stress key concepts.
    - Speak using gestures and facial expressions.
    - Pause frequently to allow time between statements for information to be processed and consolidated.
    - Translate abstract concepts into more concrete, meaningful examples.
- Avoid excessive lecturing. Use teaching methods that enhance learning. (p. 138)
- Encourage student participation to promote involvement with the lesson.
    - Ask how the new information is related to existing knowledge and personal life experiences.
    - Prompt thinking and discussion by posing questions and asking for opinions.
        - Ask open-ended questions beginning with "how," "why," or "what" to prompt thinking.
        - Pause for several seconds to allow time for processing.
        - Acknowledge correct responses. Respond and paraphrase answer. Avoid only saying "Good!" or "That's right."
    - Seek clarification of what has been presented if the student appears to not be comprehending.
    - Allow and encourage questions to be asked during the lesson.
- Use cue words or phrases such as "Listen carefully." "Don't forget that _____. "It's important to know that _____." "This will be on the test _____." "In conclusion, _____."
- Repeat, rephrase, or summarize information periodically to stress its importance.
- Emphasize answers to teacher-prepared question guides.
- Encourage the use of a <u>notetaking strategy</u>. (pp. 259-266)
- Supplement oral lessons with <u>visual aids</u>.
    - Write on the board, overhead projector, or interactive whiteboard. Highlight, underline, or frame important information with different colors.
    - Use graphic organizers to demonstrate compare/contrast, problems/solutions, opinions/facts.

Section IV

- Draw directional arrows to show cause-and-effect relationships.
- Create a timeline to highlight temporal events.
- Provide a partial outline or mind map to be filled in as the information is presented.
- Furnish a template of an organizer to be completed during the lesson.

After Oral Lesson:

- Stress the importance of summarizing or restating in a few words the most important information presented (key concepts, related facts, and conclusions).
- Recommend reviewing notes, filling in missing information, and asking questions when the notes are incomplete or the material is not understood.
- Suggest organizing the information into a mind map, written list, table, chart, or diagram.
- Answer and discuss questions prepared by the teacher.
- Encourage generating questions to ask other students.
- Formulate a list of questions about the material that will be covered in the following lesson.

> **Tics/obsessions/compulsions, underarousal/slow processing speed, inattention/impulsivity/hyperactivity, executive dysfunction, and/or memory problems frequently interfere with the ability to derive meaning from orally presented information.**

UNDERAROUSAL/SLOW COGNITIVE PROCESSING SPEED

The following behaviors serve as general indicators. The student will not exhibit every characteristic listed. These behaviors may also be indicative of other problems.

Appearing not to be listening
Being slow to understand instructions/explanations
Having difficulty keeping up with lectures and taking notes
Being reluctant to participate in class discussions
Needing additional time to think before answering questions
Asking "What?" frequently

Interventions

Review interventions for Underarousal and Slow Processing Speed in Chapter 10.

- Present material at a slower-than-normal rate or pause frequently to allow time between statements for the information to be processed. Fast-paced instruction may be difficult to understand because additional time is required to register and process the material.
- Write key concepts on the board, overhead transparency, or interactive whiteboard.
  - Use different colored pens or pencils to highlight or underline important points.
  - Frame main points with circles, squares, rectangles, and/or ovals.
- Provide additional instruction.

- Repeat, rephrase, or summarize information periodically.
- Encourage the student to ask questions to help clarify information that was missed.
- Be sensitive if the student responds slowly when answering questions or frequently asks "What?" in order to postpone answering until the question is processed.
  - Pose a question to the class, call upon another classmate, then ask the student to respond.
  - Pause for 5-10 seconds for the student to think and formulate a response.
  - Use the concept of a "lifeline" if a question is not readily answered. Allow the student to select a "lifeline" (peer whom the student thinks may know the answer). Before acknowledging the correctness of the answer, ask the student whether the answer will be accepted or rejected and another lifeline chosen. (2)
  - Paraphrase the question if the student is unable to respond.
  - Ask another classmate the question if student becomes anxious and hesitates too long.
  - Pre-establish a cue with the student to indicate that a question will be asked in a few minutes. This gives the student time to formulate a response.
  - Pass out in advance a list of questions or topics that will be discussed during the following lesson.
- Provide in advance a partial outline or photocopy of the teacher's notes. Ask the student to fill in the outline or notes as the information is delivered.

INATTENTION/IMPULSIVITY/HYPERACTIVITY

The following behaviors serve as general indicators. The student will not exhibit every characteristic listed. These behaviors may also be indicative of other problems.

Appearing to not be listening
Having difficulty focusing in large group situations
Being easily distracted during listening activities
Having problems understanding fast-paced lessons
Missing important details
Being unable to answer simple or complex questions
Having difficulty participating in classroom discussions
Asking excessive number of questions or frequently asking "What?"
Needing repetition of phrases/sentences/instructions/information
Seeming confused/hesitating after being given multi-step directions
Having difficulty following multi-step instructions
Completing assignments incorrectly
Requiring additional explanations to finish assignments
Talking to others during listening activities
Answering a question before entire question has been posed
Becoming frustrated/upset when listening becomes difficult
Interrupting oral lesson with inappropriate humor
Disturbing lecture by repeatedly sharpening a pencil
Staring out the window while teacher is talking
Moving around the room when required to be seated
Playing with objects during lectures
Losing temper when required to listen to a prolonged lectures
Responding inappropriately in presence of background noise

Section IV

Interventions

Review interventions for Inattention, Impulsivity, and Hyperactivity in Chapter 12.

- Check comprehension if the student is exhibiting inappropriate behaviors that interfere with listening.

- Use cue words or filler sentences to attract attention before imparting important information, for example, "Listen," "Ready," "I am going to begin the lesson now. I need everyone's attention." "What I'm going to say next is important."

- Introduce novelty or do something unusual (e.g., show pictures, illustrations, photographs, and objects; make sudden noises or movements; add color; interject humor or music).

- Move around the classroom to increase attention but remain near the student when cueing, redirection, or reinforcement is needed. Avoid pacing back and forth.

- Encourage student participation in oral lessons.

- Divide listening activities into short instructional segments. The student may lose interest or have difficulty paying attention when confronted with extended listening periods. Follow with less demanding activities.

- Allow for fluctuations in attention by repeating information.

- Instruct the student to "listen" for key information such as who, what, when, where, how, and why.

- Rephrase information.

- Periodically pause and request that the information be paraphrased or summarized.

- Privately prearrange with the student a nonpunitive hand gesture or signal to be used during listening activities as a reminder to refocus attention.

- Provide in advance a partial outline or photocopy of the teacher's notes. Ask the student to fill in the outline or notes as the information is delivered.

EXECUTIVE DYSFUNCTION

Review interventions for Executive Dysfunction in Chapter 13.

IMPAIRED PROBLEM SOLVING
(TASKS/ACTIVITIES/SITUATIONS)

- Provide a template of a problem solving strategy such as "**GET A CLUE**" or "**PLAN**" or another strategy to enhance listening comprehension. Be sure the strategy includes steps for goal setting, planning (generating ideas, solutions; analyzing proposed ideas, solutions; prioritizing; organizing; sequencing; managing time), initiating, and self-monitoring. (Appendix pp. 374–375)

- Model and demonstrate how to use problem solving strategies. (p. 108)

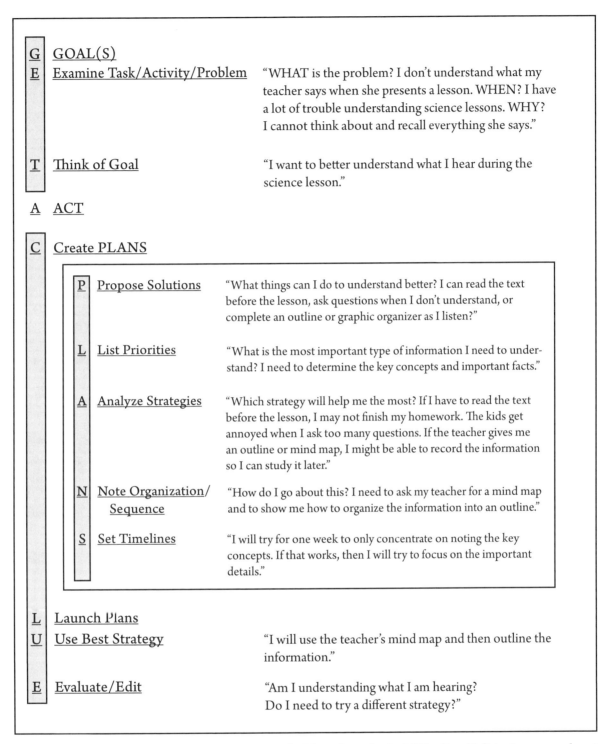

Figure 16.1. GET A CLUE – Cognitive strategy used with student who had difficulty with listening comprehension

Some students may not be able to follow the complexity of this strategy unless taught in incremental steps that must be mastered before continuing to the next step. Other students may need to learn a more simplified version "**PLAN**." If so, use "**GET A CLUE**" as a structure for discussing and teaching ways to solve tasks, activities, and problem situations.

Section IV

P	Propose Goal	"I need to develop a plan to improve my ability to understand what my teacher says when she presents a lesson."
L	List and Analyze Strategies	"What things can I do to understand better? I can read the text before the lesson, but I might not be able to finish my homework. I can ask questions when I don't understand, but the kids get annoyed when I ask too many questions. If the teacher gives me a mind map, I can record the information so I can study it later."
A	Apply Best Strategy	"I will use the teacher's mind map."
N	Notice Errors and Edit	"Am I understanding what I am hearing? Do I need to try a different strategy?"

Figure 16.2. PLAN – Cognitive strategy used with student who had difficulty with listening comprehension

Difficulty Setting Goals

The following behaviors serve as general indicators. The student will not exhibit every characteristic listed. These behaviors may also be indicative of other problems.

Being unaware of listening comprehension problem that needs to be solved
Having no concept of what it means to be able to understand and recall orally presented information
Overlooking need to set goal to achieve better listening comprehension

Interventions

- Define listening comprehension. Discuss <u>when</u>, <u>where</u>, <u>how</u> it is used and <u>why</u> it is critical to learning.

- Have the student self-evaluate listening comprehension, identify strengths and weaknesses, and determine which skills need improvement.

- Teach, prompt, and cue the student to stop and to set goals.

- Provide assistance until goals can be set independently.

Difficulty Planning

Difficulty Proposing and Analyzing Ideas/Solutions/Strategies

The following behaviors serve as general indicators. The student will not exhibit every characteristic listed. These behaviors may also be indicative of other problems.

Lacking skills to generate/brainstorm ideas/solutions/strategies
Using trial-and-error approach to achieving the goal
Having trouble identifying the who, what, when, where, how, and why of the problem
Needing help to analyze proposed strategy to carry out goal

Interventions

- Provide assistance in generating as many practical ideas as possible (e.g., read text or watch video related to the topic prior to lesson, ask questions when not understanding, complete graphic organizer during the lesson).
- Discuss both the positive and negative outcomes and consequences of each idea.
- Choose the best strategy.

Difficulty Prioritizing

The following behaviors serve as general indicators. The student will not exhibit every characteristic listed. These behaviors may also be indicative of other problems.

> Having trouble recognizing key vocabulary in the lesson
> Having difficulty identifying relative importance of oral information
> Being unable to determine main idea/important facts, particularly if embedded within lengthy lesson

Interventions

- Discuss key vocabulary words.
- Emphasize cue words or phrases such as "Listen carefully," "The next three facts are very important."
- Tell the student what to listen for (answers to questions, main ideas, related facts) prior to delivering information. "The most important ideas are _____." "The main point is _____."
    - Stress what is most important about the information to be presented.
    - Cue listening for who, what, when, where, how, and why.
- Repeat, rephrase, or summarize key ideas frequently.
- Provide a lettered or numbered outline that lists important concepts and facts being discussed.
- Supply a lettered or numbered mind map to illustrate main ideas and important details. (Appendix p. 382)
- Prepare a list of questions that assess key concepts to be asked after the lesson.

Difficulty Organizing/Sequencing

The following behaviors serve as general indicators. The student will not exhibit every characteristic listed. These behaviors may also be indicative of other problems.

> Requiring additional instructions to complete a sequential task
> Remembering facts in the incorrect order
> Having trouble following multi-step directions
> Following only the first or last part of multi-step instructions

Section IV

Interventions

- Design well-organized lessons or lectures that are easy to understand yet present important ideas and information.

- Organize and sequence verbally presented information with graphic organizers. (p. 115)

- Stress sequencing words when speaking such as "before," "after," "first," "second," "next," "then," and "finally."

- State directions one step at a time. Pause after each step to allow for processing. Say, "Take out your science book." (pause) "Turn to page 55." (pause) "Answer questions 1-5." Avoid saying "Now take out your science book, turn to page 55, and answer questions 1-5."

- Write and number the sequence of directions and information on a board or overhead projector as they are presented.

IMPAIRED SELF-MONITORING/USE OF FEEDBACK/SELF-CORRECTION

The following behaviors serve as general indicators. The student will not exhibit every characteristic listed. These behaviors may also be indicative of other problems.

Not knowing how to monitor comprehension
Being unaware of losing focus and concentration and thus not processing what is heard
Neglecting to engage in self-questioning to determine understanding
Lacking skills to know how and when to ask the teacher to repeat
Being reluctant to repeatedly ask for repetition
Failing to reread and review notes

Interventions

- Promote <u>self-awareness</u> of listening skills.

  Suggest that the student:

  - identify and list personal strengths.

  - analyze challenges or weaknesses that interfere with listening.

- Teach <u>self-questioning</u>.

  - Explain the purpose of self-questioning and how it helps monitor comprehension of an oral lesson.

  - Help generate questions such as:

    - "Am I listening as the teacher asked me to do?"

    - "What did the teacher mean by that word/phrase/sentence?"

    - "Does what the teacher is saying make sense to me?"

    - "I don't understand. What should I do? Do I need to ask the teacher to repeat or listen further for clarification?"

  - Prepare a list of the student's self-generated questions to serve as a visual reminder.

    - Add a prominent reminder that it is "OK" to ask questions.

    - Place the questions in the student's strategy ("trick") book. (p. 64)

Chapter 16

MEMORY PROBLEMS

Review interventions for Memory Problems in Chapter 14.

SHORT-TERM MEMORY PROBLEMS

Difficulty with Working Memory

The following behaviors serve as general indicators. The student will not exhibit every characteristic listed. These behaviors may also be indicative of other problems.

- Appearing confused during oral lessons
- Misunderstanding multi-step/unfamiliar/complex verbal material
- Having problems understanding fast paced lessons
- Needing repetition of phrases/sentences/instructions/information
- Being unable to follow topic shifts during lessons
- Becoming frustrated/overwhelmed when confronted with verbal tasks
- Having trouble understanding cause-and-effect
- Losing information heard at the beginning of a teacher's explanation while listening to the rest of it
- Asking excessive number of questions
- Answering questions incorrectly
- Having trouble remembering question while trying to recall answer
- Raising hand and forgetting question or answer before being called upon
- Needing clarification of oral instructions
- Following only first or last step of directions
- Being unable to paraphrase/summarize verbally presented material
- Having difficulty listening to lesson and taking satisfactory notes

Research suggests that students with **ADHD** have difficulty with listening comprehension tasks that require working memory, even though their receptive language skills are normally developed. While they appear to be able to understand factual details, they have difficulty comprehending complex verbal information such as that presented during classroom lessons. (3)

Interventions

- Remember that working memory during listening activities is impacted by the <u>amount</u>, <u>rate</u>, and <u>complexity</u> of the information presented.
    - Use clear and direct language that is easy to follow.
    - Simplify vocabulary and use words that the student is most likely to know.
    - Present material at a slower pace to allow time for processing.
    - Omit irrelevant information and include only details that are relevant to the topic being discussed.
    - Pause frequently to allow for the information to be processed in the workspace.
    - Determine the student's auditory memory span. Do not present information in excess of the verbal memory span as the student will have difficulty maintaining the information in working memory.
        - 🐾 *As mentioned previously (p. 35), the ability to hold learning material in working memory is limited to 3-7 items and depends on the age of the student.*
    - Divide lessons into segments with breaks in between. Plan the length of the segment based on the age of the student and the complexity of the material.

Section IV

- Incorporate activities that expand the workspace available for processing.

  - Make <u>associations</u> between new information and existing knowledge.

    - Encourage the connection of an abstract concept with a previously learned meaningful experience. For example, relating Shakespeare's play *Romeo and Juliet* with Stephen Sondheim's musical *West Side Story* places the play in the vernacular, both culturally and linguistically.

  - Group facts into <u>categories</u> (chunks or small, meaningful units). For example, names, dates, and places are easier to remember if they are placed in groups rather than in one long list. The number of chunks should match the capacity of the student's verbal memory span.

  - Present unfamiliar or complex information with the use of visual aids (e.g., diagrams, illustrations, graphic organizers) to reduce the demands placed on working memory.

- Implement strategies to circumvent the working memory and handwriting problems associated with notetaking. (p. 68)

  - *Notetaking may be very stressful for many students. To be able to take notes, they must simultaneously pay attention, listen, remember accurately, summarize, write in an organized and legible form, and process the ongoing lesson.*

CHAPTER 17
BASIC READING SKILLS

Dyslexia, a reading learning disability is defined as "a language-based disorder characterized by difficulties in the development of accurate and fluent single word decoding skills, usually associated with insufficient phonological processing and rapid naming abilities. These difficulties in single word decoding are often unexpected in relation to age and other cognitive and academic abilities; they are not the result of a generalized developmental disability or sensory impairment." (1)

On April, 13, 2000, a Congressionally mandated independent panel, the National Reading Panel, released a report entitled <u>Teaching Children to Read</u>. (2) After a comprehensive review of approximately 100,000 research studies, the panel determined the most effective methods for teaching reading. Reading instruction should include the following:

- **Phonemic Awareness** – knowledge that spoken words are comprised of individual speech sounds (phonemes) and combinations of speech sounds. The panel concluded that students should be <u>explicitly</u> and <u>systematically</u> taught to manipulate the sounds in spoken words. Phonological awareness was considered to be a core component of daily classroom reading instruction.

- **Phonics** – process of associating sounds with the letters of the alphabet. Research indicated that the greatest improvements in reading resulted from an organized, planned sequence of phonics instruction that taught students how to blend sounds to form words. It was recommended that teachers use <u>research-based instructional methods</u> that have been proven to be effective rather than programs that do not directly focused on training in phonemic awareness and phonics.

- **Fluency** – ability to read words accurately, rapidly, and with proper phrasing and intonation. The panel concluded that <u>reading aloud</u> to either a teacher, parent, or peer who provided appropriate feedback improved word recognition skills, fluency, and comprehension. Research results were inconclusive regarding silent reading. It was recommended that silent reading be used in combination with other types of reading instruction.

- **Comprehension** – ability to understand what is read. The panel determined that three areas were important to develop reading comprehension: <u>vocabulary development</u>, <u>text comprehension</u>, and <u>strategy instruction</u>. Vocabulary should be directly and indirectly taught as words are confronted in text. Repetition and multiple exposures to vocabulary words and the use of computer programs designed to enhance vocabulary development were recommended. Graphic and semantic organizers, understanding of text structure (narrative and expository), and summarization skills were found to improve reading comprehension.

- **Computer Technology** – computer utilization to teach reading. Three areas that proved useful included: addition of speech to computer presented reading programs, hypertext (highlighted text linked to definitions or related text), and word processing (reading instruction combined with writing instruction).

Section IV

A reading disorder is estimated to occur in approximately one out of every five school age children. (3) 23% of clinically referred students with **ADHD** (4) and 1% of students with **TS** (5) have been found to have difficulty reading words presented in isolation.

> *The frequency of reading disorders for students with **ADHD** and/or **TS** is consistent with or below that found in the general population. Therefore, comprehensive interventions for teaching phonological awareness and decoding skills are beyond the scope of this book. Recommendations will address the impact of inattention, slow processing speed, executive dysfunction (difficulty with self-regulation, sequencing, initiation, and self-monitoring), and memory problems on the acquisition of word recognition skills of students with **ADHD**, **TS**, and/or **OCD**.*

General Recommendations

Review Classroom and Individual Student Interventions in Chapter 8 and Chapter 9.

- Recommend a psychoeducational or neuropsychological evaluation if the student is having difficulty acquiring basic reading skills.

    > *Research has identified several different subtypes of reading disabilities. The most common subtypes include deficits in phonological awareness, verbal short-term memory, and speed of processing. Other language and cognitive skills vary in their impact on reading ability. A small percentage of students have visual processing problems. (6) Therefore, in-depth evaluations are considered essential to determine the specific nature of the reading problems.*

    > *A comprehensive assessment is also required as some students with **TS** and/or **OCD** may appear to have reading disabilities when, in fact, their reading problems are secondary to tics and obsessions and compulsions which interfere with reading.*

- Recognize that the student who has difficulty with reading sometimes reacts by avoiding reading. Encourage independent reading. Reading material should be relatively easy and at the independent level. For such reading, not more than one unknown word should appear in 100 or 200 running words.

- Be aware that the student with **ADHD**, **TS**, and/or **OCD** may be eligible to borrow taped texts from the Recordings for the Blind and Dyslexic (RFB&D). RFB&D, a nonprofit organization, is the largest educational library for students who are visually impaired or have learning disabilities. Recorded books are available to students (kindergarten to post-graduate levels) and professionals with certified disabilities that make reading difficult. Books cover a broad range of subjects (e.g., history, literature, mathematics, science). To listen to the digitally recorded books, students need portable CD players equipped to play RFB&D's books or standard multi-media computers equipped with CD-ROM drives and specialized software. Playback hardware and software are available through RFB&D for nonprofit sale. (7)

    > *Books on tape bypass difficulty mastering decoding skills and allow vocabulary and comprehensions skills to advance until reading is automatic.*

- Evaluate the student's learning style preferences for reading materials and design lessons accordingly. (8, 9, 10, 11)

    ○ Ask the student with auditory strengths to read aloud, dictate stories to be transcribed onto paper and then read orally, or to listen to books on tape while reading along with the words.

    ○ Present the student with a visual-spatial learning style reading materials with pictorial content (e.g., pictures with captions, cartoons, age-appropriate magazines, comic books, computer software and games).

- Ask the <u>kinesthetic</u> (tactile) learner to form letters and words with sand, clay, paint, or shaving cream on Formica; to feel and say letters and words made from felt or sandpaper; to use sidewalk chalk to write on the cement pavement while saying sounds, or to write on a computer.
- Offer the <u>logical</u> thinker a reading program based on word patterns (e.g., use flannel or magnetic letters and demonstrate how the letters can be shifted to make different words).
- Recommend that the student who prefers to learn <u>interpersonally</u> read with a partner or in a small group.
- Permit the <u>intrapersonal</u> learner to read independently.
- Combine different learning styles during reading instruction.

- Provide individualized instruction. Significant reading improvement often results from intense instruction and positive, corrective feedback.
- Use <u>researched-based</u> reading programs that teach phonemic awareness, phonics, and fluency.
- Arrange for paraprofessionals, adults volunteers, or older students to supplement reading instruction.

> Tics/obsessions/compulsions, underarousal/slow processing speed, inattention/impulsivity/hyperactivity, executive dysfunction, and/or memory problems frequently interfere with the ability to acquire effective and efficient basic reading skills.

UNDERAROUSAL/SLOW COGNITIVE PROCESSING SPEED

Speed of processing significantly impacts the acquisition of basic reading skills. (12, 13) Reduced processing speed interferes with the ability to automatize reading recognition skills so that words can be read rapidly and accurately with little conscious effort directed toward the mechanics of reading. Reduced fluency in turn affects reading comprehension.

The following behaviors serve as general indicators. The student will not exhibit every characteristic listed. These behaviors may also be indicative of other problems.

Being slow to decode words
Requiring considerable repetition to recognize words easily
Having a slow reading rate
Lacking fluency and expressiveness when reading orally
Reading orally word-by-word/haltingly/laboriously
Having difficulty finishing lengthy reading assignments
Pretending to read when reading silently
Exhibiting disinterest in reading library books
Reading less than peers

Interventions

Review interventions for Underarousal and Slow Processing Speed in Chapter 10.

- Assign reading activities at a lower skill level when developing accuracy and fluency.

Section IV

- Provide frequent practice <u>reading aloud</u> to enhance fluency.

  Ask the student to:
  - preview material prior to reading orally.
    - read passage silently.
    - ask for unfamiliar words to be identified.
    - listen as the teacher reads the selection and models the appropriate reading rate with proper phrasing and intonation.
    - listen to and read along with a tape or CD recording of the material.
  - read in a <u>small group</u> with other students who have similar reading problems.
    - 🐾 *Do not force the student to read aloud in front of the entire class. The experience of not reading well will generate a high level of anxiety and a dislike for reading.*
  - read with a partner (teacher, aide, parent, older student).
    - listen as partner reads a passage or page.
    - take turns reading orally and listening.
    - read in unison.
  - read the passage alone.
  - read to a younger student.

- Set goals with the student for increasing reading speed. Graph progress and compare individual performance across time.

- Use <u>repeated reading</u> to improve accuracy and reading rate. Repeated reading (reading the same words or passages over and over) has been found to increase word recognition and reading speed. (14)

  🐾 *Automaticity allows the student to focus on understanding.*

  - Ask the student to repeatedly read for one minute a list of words that can be phonetically decoded or a list of high frequency words.
    - Record the number of words read correctly.
    - Discuss and reread missed words.
  - Provide an <u>instructional</u> level passage (3-7 words out of 100 words are unfamiliar). (15)
    - Record amount of time needed to complete selection.
    - Have the passage reread subvocally to practice difficult words.
  - Suggest rereading the lists or passages until predetermined goals are achieved.

- Make a tape recording of the student reading. Play it back and have the student listen while following the text.

Chapter 17

INATTENTION/IMPULSIVITY/HYPERACTIVITY

The following behaviors serve as general indicators. The student will not exhibit every characteristic listed. These behaviors may also be indicative of other problems.

- Appearing not to listen
- Daydreaming/staring into space
- Becoming distracted during reading lesson
- Having difficulty concentrating during instruction
- Losing place/skipping lines/omitting or substituting words when reading
- Needing frequent repetition
- Exhibiting variable performance from day to day
- Exhibiting inappropriate behaviors that interfere with reading
- Talking to others during reading activity
- Having difficulty waiting turn in reading group
- Rushing impulsively through reading lesson
- Becoming frustrated/upset when encountering difficult words

Reading competence is significantly impacted by the inattention associated with **ADHD**. (16)

Interventions

Review interventions for Inattention, Impulsivity, and Hyperactivity in Chapter 12.

- Be aware that the student who is expending so much cognitive energy struggling to decode words may be unable to sustain attention.
- Schedule, if possible, reading instruction when the student is most alert.
- Limit the size of the reading group so the student is not distracted by other students.
- Call on the student to read near the beginning of the reading activity if the student has difficulty waiting.
- Present multi-sensory reading activities to gain attention.
- Structure the reading assignment for success.
- Select reading materials according to the student's interests and reading ability.
- Intervene if the student has difficulty tracking (loses place, skips lines, and omits or repeats words when reading aloud). (17)
    - Suggest using a finger to assist tracking.
    - Provide a tachistoscope (a reading window) to reduce the amount of page available to the eye.
    - Offer a bookmark, ruler, paper strip, or index card to be used while moving down the page.
    - Provide a colored plastic overlay which can be cut from plastic report covers. Allow the student to choose the color.
- Define appropriate reading behavior.
- Limit the size of the reading group.

Section IV

- Teach the student who reads too quickly and impulsively to read at a slower pace. (17)

  - Highlight punctuation marks with visible ink. Use yellow for commas to represent "yield signs" and red for periods to represent "stop signs."

  - Suggest taking a short breath at each comma and a regular breath at the end of each sentence.

  - Recommend silently counting to one after a comma and to two after a period. Or, depending on the learning style and interest of the student, relate commas and periods to half rests and whole rests from music.

  - Cue the student to wait after the period by raising a hand and to continue by putting the hand down.

  - Use a tape recorder to provide feedback and comparison.

- Slow the pace of reading by asking the student to read aloud.

EXECUTIVE DYSFUNCTION

Review interventions for Executive Dysfunction in Chapter 13.

Difficulty Sequencing

The following behaviors serve as general indicators. The student will not exhibit every characteristic listed. These behaviors may also be indicative of other problems.

Being unable to decode unfamiliar words
Having difficulty synthesizing the sounds of letters into words
Forgetting order of letters in words
Omitting/substituting sounds in words
Misreading words

Interventions

- Use a <u>research-based teaching</u> program that introduces learning material in a systematic, step-by-step fashion. The lessons should be sequentially presented so that the student proceeds in a sequence of small steps, each one built upon previously mastered skills.

- Develop awareness of the number of syllables in a word by tapping them. After the student can determine the number of syllables in a word, ask for syllables to be combined into a whole word.

- Teach the student how to recognize the number of individual sounds in a word once the number of syllables can be identified. After the student can distinguish the sounds, ask for them to be blended into the word.

- Combine auditory and visual sequences simultaneously. The student with auditory strengths may be able to recall the order of letters seen in words if the sounds are heard at the same time. The student with visual strengths may be able to retain an auditory sequence if the visual pattern is shown.

Chapter 17

INITIATION/EXECUTION DIFFICULTIES

The following behaviors serve as general indicators. The student will not exhibit every characteristic listed. These behaviors may also be indicative of other problems.

    Appearing hypoactive/lacking energy/uninterested in reading
    Seeming "lazy" or "unmotivated"
    Procrastinating/hesitating/avoiding beginning reading
    Requiring repeated encouragement and direction

Interventions

- Always provide reading materials at the level where the student can be successful.

- Present teacher-directed and teacher-monitored reading lessons at the <u>instructional</u> level (3-7 words out of 100 words are unfamiliar). (15)

- Determine whether the student feels capable of performing the reading activity. Often the teacher is unaware that the student is not willing to admit that reading is too difficult.

- Assign only one part of the reading lesson at a time. Modifying the amount of work and offering breaks reduces the anxiety and frustration associated with lengthy tasks.

- Read aloud the first sentence of the reading passage.

IMPAIRED SELF-MONITORING/USE OF FEEDBACK/SELF-CORRECTION

The following behaviors serve as general indicators. The student will not exhibit every characteristic listed. These behaviors may also be indicative of other problems.

    Being unaware of losing focus and concentration
    Neglecting to stop and reread an unfamiliar word
    Losing place/skipping lines/omitting or substituting words
    Making careless errors when reading aloud
    Having difficulty knowing when help is needed

Interventions

- Suggest reading orally. Reading aloud forces the student to slow down, listen to the words, and self-monitor.

- Tape record oral reading. Have the student listen to the tape and identify mistakes while reading along with the book.

- Provide feedback on reading errors and successes.

- Emphasize successes to build self-esteem.

- Teach strategies for determining when it is appropriate to ask for assistance.

Section IV

MEMORY PROBLEMS

SHORT-TERM MEMORY PROBLEMS

Review interventions for Memory Problems in Chapter 14.

Difficulty with Working Memory

The following behaviors serve as general indicators. The student will not exhibit every characteristic listed. These behaviors may also be indicative of other problems.

> Having difficulty quickly decoding words
> Being unable to hold sounds in memory while decoding rest of word
> Lacking automatic word recognition skills

Students with word recognition deficits often have working memory problems. (13, 18) Reduced reading efficiency is exhibited when students are required to perform simultaneously the multiple skills involved in reading. When reading a word, students must be able to pay attention and visually perceive and recognize the letters. They must retrieve from memory sound-symbol associations and hold them in working memory while the rest of the word is decoded. Then the sounds must be blended to form the word.

Interventions

- Increase <u>automaticity</u> of phonemic awareness and word recognition skills. (19)

  - *If decoding skills have not been mastered at an automatic level and demand more effortful processing, less workspace will be available for the more complex task of understanding the reading materials.*

  - Use a cognitive-based decoding approach to give meaning to abstract sounds (e.g., "Mother Vowel" in Appendix pp. 376–377).

  - Limit the number of sound-symbol relationships presented together.

  - Make sure that previous decoding skills have been mastered before introducing new skills.

    - *Mastery is defined as knowing the sounds <u>90%</u> of the time over an extended period.*

  - Provide repeated exposures to words.

  - The average student needs approximately 20 repetitions of unfamiliar words to rapidly and accurately recognize them. (20) The student with decoding problems requires many more repetitions.

  - Ensure that word recognition skills are continually reviewed. Most forgetting occurs within a few minutes following learning. (p. 143) If drill is used, it should be provided in a game format to lessen disinterest.

  - Provide for overlearning by creating regular opportunities throughout the day for reading decodable words.

- Limit demands placed on the capacity of working memory. (p. 36) Reduced capacity may be associated with word recognition problems. (18)
  - Break reading lesson into short segments.
  - Avoid introducing several sound-symbol relationships simultaneously. Wait for the first one to be mastered before teaching the next one.
  - Present unfamiliar sounds and letters with the use of visual aids.
  - Allocate time for verbal rehearsal during the lesson in order to prolong the sounds in working memory.
    - Allow subvocalization.
    - Repeat sounds frequently.
  - Combine as many sensory modalities as possible (verbal, visual, tactile, motor). For example, ask the student to trace the letters in a word and pronounce the sounds.
- Be aware that working memory problems result not only from trouble maintaining several pieces of information during processing (each individual sound as the word is being decoded), but also difficulty automatically retrieving information from long-term memory (recalling sounds associated with the letters) to use during processing.

LONG-TERM MEMORY PROBLEMS

Difficulty Encoding/Consolidating (Learning)

Basic reading skills include not only phonemic awareness and fluency but encoding, storage, and retrieval of sound-symbol relationships. Consolidation deficits lead to inaccurate recall of the sounds during the decoding process.

The following behaviors serve as general indicators. The student will not exhibit every characteristic listed. These behaviors may also be indicative of other problems.

    Having difficulty mastering sound-symbol relationships
    Needing additional instruction
    Relying only on rote memory to learn decoding skills
    Pausing for a long time when encountering words
    Forgetting sounds and words learned yesterday
    Requiring excessive number of exposures to words to recognize them easily and automatically

Interventions

- Discourage rote memorization.
  - 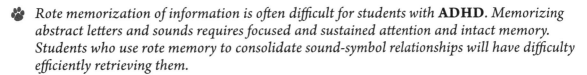 *Rote memorization of information is often difficult for students with **ADHD**. Memorizing abstract letters and sounds requires focused and sustained attention and intact memory. Students who use rote memory to consolidate sound-symbol relationships will have difficulty efficiently retrieving them.*

Section IV

- Use a <u>research-based teaching program</u> that introduces learning material in a systematic, step-by-step fashion such as Orton-Gillingham. The lessons should be sequentially presented so that the student proceeds in small steps, each one built upon previously mastered skills.

  🐾 *Teach the parents how to use the same method of reading instruction that is being used in the classroom.*

- Systematically introduce word recognition skills so that errors are <u>minimized</u>. (21, 22) "Errorless learning" has been found to be more effective than "trial-and-error" learning. (22) Preventing errors during the learning process and practice sessions will keep the student from repeating and, thereby, encoding incorrect sound-symbol relationships.

  🐾 *Students with **ADHD** often do not learn from their mistakes due to inattention and inefficient working memory. The student with **OCD** may become "stuck" on an incorrect sound-symbol association.*

  ○ Sit with the student as a passage or page is read aloud.

  ○ Immediately correct a missed word and proceed.

  ○ Review missed words at the end of the selection.

- Use teaching techniques that make sound-symbol associations more concrete.

  ○ Link the letter-sound combinations to meaningful stimuli (pictures, stories, rhymes).

  ○ Use color coding to aid recognition (consonants – yellow; vowels – red; blends – green).

  ○ Represent phonemes, syllables, and phrases with moveable blocks, tiles, or magnetic strips. Have the student add, omit, substitute, and rearrange the phonemes in words or the phrases in sentences.

  ○ Supplement with visual materials (e.g., pictures, drawings).

- Teach a set of <u>basic sight words</u> - common words such as "the", "come", "have", "was", "here", and "do" - most of which cannot be decoded using phonic rules [e.g., Dolch Basic Sight Words (Appendix p. 378)].

  🐾 *Approximately 100 words comprise 50% of the words in textbooks. (23) It is crucial that these high-frequency words be memorized and recognized immediately upon "sight."*

  ○ Ensure that not more than one out of 100 words in the passage is unknown.

  ○ Use "backward chaining" (source unknown) to imprint sight words. Initially, the entire word is shown. Remove the last part of the sequence and ask the student to remember the letter and state the word. A letter is removed at each successive lesson. The gradual removal of letters reduces the chance for errors. (17)

  Example: If the student is having difficulty learning the word "who," write the word on a board, in shaving cream spread on a Formica surface or desktop, on a white board with a dry erase marker, on a transparency with an overhead marker, or on a window with an erasable marker. (The visual and tactile input provided by these media increases attention to task and improves storage and retrieval.) Erase the last letter. Have the student write the "o" and say and spell the whole word. When the student is successful, erase the last two letters. Have the student rewrite the "h" and "o" and say and spell "who." Have the student say and spell the words orally during each step. Once the student can write the entire word from memory, introduce another sight vocabulary word. Once mastered, recheck weekly.

- - Use repetition, drill, and practice to master high frequency words.
  - Use flash cards. The utilization of flash cards incorporates both the auditory and visual modalities.
  - Design and play word games. Games provide immediate reinforcement and drill without being boring.
- Reinforce learning by encouraging the use of computer software specifically designed to promote acquisition of basic reading skills.

Difficulty Retrieving (Recalling)

The following behaviors serve as general indicators. The student will not exhibit every characteristic listed. These behaviors may also be indicative of other problems.

> Having trouble recalling sounds associated with letters
> Being unable to quickly recall basic sight words

Research has documented the close relationship between reading and rapid naming or rapid automatic retrieval of words. Students who have impaired rapid naming skills often have difficulty reading fluently. (24)

Interventions

- Consult recommendations for Retrieval. (pp. 144-145)
- Use strategies to organize information in an easily retrievable form.
- Provide phonetic cues.
  - Say the beginning consonant sound of the intended word.
  - Provide a word fragment containing one or more of the beginning syllables.
- Present associative cues.
  - Use an associated word which belongs to the same semantic (conceptual) class as the cue.
- Offer sentence completion cues.
- Allow extra time if the student responds slowly.

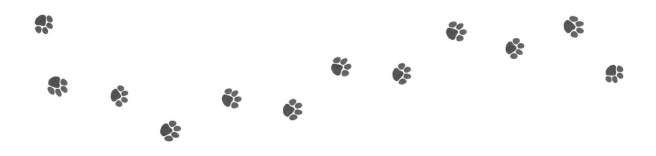

CHAPTER 18

READING COMPREHENSION

The majority of students with **ADHD**, **TS**, and/or **OCD** acquire age-appropriate basic reading skills. However, clinical and teaching experience suggests that they at times encounter problems with the comprehension and recall of reading materials. A reading comprehension problem is estimated to occur in approximately 20% of clinically referred students with **ADHD**. (1) The frequency of the disability has not been assessed for students with **TS** and **OCD**.

The congressionally mandated National Reading Panel determined that three areas are important for reading comprehension: vocabulary development, text comprehension, and strategy instruction. The panel advised teachers to directly and indirectly teach vocabulary as words are confronted in text. Repetition and multiple exposures to vocabulary words and computer programs to promote vocabulary development were recommended. Understanding of text structure (narrative and expository), summarization skills, and graphic and semantic organizers were found to enhance reading comprehension. (2)

> *Students with **ADHD**, **TS**, and **OCD** typically possess age adequate vocabularies. Therefore, interventions for the remediation of vocabulary deficits are beyond the scope of this handbook. Vocabulary development, as suggested by the panel, should always be an important component of reading instruction. The reading comprehension problems of these students are secondary to underarousal/slow processing speed, inattention, executive dysfunction, and/or memory problems.*

General Recommendations

Review Classroom and Individual Student Interventions in Chapters 8 and 9.

- Determine whether the student's phonemic awareness, decoding skills, and reading fluency have been mastered.

  > *Understanding is often compromised when the student struggles to sound out words or reads slowly.*

- Be aware that some students with **TS** and/or **OCD** may appear to have reading comprehension problems when, in fact, their reading problems are secondary to tics, obsessions, and compulsions that interfere with reading.

- Evaluate the student's learning style preferences (pp. 65-67) and design reading comprehension lessons accordingly. (3, 4, 5, 6)

  - Ask the student with auditory strengths to read aloud, to listen to books on tape, or to put graphically presented information into words.

  - Have the student with a visual-spatial learning style watch movies related to the topics, use graphic organizers, draw pictures of the sequences of events in stories, or create posters or collages.

  - Ask the kinesthetic (tactile) learner to act out stories, to give demonstrations related to the text, or to build models of the scenes described in the stories.

  - Suggest that the logical thinker use categorization, connect ideas and draw conclusions ("If _____, then _____."), make predictions, use Venn diagrams to demonstrate similarities and differences, or use timelines to show series of events.

Section IV

- Recommend that the student who prefers to learn <u>interpersonally</u> read with a partner or in a group assigned to discuss characters, main ideas, relevant details, and other important elements of the reading materials.

- Permit the <u>intrapersonal</u> learner to read independently and choose the formats for demonstrating comprehension of the reading assignments.

- Integrate several different learning styles during reading comprehension instruction.

- <u>Always</u> provide work at the appropriate <u>instructional level</u>.

    - 🐾 *Research suggests that when students are presented reading comprehension tasks at the proper <u>instructional level</u> (3-7 words out of each 100 words are unfamiliar), attention to task, work completion, and comprehension are enhanced. Understanding and task completion are adequate when assigned learning materials at the <u>independent</u> level (only 3 words out of 100 words have not been mastered). In contrast, when students are provided work at the <u>frustration</u> level (10 words out of 100 words are unknown), learning and on-task behaviors are negatively impacted. (7)*

    - Present teacher-directed and teacher-monitored lessons at the <u>instructional</u> level.

    - Assign unmonitored seatwork and homework at the <u>independent</u> level.

    - Assign no work at the <u>frustration</u> level.

- Teach reading comprehension in a group that is different from the oral reading group.

    - 🐾 *Some students in the oral reading group might not need instruction in reading comprehension or might require a different level of comprehension instruction.*

- Read aloud to the class every day and model comprehension strategies.

- Select reading materials according to the student's interests (e.g., animals, sports, mechanics, cars). If a book appeals to the student, it may spark an interest in reading and provide motivation to improve reading comprehension.

- Use a variety of texts (e.g., picture books, short stories, poems, comics, articles from newspapers, high interest magazines, and web sites).

    - 🐾 *Remember – reading is reading!*

- Schedule one period each day for pleasure reading. De-emphasize skill-related activities and stress reading for enjoyment.

    - Create a comfortable reading area furnished with carpet, pillows, and beanbags.

    - Supply the reading center with a variety of short, interesting books.

    - Encourage use of this area at the designated time and as reinforcement when assignments are completed.

- Reinforce learning with the use of computer software specifically designed to improve reading comprehension skills.

- Recommend listening to books on tape. (p. 166) Recordings can be used when the student with **ADHD** has difficulty sitting still long enough to read. Taped books are particularly helpful if the student with **TS** has eye tics or the student with **OCD** has a compulsion to read backwards, count words, or read words, lines, or paragraphs over and over again. Audio text has been found to significantly enhance a student's acquisition of content materials. (8)

    - *Clinical and teaching experience indicates that students with reading comprehension problems who listen to books on tape expand their vocabularies and score higher on the verbal section of the SAT and on the ACT.*

    - Prepare and provide teacher- or parent-recorded reading materials.

- Ask an aide or compatible peer to read to the student.

- Recommend individualized instruction from a learning disability teacher who is trained to remediate reading comprehension problems.

> Tics/obsessions/compulsions, underarousal/slow processing speed, inattention/impulsivity/hyperactivity, executive dysfunction, and/or memory problems frequently interfere with the ability to derive meaning from written text.

UNDERAROUSAL/SLOW COGNITIVE PROCESSING SPEED

The following behaviors serve as general indicators. The student will not exhibit every characteristic listed. These behaviors may also be indicative of other problems.

Lacking persistence when reading
Possessing age-appropriate decoding skills, but unable to finish reading assignment in allotted time
Being slow to grasp main ideas and related facts

Interventions

Review interventions for Underarousal and Slow Processing Speed in Chapter 10.

- Adjust the demands of tasks if they are not congruent with the student's arousal level.

    - Assign short segments of work with mobility breaks in between (e.g., read 10 pages and stand up and stretch).

    - Vary pace and change activities frequently.

    - Suggest working on a reading comprehension program on the computer to increase interest and arousal.

- Discuss important concepts prior to reading.

    - Write main ideas and important facts on a board, overhead transparency, or electronic whiteboard.

    - Highlight, underline, or frame key points using different colors. Always use same colors (e.g., main ideas – red, important details – yellow).

- Provide partial outlines to be filled in as material is read.

- Waive time limits or provide sufficient time for the assignment to be completed.

Section IV
INATTENTION/IMPULSIVITY/HYPERACTIVITY

The following behaviors serve as general indicators. The student will not exhibit every characteristic listed. These behaviors may also be indicative of other problems.

- Appearing to exert little effort
- Becoming distracted during reading process
- Needing reminders to persist on reading assignment
- Losing place when reading orally
- Ignoring punctuation/skipping or substituting words/phrases/lines
- Having difficulty following along as others read aloud
- Subvocalizing during silent reading
- Overlooking important details
- Having to repeatedly reread passage/chapter to understand/remember
- Requiring high interest reading materials to remain on-task
- Disliking/avoiding reading for pleasure
- Rushing impulsively through reading assignment
- Talking to others during reading activity
- Having difficulty waiting turn in reading group
- Responding to comprehension question before reading entire question
- Answering comprehension questions before they are finished being asked
- Becoming frustrated/upset when encountering difficult words/text

Inattention has a significant influence on reading comprehension and attitudes toward reading. (9)

Interventions

Review interventions for Inattention, Impulsivity, and Hyperactivity in Chapter 12.

- Provide reading materials that can be read at the <u>independent</u> level. (p. 64) All the vocabulary words and sight words should be understood at the mastery level. Complete ease of reading allows attention to be focused on comprehension and promotes on-task behavior.

- Select reading materials according to the student's interests and reading ability.

- Encourage reading aloud to slow the pace of the impulsive reader.

- Divide reading assignments into short segments. The student may lose interest or have difficulty maintaining attention when given long reading materials. (10)

  - Assign one part at a time.
  - Permit the restless student to move after each reading segment (e.g., sharpen a pencil, walk to the water fountain).
  - Gradually increase the length and difficulty of the reading material as success is demonstrated.

- Provide a bookmark, ruler, paper strip, or index card to use while moving down the page.

- Furnish in advance a list of specific questions to be answered.

  - Begin by asking comprehension questions about short paragraphs.
  - Recommend highlighting or underlining answers to the questions.
  - Suggest rereading the passage if the answers cannot be located.

- Hand out a partial outline to be completed as the text is read.

- Recommend using different colored highlighters with visible ink to note the main ideas and supporting details. Use the same colors each time a passage is read.
- Pause during reading and ask for key concepts and important facts to be paraphrased or summarized.
- Limit the size of the reading group so the student has more opportunities to read and answer questions rather than needing to wait to respond.
- Call on the student to read near the beginning of the reading activity if there is a problem taking turns.
- Allow walking while reading if walking increases attention.
- Suggest going to a quiet spot to read aloud during silent reading periods. Subvocalization focuses attention on the task.
- Assign a compatible peer to act as a reading "buddy."

EXECUTIVE DYSFUNCTION

Review interventions for Executive Dysfunction in Chapter 13.

IMPAIRED PROBLEM SOLVING
(Tasks/Activities/Situations)

- Provide a template of a problem solving strategy such as "**GET A CLUE**" or "**PLAN**" or another strategy to enhance reading comprehension. Be sure the strategy includes steps for goal setting, planning (generating ideas, solutions; analyzing proposed ideas, prioritizing; solutions; organizing; sequencing; managing time), initiating, self-monitoring, and self-correcting. (Appendix pp. 374–375)
- Model and demonstrate how to use the strategy for problem solving. (p. 108)

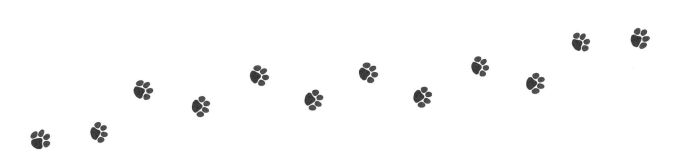

Section IV

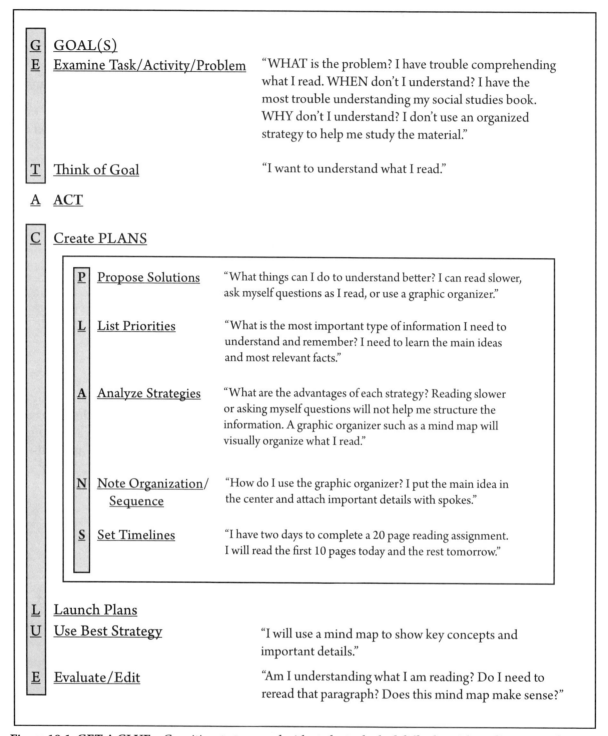

Figure 18.1. GET A CLUE – Cognitive strategy used with student who had difficulty with reading comprehension

Some students may not be able to follow the complexity of this strategy unless taught in incremental steps that must be mastered before continuing to the next step. Other students may need to learn a more simplified version "**PLAN**." If so, use "**GET A CLUE**" as a structure for discussing and teaching ways to solve tasks, activities, and problem situations.

P	Propose Goal	"I need to develop a plan to improve my reading comprehension."
L	List and Analyze Strategies	"What things can I do to understand better? I can read slower or ask myself questions as I read, but those ideas will not help me structure the information so I can understand it more easily. I can use a graphic organizer to depict the information."
A	Apply Best Strategy	"I will use my teacher's mind map."
N	Notice Errors and Edit	"Am I understanding what I am reading? Do I need to try a different strategy? Do I need to reread that paragraph? Does this mind map make sense? Is it correct?"

Figure 18.2. PLAN – Cognitive strategy used with student who had difficulty with reading comprehension

Difficulty Setting Goals

The following behaviors serve as general indicators. The student will not exhibit every characteristic listed. These behaviors may also be indicative of other problems.

Being unaware of reading comprehension problem that needs to be solved
Having no concept of what it means to be able to understand and recall reading materials
Overlooking need to set goal to achieve better reading comprehension

Interventions

- Define reading comprehension. Discuss <u>when</u>, <u>where</u>, <u>how</u> it is used and <u>why</u> it is critical to learning.

- Have the student self-evaluate mastery of reading comprehension, identify strengths and weaknesses, and determine which skills need improvement.

- Teach, prompt, and cue the student to stop and set goals.

- Provide assistance until goals can be set independently.

Difficulty Planning

Difficulty Proposing and Analyzing Ideas/Solutions/Strategies

The following behaviors serve as general indicators. The student will not exhibit every characteristic listed. These behaviors may also be indicative of other problems.

Lacking skills to generate/brainstorm ideas/solutions/strategies
Using trial-and-error approach to achieving goals
Having trouble identifying the who, what, when, where, how, and why of the problem
Needing help to analyze proposed strategy for carrying out goal

Section IV

Interventions

- Provide assistance in generating as many practical ideas as possible (e.g., read slower and more carefully, use self-questioning while reading, fill in a graphic organizer).

- Discuss both the positive and negative outcomes and consequences of each idea.

- Choose the best strategy.

Difficulty Prioritizing

The following behaviors serve as general indicators. The student will not exhibit every characteristic listed. These behaviors may also be indicative of other problems.

Having difficulty determining relative importance of information
Comprehending only general ideas rather than key concepts
Missing important details
Overlooking significance of main characters and their relationships to other characters
Having difficulty determining author's purpose and opinions
Reading least important part of assignment first
Misunderstanding importance of highlighting material

Interventions

- Provide an outline or chart listing most salient points of assignment.

    o Make sure the main ideas and characters are listed and emphasized.

    o Enumerate pertinent information (e.g., characters' names and relationships to other characters, key concepts, important details).

    o Have the student complete the outline or chart as important information is located.

- Emphasize the relevance of identifying the main ideas.

    o Recommend reading the title of the story in the text and trying to predict the plot or content.

    o Read a short passage and ask for different titles.

    o Suggest reading a paragraph and highlighting or underlining the first sentence, additional sentences that appear important, and the last sentence. Have the marked sentences reread and the one that represents the main idea selected.

    o Recommend reading the passage, highlighting important facts, and forming a sentence that states the main idea when the key concept is not directly stated.

- Provide practice locating important details related to major ideas.

    o Assign a reading passage with sentences containing details that are related and unrelated to the key concept. Ask the student to choose those facts associated with the main idea.

    o Assign a reading passage. Ask the student to identify and paraphrase the main idea and two details.

    o Provide a graphic organizer to help determine the main idea and its details.

- Teach selective <u>highlighting or underlining</u> of words, phrases, vocabulary, and concepts that are important for comprehension.
    - Project a photocopied passage on an overhead or electronic whiteboard. Model and demonstrate highlighting and underlining.
    - Provide a copy of the same text to be highlighted or underlined.
    - Recommend using different colored pencils or markers to emphasize key concepts and supporting details. Stress selecting only words and phrases, not entire sentences and paragraphs.
    - Suggest drawing shapes around important information such as circles (main ideas), boxes (subtopics), ovals (related facts), and rectangles (vocabulary), and underlining (definitions).
    - Use the same colors or shapes with all reading comprehension assignments.
    - Practice highlighting for different purposes (e.g., cause-and-effect, compare and contrast, opinion and facts).
- Teach and practice <u>summarization</u>.

    Ask the student to:
    - briefly describe a story, movie, or TV program.
    - write a classified ad for the school newspaper.
    - send a telegram to another student.
    - read a short passage and create a title.
    - read a selection, pausing after each paragraph to summarize the key concept in one sentence.
    - extract and state in two or three sentences the main idea and important details in a passage.
    - identify the who, what, when, where, how, and why of a story.
    - highlight or underline a passage and reread the marked sentences, then write a summary paragraph without looking at the paper. If necessary, keep looking back at the highlighting until the most important ideas and facts are included. Gradually reduce reliance on highlighted points.
    - write successively shorter summary paragraphs (e.g., reducing a half page summary to three paragraphs, one paragraph, two or three sentences, and finally one sentence).
    - make an outline.
- Provide instruction for interpreting <u>opinions/facts</u> essays.
    - Teach the difference between opinions and facts (e.g., facts can be confirmed, opinions cannot).
    - Critique ads for products in magazines and commercials on TV.
    - Analyze exaggerations, false claims, distortions of facts, and errors.

Section IV

Difficulty Organizing

The following behaviors serve as general indicators. The student will not exhibit every characteristic listed. These behaviors may also be indicative of other problems.

   Being unable to break down reading assignments into manageable units
   Lacking organized structure for studying information in narrative and expository texts
   Using disorganized approach to derive meaning from reading materials

Interventions

- Teach <u>text structure</u> (narrative and expository) to facilitate reading comprehension.

    🐾 *Many students with executive dysfunction do not spontaneously use organized approaches to enhance reading comprehension.*

   Use the following progression of instruction when teaching:

   - Provide clear, explicit instructions. Point out <u>when</u> and <u>where</u> to use the different text structures.

   - Model or demonstrate <u>how</u> to use the approaches. Use an LCD projector with Power Point, electronic whiteboard, or other multi-media aid. Verbalize each step of the process.

   - Supply a visual cue card that indicates how to apply the structure.

      🐾 *Visual reminders ameliorate demands placed on working memory.*

   - Assign practice lessons and offer positive corrective feedback.

   - Encourage working independently without a visual cue when the format has been mastered.

   - Review and reteach as needed.

   - Have the student add the text structures to the "trick" book. (p. 64)

   - Suggest referring to the book when the format is not recalled.

- Plan organized lessons to enhance understanding of <u>narrative reading materials</u>. Stories and plays typically include descriptions of characters, setting, problems, sequence of events, and outcomes.

Before Reading:

   - Recommend watching a video or movie about the assigned book. This will provide a context in which the story can be understood and remembered.

   - Suggest purchasing a published study guide to obtain an overview of the characters, settings, problems, and solutions.

   - Discuss the title, look at the pictures, and predict what might happen in the story.

186

During Reading:

- Pose <u>factual</u> and <u>interpretive</u> questions to elicit comprehension. Factual questions address the <u>who</u>, <u>what</u>, <u>when</u>, and <u>where</u> of the story while interpretive questions seek answers to the <u>how</u> and <u>why</u>.

  - 🐾 *The majority of questions posed by teachers are literal in nature, requiring only recognition (locating information) or recalling facts from memory.*

  - <u>Who</u> were the main characters?
  - <u>Who</u> were the other characters?
  - <u>What</u> happened in the story?
  - <u>When</u> did the story take place?
  - <u>Where</u> did the story occur?
  - <u>Why</u> was there a problem?
  - <u>How</u> was the problem solved?

- Suggest creating images or pictures in the mind, thinking about the words used to describe them, and relating what is seen, heard, and felt.
- Provide a story organizer to be completed as the story is read. (Appendix pp. 379–380)
- Use a sequencing chain to show the order of events and the outcome. (Appendix p. 381)

After Reading:

- Discuss the "beginning" (characters, setting), "middle" (what happened), and "end" (outcome) of the story.
- Ask for different endings to the story and explanations as to why they might be better.
- Use a story organizer to consolidate the elements of the story.

- Provide a meaningful structure for understanding <u>expository text</u>. As students progress through school, reading increasingly involves reading expository texts (textbooks, reference materials).

Before Reading:

- Furnish short, nonfiction reading materials to teach expository comprehension strategies (e.g., articles and editorials in newspapers, magazines, trade manuals).
- Do a hands-on or experiential learning activity (e.g., science experiment, field trip).
- Encourage listening to or looking at a video or multi-media presentation of the topic to be studied (e.g., watching the movie *Apocalypse Now* before reading *Heart of Darkness* for a literature class). This will provide an overview or context in which the reading material can be understood.

  - 🐾 *Some students are global learners and cannot understand the parts until they understand the whole.*

- Brainstorm or activate the student's existing knowledge and personal experiences as they might relate to the text.

Section IV

- Define <u>vocabulary</u>.
    - Relate definitions to something meaningful to the student.
    - Hand out a prepared sheet with proper spellings and acceptable definitions. Allow it to be used while reading.
- Present an overview of the chapters and book. (11)

Ask the student to:

- read the <u>title</u> as it generally reveals the main idea.
- read the <u>table of contents</u> to obtain an outline of the book. Observe how the material is organized by chapters with sections and subsections.
- read the <u>headings and subheadings</u> of each section.
- focus on <u>italicized words</u>, bold face print, bullets, etc. that indicate key concepts.
- look at and discuss all <u>charts</u>, <u>graphs</u>, <u>captions</u>, and <u>illustrations</u>. Recognize the purpose of the graphic aid, identify the parts, and determine the relationship between the parts. Make interpretations and draw conclusions based on the graphic aids.
- formulate questions based on the title, headings, subheadings, and graphic materials.
- predict the content of the text.
- generate questions to be answered while reading the text.

- Ask the student to read the chapter <u>introduction</u> and then the <u>summary</u>.
- Recommend reviewing the <u>questions</u> at end of section or text and the teacher-prepared study questions immediately prior to reading the chapter.

During Reading:

- Suggest reading one section at a time.

Ask the student to:

- pause periodically to review the main idea and supporting details. Stress that the first sentence of a paragraph usually indicates the main idea of the paragraph.
    - *Many students continue reading the entire assignment without stopping to think about the information.*
- complete a teacher-prepared outline.
- locate and mark answers to teacher-prepared questions.
- look for and note answers to self-generated questions.
- underline with a pencil, mark with different colored highlighters, or make notes in the margins of the book to indicate key concepts and supporting details. Highlight or underline only words or phrases, not entire sentences and paragraphs. What is noted can then be easily reread.
    - *Recommend that the parents purchase an additional set of books or obtain permission to photocopy the material so that important information can be highlighted, underlined, or noted.*

- Structure concepts and facts visually by using a graphic organizer suitable for the type of expository text being read. (Appendix pp. 382–388) Research studies examining the effects of graphic organizers on reading comprehension indicate that their use enhances the teaching and understanding of reading materials. (12)

  - *The graphic organizer can be used as a pre-reading, during-reading, and post-reading instructional technique.*

  - *Use the same narrative and expository graphic organizers for reading comprehension and written expression so the student is not required to learn and recall many different ones.*

  Ask the student to:

  - create a mind map to summarize the text. (Appendix p. 382)

  - organize information into written lists, tables, charts, or diagrams.

  - use a Venn diagram with two or three overlapping circles that demonstrate the comparison (similarities/differences) between two or three characters, ideas, events. (Appendix pp. 384–385)

  - use a sequencing chain or horizontal line to demonstrate the stages of something (life cycle), steps of a procedure (science experiment), or series of historical events. (Appendix p. 381)

  - use a timeline to show the occurrence of historical events, ages, degrees of meaning, rating scales.

  - use an opinion/fact chart to note the differences between ideas. (Appendix p. 386)

  - use a circle to depict a cycle of self-reinforcing events such as life cycles, cycles of achievement and failure, or weather conditions. (Appendix p. 387)

  - use computer-generated graphic organizers from such programs as *Inspiration* or *Kidspiration*. (13)

- Repeat the above steps for each section.

- Encourage thinking by asking probing questions that stimulate critical analysis, interpretation, and generalization of ideas.

After Reading:

Ask the student to:

- reread the chapter summary.

- summarize or restate succinctly the most important information (key concept, related facts, conclusion).

- use graphic organizers to summarize the information. (p. 115)

- review all the questions at the end of the chapter or unit and teacher-prepared questions, looking up the answers if necessary.

- generate questions to ask other students.

- discuss and evaluate the reading assignment.

- place visual cue cards listing the necessary steps for studying narrative and expository reading materials in the student's strategy ("trick") book (p. 64).

Section IV

Difficulty Sequencing

The following behaviors serve as general indicators. The student will not exhibit every characteristic listed. These behaviors may also be indicative of other problems.

    Forgetting sequence of events or plot of story while reading
    Placing information in incorrect order

Interventions

- Demonstrate how to arrange a series of pictures into a logical sequence. Have the student verbalize the story associated with each picture. Then provide a set of pictures to be reordered.

- Ask the student to tell the story.

- Encourage looking at the pictures in the reading material to assist with the visual sequencing of the materials.

- Teach cue words that indicate sequences in reading materials such as "first," "second," "next," "then," and "finally."

  Using cue words, ask the student to:
  - read a passage and highlight or underline the cue words.
  - read a short story and retell it.

- Remind the student to think about the "beginning," "middle," and "end" of reading materials.

- Provide instructions on how to make something. Have the student read the directions and make the object.

- Make sentence strips to be read and sequentially ordered.

- Read a brief, unfinished story and ask the student to make up the story sequence. Read the story and compare with the student's response.

- Pause at intervals during reading and ask what will happen next.

- Assign reading a story and numbering the events in the story.

- Suggest acting out the order of events in a story.

- Use a flow chart or timeline to visualize a sequence. (10)

Difficulty Managing Time

The following behaviors serve as general indicators. The student will not exhibit every characteristic listed. These behaviors may also be indicative of other problems.

    Having difficulty setting/following a schedule to complete reading assignments
    Underestimating amount of time needed to complete task
    Starting reading assignment at last minute
    Being unable to meet deadlines for turning in assignments
    Needing extra time to finish reading

Interventions

- Structure the time allotted to reading sessions.
    - Determine the amount of time the student is able to exert full attention and concentration.
    - Schedule several short sessions rather than one long session.
    - Allow movement during breaks to increase alertness.
- Be aware that the "internal clock" of the impulsive student may be faster than that of the nonimpulsive student. The student is more likely to perceive time as moving slowly and rush to complete reading assignments, often overlooking important information. On the other hand, the student with a slower cognitive pace may think there is ample time and fail to finish the assignment within the limits.
- Divide the reading assignment into manageable stages and determine a timetable for completing each part.
    - Assign one step at a time with a specific deadline.

        Step I   – watch video about assigned topic and read study guide.
        Step II   – read assignment.
        Step III – complete graphic organizer.
        Step IV – answer teacher-prepared questions.

    - Monitor progress and do not allow movement to the next step until the current step is completed.
    - Offer positive reinforcement as each stage is completed.

INFLEXIBILITY

The following behaviors serve as general indicators. The student will not exhibit every characteristic listed. These behaviors may also be indicative of other problems.

Exhibiting rigid, concrete thinking
Perseverating (becoming "stuck" on one idea/detail)
Having difficulty making inferences
Being unable to identify cause-and-effect
Overlooking the need to envision or predict the outcome of events

Interventions

- Teach the student how to make <u>inferences</u>. (10)
    - Teach inferential comprehension separately from basic reading skills.
    - Point out that inferences are ideas that are based on the text but not directly stated.
    - Help connect the student's current knowledge with clues or other facts to "read between the lines" and draw logical conclusions.
    - Brainstorm what might be meant by a statement or action.
    - Associate the inference with another situation that the student has previously experienced.
    - Demonstrate how to find support in the text for the inferences and conclusions that are drawn.

Section IV

- Provide instruction on how to make <u>predictions</u> based on existing knowledge.
  - Present a picture and encourage guessing what might have occurred before the picture.
  - Show a picture in a book. Ask the student to predict the outcome of the event depicted. Read the story and confirm or change the prediction.
  - Pause at key points in the story and ask, "<u>What</u> do you think will happen next?" "<u>Why</u> do you think that will occur?" Encourage accessing prior knowledge and using that information to think about what will happen.
  - Read several parts of a sequential story and have the student predict the finish.
  - Ask for an alternative solution to the outcome of an event.
  - Photocopy a story. Delete the ending. Have the student guess the outcome. Read the original conclusion and compare it with the prediction.

- Teach the interpretation of <u>cause-and-effect</u> situations.
  - Use initially cause-and-effect relationships that are familiar to the student.
  - Teach cue words indicating cause-and-effect such as "since", "therefore", "because", "before/after", "when", "if/then", and "as a result of."
    - Ask the student to highlight or underline cue words in cause-and-effect sentences.
    - Provide cause-and-effect sentences missing the cue words. Have the student insert the omitted words.
  - Show pictures of cause-and-effect situations. Discuss the causes and the effects.
  - Discuss real-life cause-and-effect examples.
  - Suggest identifying sentence parts with (C) for cause and (E) for effect.
  - Furnish statements of cause and ask the student to complete them with possible effects.
  - Teach inferential and nonsequential cause-and-effect materials.
  - Provide a Venn diagram with the cause in the center circle and request that the overlapping circles be filled in with possible effects.
  - Furnish a graphic aid to assist visualization of cause-and-effect. (Appendix p. 388)

- Teach comprehension of <u>compare and contrast</u>.
  - Use a Venn diagram to visually depict the similarities and differences between two or more people, places, events, concepts, etc. (Appendix pp. 384–385)

Chapter 18

INITIATION/EXECUTION DIFFICULTIES

The following behaviors serve as general indicators. The student will not exhibit every characteristic listed. These behaviors may also be indicative of other problems.

> Appearing hypoactive/lacking energy/uninterested in reading
> Seeming "lazy" or "unmotivated"
> Procrastinating/hesitating/avoiding beginning reading activity
> Requiring repeated encouragement/direction to start/finish assignments
> Initiating/completing assignment after observing another student

Interventions

- Provide reading tasks with which success can be experienced.

- Always assign work at the appropriate instructional level. (p. 178)

  - *Check the reading level of textbooks. Content area texts are often not written at the instructional level but at the frustration level.*

- Determine whether the student feels capable of performing the reading assignment. Often the teacher is unaware that the student is not willing to admit that the reading task is too difficult. This is particularly evident in middle and high school classes which expect more in-depth reading comprehension. (10)

  - Provide easier reading materials related to the same subject.

  - Use multi-media presentations prior to reading to visually enhance comprehension.

- Check understanding of the directions related to the reading task before allowing the student to begin working.

- Break reading assignments into several parts. The student tends to become discouraged and frustrated when confronted with long reading assignments and then is unable to overcome the inertia caused by feeling overwhelmed.

- Read aloud the first paragraph of the reading assignment.

- Teach the student how to ask for help. (p. 126)

IMPAIRED SELF-MONITORING/USE OF FEEDBACK/SELF-CORRECTION

The following behaviors serve as general indicators. The student will not exhibit every characteristic listed. These behaviors may also be indicative of other problems.

> Being unaware of losing focus and concentration
> Continuing to read even though material has not been understood
> Missing important details
> Misreading words
> Being unable to answer questions about material that was just read
> Lacking the skills to know how and when to reread
> Overlooking the need to stop, clarify thinking, and then reread
> Forgetting to engage in self-questioning to assess understanding

Section IV

Interventions

- Teach self-monitoring and self-correction using materials at the <u>instructional level</u> (3-7 out of 100 words not mastered) so that some comprehension problems will be encountered.

- Suggest reading orally. Reading aloud forces the student to slow down, listen to information, and self-monitor.

- Recommend identifying while reading the primary details: who, what, when, where, how, and why.

- Propose highlighting and color coding main ideas and details. Use the same colors with all reading materials.

- Teach <u>self-questioning</u>.

  ○ Explain the purpose of self-questioning and how it will help monitor understanding of the reading materials.

  ○ Model or demonstrate how to use self-questioning.

  ○ Help the student generate questions such as:

    - "What did the teacher ask me to do? Find the main idea and important facts? Make a mind map? Answer the questions?"

    - "Do I know how to do that?"

    - "What does this word/phrase/sentence mean?"

    - "Does this paragraph make sense to me?"

    - "Am I paying attention and remembering what I just read?"

    - "What is going to happen next?"

    - "Do I understand? I don't understand. What should I do? Do I need to reread or read further for clarification?"

    - "Have I finished what I was supposed to read?"

  ○ Prepare a list of the student's self-generated questions to serve as a visual guide and cue.

  ○ Place a list of the questions in the student's strategy ("trick") book. (p. 64) Suggest referring to the list when the questions are not recalled.

- Request that a story be retold so that the student can determine whether the material was understood.

- Encourage periodic self-review by paraphrasing or summarizing.

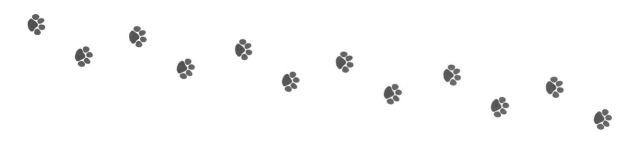

- Furnish in advance a list of questions for the student to answer after the reading is completed. If the student does not know the answers, suggest rereading the material.
  - Ask questions that contain identical wording found in the text.
  - Recommend underlining or noting the page number where an answer can be located.
  - Pose questions that cue meaning and permit correction of erroneous answers.
  - Design questions for which the answer is in the text but is not directly stated. This type of question requires engagement of existing knowledge and connects that information with the reading material.
- Tape-record oral reading. Have the student listen to the tape while reading along with the text and identify errors that impact comprehension (e.g., misreading words, omitting words, skipping lines).
- Suggest predicting the number of times it will be necessary to reread passages. Keep a record and compare performance across time.
- Provide feedback on reading errors and successes. Emphasize <u>successes</u> to build self-esteem.

MEMORY PROBLEMS

Review interventions for Memory Problems in Chapter 14.

SHORT-TERM MEMORY PROBLEMS

Difficulty with Working Memory

The following behaviors serve as general indicators. The student will not exhibit every characteristic listed. These behaviors may also be indicative of other problems.

Forgetting main ideas/details, while sounding out words
Forgetting key concepts/facts read at beginning of a page/chapter, while reading remaining text
Having difficulty holding in mind the sequence of the story
Forgetting the plot of the story while reading
Being unable to follow appropriate text structure to guide reading
Becoming overwhelmed when confronted with lengthy reading materials
Having trouble retelling/paraphrasing/summarizing material
Being unable to think about cause-and-effect situations
Being unable to predict the outcome of events
Having difficulty analyzing author's purpose/opinions
Forgetting today reading material that was recalled yesterday

A significant relationship has been identified between working memory and reading comprehension. (14, 15)

Section IV

Interventions

- Divide reading task into small segments.
- Teach strategies that enhance the <u>capacity</u> of working memory.
  - Use <u>association</u>.
    - Help link new information with existing knowledge and personal life experiences.
    - Encourage the connection of an abstract concept with a previously learned, meaningful experience. For example, relating Shakespeare's play *Romeo and Juliet* with Stephen Sondheim's musical *West Side Story* places the play in the vernacular, both culturally and linguistically.
  - Encourage <u>verbal rehearsal</u>.
    - Allow subvocalization (whispering under breath).
    - Suggest frequent repetition of main ideas and relevant facts.
    - Stress the need to spend as much time reciting as reading.
    - Encourage reciting while covering or looking away from the material.
    - Recommend the use of inflection while reciting aloud.
    - Emphasize paraphrasing or summarizing the material at intervals.
  - Teach <u>categorization</u> skills (putting new information into existing categories).
    - 🐾 *Categorization also enhances efficient word retrieval.*
    - Demonstrate how to consolidate facts into categories or chunks (memory units). For example, names, dates, and places are easier to remember if they are grouped together into small, meaningful units that are related to each other rather than one long list. The size of the chunk should match the capacity of the student's verbal memory span. The ability to process information in working memory decreases significantly as the student tries to process more than the memory span can retain.
  - Emphasize <u>visualization</u>.
    - Have the student with nonverbal strengths create images of a series of pictures that depict the material. The pictures need to be absurd or unusual to promote recall.
      - 🐾 *Before starting, make sure that the student can visualize (make a mental picture).*
    - Recommend drawing pictures that reflect important information to be held in working memory.
    - Use graphic organizers for narrative and expository text structure to enhance the capacity of working memory. (Appendix pp. 379–388)

Chapter 18

LONG-TERM MEMORY PROBLEMS

Difficulty Encoding/Consolidating (Learning)

The following behaviors serve as general indicators. The student will not exhibit every characteristic listed. These behaviors may also be indicative of other problems.

> Having difficulty associating new information with existing knowledge/personal experiences
> Being unable to learn/select/use encoding strategies
> Relying only on rote memory to remember reading materials
> Storing/filing information in a disorganized manner
> Needing additional instruction to master new information
> Forgetting today reading material learned yesterday
> Having trouble when required to recall cumulative materials

Students with **ADHD** frequently do not use organized and efficient strategies to encode information into long-term memory. Investigators suggest that, while they know encoding strategies, are capable of using them, and know they "should" be used, they utilize superficial strategies, spend less time studying, put forth less effort (skim rather than reread) when confronted with complex reading materials. (16, 17)

Interventions

- Encourage the use of strategies and different text structures to encode information presented in reading materials. Explain <u>why</u> it is important to utilize them and <u>when</u> and <u>how</u> they will improve learning and recall.

- Structure reading lessons to facilitate encoding.
    - Recommend listening to a tape or watching a video or movie (video from a science series, movie of a famous novel) before reading. This provides an overview, or context, in which the material can be understood and learned.
    - Discuss the meaning of unfamiliar vocabulary words before reading.
    - Divide the reading task into segments.
    - Extract and write down key information to be remembered, such as who, what, when, where, how, and why.
    - Suggest highlighting, underlining, or color coding important ideas and facts for emphasis.
    - Provide graphic organizers. (Appendix pp. 379–388)

- Recommend using verbal (p. 141) and/or visual (p. 142) strategies to encode main ideas and relevant details.

- Teach effective <u>study skills</u>.

    Suggest that the student:

    - review new information immediately, even if just for 5 minutes. (p. 143)

        > *Most forgetting occurs in the first few minutes after the information is learned. This quick review helps ensure that learning is permanent and saves time. Studying the material at a later time requires relearning, not just reviewing.*

    - paraphrase or summarize information at the end of each paragraph, page, and section of a chapter.

Section IV

- state main ideas and important details while covering or looking away from the material.
- spend as much time reciting as reading.
- use inflection while repeating aloud.

○ spend extra time studying the middle sections of reading materials. Beginnings and endings are more easily remembered. Middle sections need extra study and emphasis. (p. 139)

○ do something different each time the material is studied (e.g., reorganize or outline the notes, color code information, or transcribe the notes onto a word processor).

🐾 *Reading notes over and over is an ineffective and inefficient means of transferring information into long-term memory.*

- Use the student's learning preferences (cognitive strengths) when designing strategies to encode reading materials.

Difficulty Retrieving (Recalling)

The following behaviors serve as general indicators. The student will not exhibit every characteristic listed. These behaviors may also be indicative of other problems.

Having trouble recalling reading material when asked questions in class, even when student has raised hand to respond
Being unable to answer test questions, even when material has been learned
Requiring extended time to complete tests on reading materials
Exhibiting discrepancy between what parents report and what student produces on tests

Interventions

- Use strategies to organize reading materials in an easily retrievable form (e.g., categorization, verbal and visual strategies).

- Allow extra time to respond to questioning.

- Place more emphasis on assessing understanding of concepts than recall of specific facts.

- Permit demonstration of what has been learned in an alternate form (e.g., give a presentation or demonstration; make a poster, diagram, timeline; write a newspaper article or TV report).

- Furnish in advance specific reading comprehension questions that will be asked in class or on a test.

- Use a multiple-choice or matching test format rather than a short-answer or essay format.

  🐾 *Fill-in-the-blank questions are difficult for the student who has retrieval problems. However, this problem may be circumvented with word banks from which to select answers.*

- Provide extended time for taking tests on narrative and expository reading materials.

CHAPTER 19

WRITTEN EXPRESSION/LONG-TERM REPORTS

> **MY WRITING PROBLEM**
>
> I have had trouble with writing assignments ever since I was given my first one in first grade, although since I cant recall my exact thoughts and reasons for these trouble I can only assume they were most likely similar to my writing problems now.
>
> Imagine having all the right thoughts and ideas in your head to easily get an A+ on a paper, now imagine that all these ideas have been broken apart into pieces and scattered all over your brain. Then when your brain decides it needs this information all at once these thoughts, ideas (although still in pieces) are forcing themselves simultaneously through a slender tube to be written down in an intelligent legible fashion. The tube is jammed and the thoughts are still a jumbled disorganized mess and you meanwhile are trying to somehow organize them in this crowded tube.
>
> I'll glance at the clock and realize its well after 2am and ive been working on and off since around 8 or 9pm. I decide to reread what I have written so far and relize that it sounds terrible and resembles nothing of the time and effort spent on it. Even as I write this now I am totally ready to give up just because I know I can write better than this. ...
>
> Another problem is that I overanalyze everything, which makes the simplest task into something so complex it is exhausting. Sometimes I will get so stuck in just thinking that I will psyche myself out and end up having an anxiety induced panic attack. When this occurs I will undoubtedly give up. Because I tend to shut down completely and have no chance of rebooting and getting any more work accomplished. After this happens I will get frustrated with myself for giving up and then feel guilty for allowing myself to accept failure. Then I will just end up going to bed depressed and angry that I make things so difficult on myself. It's the worst feeling knowing that I am the only one standing in my own way. I feel even worse knowing that when I am able to write a whole paper that I do write very well. I just wish that it didn't take so much out of me to write a paper.
>
> By far the worst is that once I have hand written all that I have to write and am ready to type is up on Word, I basically end up completely rewriting it over again as i go. This takes just as long, if not longer, than the initial writing process. I always try to get myself to type strictly what i have written but by some point or another I will get fed up about the way I had it written on paper and start to 'improv' it as I go.
>
> The whole writing process for me is a very tedious, lengthy, and painfully stressful. It really takes a lot out of me to put all the time, energy and effort into it and I often don't have it in me to endure such a tiresome process. I know that even when I have finished half of the paper, the process is nowhere near done and I then have to do the entire rewrite. This alone makes me even less hopeful of finishing and more likely to give up during any point of the process. Thankfully though this time after, so many weeks of it being overdue, I am done with it and can let it be one less thing for me to feel even more guilty about not completing. Sadly though I know that no matter how good this is the best I can get is a C, but I know that this is always better than getting a Zero.
>
> Just for the record I am completing this at 2:15AM.
>
> Josh, 18 yr. old college student

Figure 19.1. Written Expression Sample – Written by student with ADHD, tics, OCD, depression, and executive dysfunction

Section IV

Students in the upper elementary and secondary grades are increasingly expected to use writing to enhance learning and to demonstrate what has been mastered. Writing is a complex process requiring the integration of several different skills. Impairment in one component can interfere with progress in another. Problems may result from graphomotor impairment, inattention, executive dysfunction (difficulty planning, prioritizing, organizing, sequencing, initiating, executing, revising, editing), and/or memory deficits.

Many students struggle with written language and develop a dislike for writing and a negative perception of their ability to communicate through writing. Research suggests that approximately 75% of clinically referred students with **ADHD** and 20% of students with **TS** meet the criteria for learning disabilities in the area of written expression. (1, 2) About 25% of students with **OCD** report writing problems. (3)

General Recommendations

Review Classroom and Individual Student Interventions in Chapters 8 and 9.

- Do not allow the student with **OCD** to start any writing activity that cannot be finished in the allotted time frame. The student may be unable to change tasks or sets without subsequent anxiety which can then produce inappropriate behaviors. The student may experience a compulsive need to complete the writing assignment and be unable to be redirected.

- Establish a secure classroom environment that reduces the anxiety and stress associated with writing assignments and stimulates an interest in writing.
  - Model an enthusiastic attitude toward writing.
  - Do not grade every writing assignment.
  - Avoid returning the student's written work marked with an excessive number of corrections.
  - Refrain from asking peers to correct the student's writing to allay feelings of embarrassment.
  - Never use the writing of words, phrases, or sentences as punishment.
  - Do not display the student's writing without permission.

- Encourage divergent, creative, imaginary thinking.

- Establish an email pen pal program to practice written communication skills. (4)
  - Pair the student with another person who has good writing skills (older student, trusted relative).
  - Suggest contacting each other one or two times a week.

- Recognize that the ability to effectively express ideas in writing is affected by the volume, rate, and complexity demanded by the task.
  - Reduce the amount of writing expected.
  - Allow additional time to finish the writing assignment.
  - Emphasize only one or two basic skills on a given assignment (e.g., spelling, punctuation, grammar, word usage).

- Allocate time for daily writing instruction. Forty-five minutes per day is considered the optimal amount of time.

- Assign a short, free-writing activity such as writing in a diary or journal each day. Suggest recording events, thoughts, and feelings. These can be used as ideas for future compositions.
  - Focus on content and overlook inaccurate spelling, punctuation, and grammar.
  - Assign no grades to journal writing.

- Integrate writing instruction with other academic subjects (e.g., literature, history, social studies, science).

- Create a writing folder or notebook. The folder might contain the following:

    Laminated templates of narrative and expository writing formats
    Brainstormed list of topics
    Organizational strategies
    Self-generated revision questions
    Editing strategies
    Spelling list of basic sight vocabulary
    Spelling list of student's frequently misspelled words
    Unfinished writing assignments
    Completed writing assignments

- Recommend, when needed, individualized remedial instruction in written expression from an educational specialist specifically trained to remediate a learning disability in written expression.

- Modify expectations for <u>handwritten assignments</u>. (p. 68) (5)

  - *Research studies have consistently shown that students with **ADHD**, **TS** and/or **OCD** have neurologically-based graphomotor (handwriting) impairment. (6, 7, 8, 9) Inattention, impulsivity, poor planning, and a lack of self-monitoring also contribute to deficient handwriting skills. Graphomotor difficulties in turn interfere with the ability to express ideas in writing efficiently and effectively.*

  - Permit dictation of reports into a tape recorder or to the teacher or another adult.

    - *Teaching experience suggests that students produce better compositions when their thoughts are dictated.*

  - Assign cooperative writing projects. Have each student assume a different task (e.g., brainstormer, researcher, organizer of information, writer, editor, artist).

  - Suggest creating a model, designing a poster, making a scrapbook, giving a demonstration, or making an oral presentation instead of writing a report.

- Permit the use of a <u>computer</u>. (5)

  - *Reducing the impact of problems associated with written expression may motivate the reluctant writer.*

A computer:

  - increases interest and attention to task.

  - avoids working memory deficits.

  - allows the student to focus on the content while writing the first draft and to postpone the editing process.

Section IV

- bypasses impaired graphomotor (handwriting) skills and poor use of space on the paper.
- circumvents retrieval problems by providing word banks from which to select words.
- permits reorganization and resequencing of sentences and paragraphs.
- locates and corrects misspelled words.
- identifies grammatical errors.
- finds and corrects capitalization and punctuation errors.
- provides graphic organizers that allow the student to visually display key concepts and relevant details, reorganize ideas, and create outlines prior to writing.
- enables the student to listen to what has been written and to correct incomplete, awkward, and rambling sentences with speech synthesis software.
- allows the student to dictate essays and reports which are automatically transcribed into text with speech recognition technology. Errors can be edited with the keyboard or vocal commands.

  Voice-input software has been found to improve the quality of work for the less skilled writer. (10)

- Provide spelling instruction when spelling skills have not been mastered at an automatic level. (11) Spelling problems interfere with both the amount and quality of the writing. For example, when a student must stop to think how to spell a word, ideas that were developed and held in working memory are often forgotten.

  - Select only words that the student can read.
  - Allot 10 to 15 minutes each day for spelling.
  - Teach words that are encountered with high frequency. There are approximately 100 words that are used 50% of the time. (Appendix p. 376) Eliminate words associated with the various academic subjects (e.g., social studies, science) as they are quickly forgotten when the unit is completed.
  - Use a multi-sensory approach to teach basic sight words.

    Ask the student to:
    - look carefully at the word and say it.
    - write and simultaneously say the whole word aloud (not letters or sounds).
    - check the word.
    - cover the word and write it from memory.
    - check the spelling of the word. If the word is misspelled, repeat the sequence.

  - Teach the spelling of phonetically-based words and word parts.

    Ask the student to:
    - identify the number of syllables in a word – ("computer" has three).
    - listen carefully to the vowel sound in each syllable.
    - spell each syllable in the correct order – ("com, pu, ter").
    - read the word.

- recognize that the word was spelled phonetically but incorrectly.
- correct the spelling.
- read the corrected spelling and copy it.

○ Teach spelling rules that apply to a large number of words (e.g., when adding "ing" to a word that ends in "e," the "e" is usually dropped – "make" becomes "making" and "take" becomes "taking;" the letter "q" is always followed with "u" – "quart," "quick," "queen;" "i" comes before "e" except after "c" – "believe," "receive.").

○ Avoid teaching rules for words that have exceptions.

○ Refrain from requiring spelling words to be written a designated number of times. When words must be copied over and over again, it is difficult to think about the word or how to spell it. Furthermore, if the word is written incorrectly, it may be learned incorrectly.

> 🐾 *The student with **ADHD** and/or **TS** may develop muscle soreness and fatigue which in turn may produce inappropriate behavior. The student with **OCD** may become "stuck" and need to rewrite each word until it looks "perfect."*

- Assign instead the completion of sentences in which the spelling word is omitted.

○ Use a pretest-study-posttest rather than study-test procedure.
- Give a pretest.
- Have the student self-correct spelling test.
- Assign only the missed words to study.
- Give a posttest including both words spelled correctly and incorrectly on the pretest.

○ Stress self-correction. Self-correction is sometimes sufficient for learning to spell a word properly.

○ Assign tasks requiring the use of spelling words in <u>meaningful</u> contexts (e.g., writing words in phrases, sentences, paragraphs, essays).

○ Promote spelling fluency.
- Review and dictate the basic sight vocabulary words repeatedly.
- Dictate phrases and short sentences containing the words, increasing the pace until spelling becomes automatic.

○ Develop an individualized spelling list for the student to use when writing.

○ Place a list of the basic sight vocabulary and the student's frequently misspelled words in the writing notebook. Suggest referring to the list when the correct spelling cannot be recalled.

- Suggest using a Franklin Spelling Ace to improve spelling skills. This electronic reference device is able to verify spelling, correct misspellings, point out phonetically-based spelling errors, provide an alternative word list, and/or explain words that sound alike. A model is available that pronounces words aloud. (12)

- Recommend utilizing the computer spell checker.

Section IV

> Tics/obsessions/compulsions, underarousal/slow processing speed, inattention/impulsivity/hyperactivity, executive dysfunction, and/or memory problems frequently interfere with the ability to express one's self in writing.

UNDERAROUSAL/SLOW COGNITIVE PROCESSING SPEED

Review interventions for Underarousal and Slow Processing Speed in Chapter 10.

The following behaviors serve as general indicators. The student will not exhibit every characteristic listed. These behaviors may also be indicative of other problems.

    Appearing to have difficulty concentrating on writing assignments
    Lacking persistence
    Possessing age-appropriate writing skills, but being unable to finish writing assignment in allotted time
    Producing simplistic, concrete writing
    Being slow to recall specific vocabulary words to use
    Having trouble quickly retrieving correct spelling of words/grammar and punctuation rules
    Being unable to hold ideas in working memory while shifting back and forth between tasks that require selecting specific vocabulary words/spelling correctly/using appropriate grammar/recalling capitalization and punctuation rules/following sequence of thoughts

Interventions

- Assign writing tasks that can easily be completed.
- Modify the length and requirements of the writing assignments.
- Divide writing assignments into small, manageable sections.
- Provide frequent breaks.
- Provide a graphic organizer to visually help maintain information while writing.
- Waive time limits or provide sufficient time for the writing assignment to be completed.

INATTENTION/IMPULSIVITY/HYPERACTIVITY

Review interventions for Inattention, Impulsivity, and Hyperactivity in Chapter 12.

The following behaviors serve as general indicators. The student will not exhibit every characteristic listed. These behaviors may also be indicative of other problems.

    Becoming distracted during the writing process
    Daydreaming/staring into space/appearing to exert little effort
    Being off-task after initially starting
    Needing reminders to persist on writing assignment
    Omitting words/phrases when writing
    Making grammatical errors not evident in oral language
    Ignoring capitalization and punctuation rules
    Spelling correctly on spelling test, but incorrectly when writing
    Impulsively rushing through writing assignment
    Exhibiting inappropriate behaviors that interfere with writing
    Becoming frustrated/upset when required to write
    Not knowing how to use self-talk to control behavior when writing

Interventions

- Define appropriate writing behavior.
- Structure the writing assignment for success so that the student is able to sustain attention.
  - Assign writing tasks that focus on the student's ideas, interests, and experiences (e.g., animals, sports, cars), especially when teaching a new writing concept.
    - 🐾 *This also allows the student to use familiar content that does not interfere with learning a new skill.*
  - Divide the writing activity into segments to mitigate the loss of interest and difficulty persisting when assigned long writing tasks.
    - Assign one part at a time.
    - Permit physical movement after each segment is completed (e.g., sharpen a pencil, walk to the water fountain).
  - Gradually increase the length and difficulty of the writing assignment as success is exhibited.
- Recommend using <u>self-talk</u> to focus attention during the writing process.
- Explain how negative comments about writing impact performance (e.g., "I hate writing." "This is dumb." "I will never learn to write a report.").
  - Help the student reframe the statements ("I can write a good paper if I slow down, concentrate, and use the strategies in my 'trick' book.").
- Teach the student how to appropriately <u>ask for help</u>. (p. 126)

EXECUTIVE DYSFUNCTION

Review interventions for Executive Dysfunction in Chapter 13.

IMPAIRED PROBLEM SOLVING
(Tasks/Activities/Situations)

- Provide a template of a <u>problem solving strategy</u> such as "**GET A CLUE**," "**PLAN**," or another strategy to enhance written expression. Be sure the strategy includes steps for goal setting, planning (generating ideas, solutions; analyzing proposed ideas, solutions; prioritizing; organizing; sequencing; managing time), initiating, self-monitoring, and editing. (Appendix pp. 374–375)
  - 🐾 *Strategies have been found to help students effectively plan, organize, write, revise, and edit written work. (13)*
- Model and demonstrate how to use the <u>problem solving strategy</u>. (p. 108)

Section IV

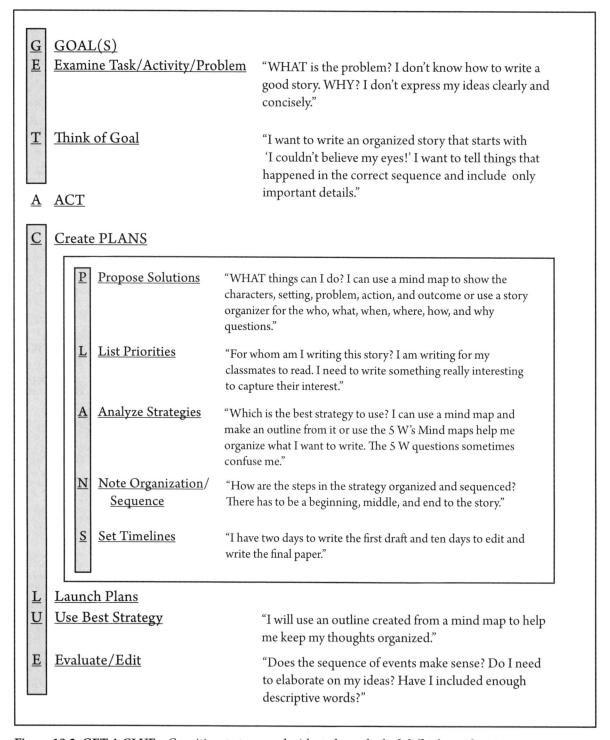

Figure 19.2. GET A CLUE – Cognitive strategy used with student who had difficulty with written expression

Some students may not be able to follow the complexity of this strategy unless taught in incremental steps that must be mastered before continuing to the next step. Other students may need to learn a more simplified version "**PLAN.**" If so, use "**GET A CLUE**" as a structure for discussing and teaching ways to solve tasks, activities, and problem situations.

P	Propose Goal	"I need to develop a plan to convey my ideas clearly and logically."
L	List and Analyze Strategies	"What things can I do? I can use a mind map to show the characters, setting, problem, action, and outcome. I can use a story organizer for the who, what, when, where, how, and why questions, but the 5W's sometimes confuse me."
A	Apply Best Strategy	"What is the best strategy to use? I can use a mind map and make an outline from it. It will help me organize what I want to write."
N	Notice Errors and Edit	"Does the sequence of events make sense? Do I need to elaborate on my ideas? Have I included enough descriptive words?"

Figure 19.3. PLAN – Cognitive strategy used with student who had difficulty with written expression

Difficulty Planning

Difficulty Proposing (Generating) Ideas

The following behaviors serve as general indicators. The student will not exhibit every characteristic listed. These behaviors may also be indicative of other problems.

Neglecting to think about what is to be written before beginning
Overlooking need to set goals to improve writing
Using trial-and-error approach to writing
Being hesitant to generate own ideas when setting goals
Having difficulty retrieving ideas and experiences from memory

Interventions

- Teach the student how to propose (brainstorm, generate) ideas for a topic.

   🐾 *Stress the importance of choosing a topic that is neither too comprehensive nor too limited. If the topic is too broad, there will be too many reference materials to read and understand, and too much information to include in the report. If the topic is too restricted, there will not be enough information to research and present.*

> **The Universe**
> **When my son with ADHD/TS/OCD was assigned his first report to write, the teacher knew the importance of selecting a topic that would be easy to write about and of not making the assignment overwhelming. She allowed everyone to select a topic of personal interest for a three page paper. My son chose "The Universe" as his topic! When questioned about the unrealistic scope of the subject, he could not understand the necessity of limiting the subject. EDF !!!**

Section IV

- activate existing knowledge and personal experiences to generate a list of topics (e.g., books/magazines, television, movies, Internet, discussions, hobbies, dreams, make-believe, memories, mysteries, music, visual arts).

- brainstorm as many practical and unusual ideas as possible.

- use a mind mapping strategy to stimulate ideas. Place a topic of interest in the middle circle. Record every idea that comes to mind, circle that word, and connect it to the closest related idea. (Appendix p. 382)

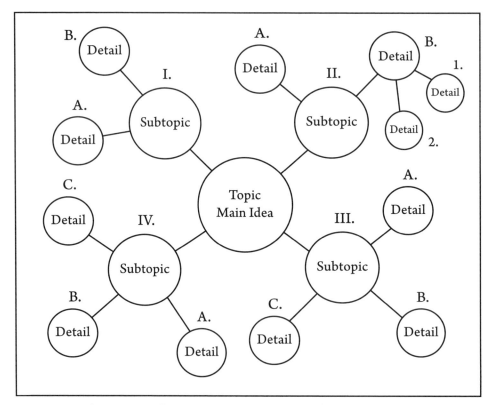

Figures 19.4. Mind Map – Visual cognitive strategy for brainstorming, organizing, outlining ideas

- generate ideas on a computer (e.g., use a mind mapping program such as *Inspiration/Kidspiration*.) (14)

- provide teacher-prepared writing prompts to stimulate ideas (e.g., "The worst/best thing that ever happened ____," "My scariest moment ____," "If only ____," "All at once ____," "Suddenly without warning ____.").

- rewrite the ending of an interesting story provided by the teacher.

- create a story that ends with a sentence provided by the teacher.

- visualize a scene for "painting a picture" with words.

- tape record proposed ideas, solutions, or strategies.

- brainstorm with a classmate who excels in generating original ideas.

• Allow a topic of self-interest to be selected.

Difficulty Prioritizing

The following behaviors serve as general indicators. The student will not exhibit every characteristic listed. These behaviors may also be indicative of other problems.

> Having difficulty deciding most relevant information to include
> Writing around a subject and never clearly stating main idea
> Including ideas only vaguely related to the topic and inconsistent with intent or structure of the writing
> Providing too much information
> Being unrealistic regarding expectations for amount of content to write (one page/five pages/ten pages)

Interventions

- Emphasize thinking about audience for whom the composition will be written (e.g., teacher, parent, classmate, sibling, editor).

- Have the student define the purpose for writing (e.g., problem/solution, explanation, opinion/persuasion, comparison/contrast, cause/effect) and then identify the most appropriate text structure for the topic.

- Suggest rank ordering the ideas. Discard those that are not relevant, or saving them in the writing notebook (p. 201) for future compositions.

Difficulty Organizing/Sequencing

The following behaviors serve as general indicators. The student will not exhibit every characteristic listed. These behaviors may also be indicative of other problems.

> Overlooking need to follow organized narrative/expository text structure
> Being unable to break down writing assignments into manageable segments
> Writing everything known about a topic without expressing ideas logically/sequentially
> Interjecting disconnected thoughts

Interventions

- Teach the structure of writing <u>narrative text</u> (stories, plays). Story structure typically includes a description of the characters, setting (time, place), sequence of events, and outcome.

    ○ Use a who, what, when, where, how, and why organizational approach.

    - <u>Who</u> is the main character in the story?
    - <u>Who</u> are the other characters?
    - <u>When</u> does the story occur?
    - <u>Where</u> does the story take place?
    - <u>What</u> happens in the story?
    - <u>What</u> is the problem?
    - <u>Why</u> is there a problem?
    - <u>How</u> will it be resolved?

    ○ Recommend thinking about and briefly relating the "beginning" (characters, setting), "middle" (problem/event), and "end" (outcome) of the story.

Section IV

- Discuss the sequence of events prior to writing (what will happen "first," "second," "next," and "finally").
- Suggest creating pictures in the mind and imagining descriptive words that depict what is seen, heard, and felt.
  - 🐾 *Some students need to be taught how to visualize.*
- Generate different endings to the story and select the best ending.
- Furnish a graphic organizer that visually structures narrative writing. (Appendix pp. 379–380)

• Explain the different structures associated with writing expository texts (e.g., description, explanation, chronology of events, cause-and-effect, compare/contrast, opinion/persuasion, problem/solution).

  - 🐾 *Expository writing is an important skill in the upper elementary and secondary grade levels as content-related academic subjects increasingly require the student to write essays and reports.*

  - Demonstrate how different graphic organizers are used for expository text to visually structure ideas, facts, and concepts.
    - 🐾 *Use the same graphic organizer for written expression and reading comprehension so the student is not required to learn and recall so many different ones.*

    Suggest that the student:
    - use a mind map to select important ideas and related facts. (Appendix p. 382)
    - use a Venn diagram of two or three overlapping circles to decide on the comparison (similarities/differences) between two or three characters, ideas, events. (Appendix pp. 384-385)
    - use a sequencing chain or horizontal line to plan stages of something (life cycle), steps of a procedure. (Appendix p. 381)
    - use a timeline to choose the order of events.
    - use an opinion/fact chart to delineate the differences between ideas. (Appendix p. 386)
    - use a circle to determine a cycle of self-reinforcing events. (Appendix p. 387)
    - use a cause and effect chart to decide on events that happen and their consequences. (Appendix p. 388)
    - outline or list the main sections and subsections.
    - use computer-generated graphic organizers from such programs as *Inspiration/Kidspiration*. (14)

  - Teach cue words associated with each type of expository text to provide coherence between the ideas being presented and the preceding idea (e.g., "like," "different," "but," "in contrast," for a compare and contrast essay; "first," "second," "third," "then," "finally" for sequential text).

• Use various examples from reading materials to demonstrate the difference between narrative and expository writing formats.

- Teach an organized, step-by-step approach for the <u>preparation for expository writing</u>.

  Suggest that the student:

  - locate <u>sources of information</u>.
    - interview other people (teachers, librarians, tutor, professional experts).
    - consult reference materials (textbooks, encyclopedias, websites, journals, magazines, newspapers).
      - 🐾 *Students with **ADHD** often utilize electronic reference materials better than other sources.*
  - use 3 x 5 or 4 x 6 spiral bound <u>index cards</u> to record information.
    - write only one idea on each card. Note the name of the author; date; title of book, magazine, or article; and publisher (name, city, state).
    - write information in own words.
    - place quotation marks around quotes. Write page number of each quote.
    - number main ideas and important facts in the sequence to be written.
    - reread the cards and color code using dots to designate different ideas.
  - complete an outline or graphic organizer for writing expository text.
    - number the main ideas and important facts in the sequence to be written in the report.
    - make an outline from the numbers.
    - paraphrase most important information on the cards and use it to expand the graphic organizer.
    - eliminate ideas that do not fit.
    - check the outline or graphic organizer to be sure that the information is balanced appropriately.
    - assign each key concept the color that corresponds to the ideas on the cards.
  - separate the cards from the spiral binding, sort them by color, and place them in the correct sequence. Make decisions concerning where to include information from cards having more than two dots.

- Teach the <u>steps for writing</u> the paper.

  Instruct the student to:

  - use the <u>computer</u> to write the first draft. Double space between the lines so that there is enough room to make revisions.
  - write the <u>title</u> at the top of the page.
  - write an <u>introductory paragraph</u> that states and defines the topic.
    - include three or four ideas or examples to be developed in the different sections of the essay.
    - try to make the reader want to read further.
    - conclude with a transition sentence that connects the <u>following paragraph</u>.

Section IV

- o develop the topic in the <u>following paragraphs</u>.
    - write a beginning or topic sentence for each paragraph, repeating keywords and ideas. Use cue words associated with the text structure (e.g., "first", "second", "next", "finally", "in my opinion", "in contrast").
- o present facts and specific examples in each paragraph to support the topic sentence.
- o move in a logical sequence from paragraph to paragraph and develop each point as it relates to the subject.
    - include a few quotations from accepted sources of information.
    - provide illustrations (maps, charts, graphs, timelines) to visually explain the content.
- o write a <u>concluding paragraph</u>.
    - restate the main idea in words that are different from those used in the first paragraph.
    - note most important facts presented in the preceding paragraphs.
    - end with a summary statement.
- o print the first draft of the paper.
    - 🐾 *Emphasize that the first draft is not expected to be the finished paper.*
- Have the student place the structures for narrative and expository writing and their corresponding graphic organizers in the writing notebook. (p. 201)

Difficulty Managing Time

The following behaviors serve as general indicators. The student will not exhibit every characteristic listed. These behaviors may also be indicative of other problems.

Having difficulty setting/following schedule for writing reports
Underestimating amount of time needed to complete writing task
Starting essays/reports at the last minute
Having trouble completing reports
Being unable to meet deadlines for turning in written assignments
Needing extra time to finish written work

Interventions

- Structure the time allotted to writing.
    - o Determine the amount of time the student is available to exert full attention and concentration. Plan accordingly.
    - o Be sure to plan movement breaks to increase alertness.

        Step I   – brainstorm and select a topic.
        Step II   – research topic.
        Step III   – plan and organize writing.
        Step IV   – write first draft.
        Step V   – revise and edit.
        Step VI   – rewrite.
        Step VII   – reread and write final paper.
        Step VIII   – present report to class.

- Divide the writing assignments into manageable stages and help the student make a timetable for completing each part.
    - Assign one step at a time with a specific deadline.
    - Monitor progress and do not allow movement to the next step until the current step is completed.
    - Offer positive reinforcement as each step is completed.
- Post instructions and due dates for completing research and written assignments on the school or class web site.
- Mail the parents a copy of the instructions and deadlines.

INITIATION/EXECUTION DIFFICULTIES

The following behaviors serve as general indicators. The student will not exhibit every characteristic listed. These behaviors may also be indicative of other problems.

Appearing hypoactive/lacking energy/uninterested in writing
Seeming "lazy"/"unmotivated"
Procrastinating/hesitating/avoiding beginning writing activity
Requiring repeated encouragement and direction to start/complete task

Interventions

- Determine performance capability. Often the teacher is unaware that students are not willing to admit that written tasks are too difficult. This is particularly evident in middle and high school classes that demand more independent and complex writing.
- Always provide writing assignments with which success can be experienced.
- Avoid requiring accurate spelling, grammar, and punctuation on the first draft. Focus on content.
- Check to make sure that the student understands the directions related to the writing assignment before beginning the task.
- Break writing assignments into several parts. The student tends to become discouraged and frustrated when confronted with lengthy writing activities and then is unable to overcome the inertia and anxiety associated with feeling overwhelmed.
- "Kick start" writing by providing the first sentence of the opening paragraph. The first paragraph is often the most difficult to write.
- Teach the student how to appropriately ask for help. (p. 126)

Section IV

IMPAIRED SELF-MONITORING/USE OF FEEDBACK/SELF-CORRECTION

The following behaviors serve as general indicators. The student will not exhibit every characteristic listed. These behaviors may also be indicative of other problems.

    Lacking the skills needed to proofread and detect errors
    Having difficulty revising (improving) simplistic, concrete writing
    Omitting words and phrases
    Being unaware that the writing does not make sense
    Spelling words correctly on spelling tests, but having difficulty spelling accurately when writing
    Knowing grammar/capitalization/punctuation rules, but being unable to apply rules when writing
    Having difficulty understanding one's writing when read aloud

Interventions

- Suggest writing the first draft on every other line or double space so corrections can easily be made.

    🐾 *Writing the first draft on the computer allows for ease of production and correction.*

- Assign the task of revising and editing a day or two after the first draft is completed. If the student proofreads immediately after writing, the intended meaning may be read instead of the actual words written. Emphasize that the first draft is not expected to be the finished paper.

- Encourage the use of a <u>self-talk strategy</u> by reading the composition aloud. Oral reading helps the student stop, listen, and monitor both the content and mechanics of the writing. Rapid, silent reading makes it difficult to identify errors.

- Separate the revision of content from the editing of mechanical errors.

- Focus on <u>content (revision)</u> before concentrating on <u>mechanics (editing)</u>.

- Provide instruction in revision (improvement) of narrative writing.
  - Furnish a list of revision questions to be answered prior to turning in the assignment. (Appendix p. 389)

Revision Checklist for Narrative Writing

First Paragraph	Did you capture the reader's attention and make the reader want to read further?	Yes	No
Character(s)	Who was the main character?		
	Who were the other important characters?		
	Did you adequately describe the characters?	Yes	No
	Did the dialogue develop the characters' personalities and advance the plot?	Yes	No
Setting	Did you tell <u>where</u> the story took place?	Yes	No
	Did you tell <u>when</u> the story took place?	Yes	No
	Did your <u>setting</u> enhance the story?	Yes	No
	Did you frequently refer to the setting?	Yes	No
	Did you use <u>descriptive words</u> to depict what was seen, heard, and felt?	Yes	No
Plot	Did you explain <u>what</u> the conflict/problem was?	Yes	No
	Did you explain <u>why</u> there was a conflict/problem?	Yes	No
	Did you provide a logical sequence of events?	Yes	No
Outcome	Did you explain <u>how</u> the conflict/problem was resolved?	Yes	No
	Did you include an appropriate ending/solution (not abrupt/leave the reader with many unanswered questions)?	Yes	No

** If you circled "No" to any of the above questions, revise that part before turning in your paper.

Adapted from Grace Haygood's "Checklist for Fictional Piece" 2003.

Figure 19.5. Revision Checklist for Narrative Writing

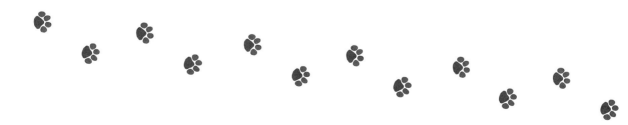

Section IV

- Provide instruction in <u>revision</u> (improvement) of <u>expository writing</u>.
    - Furnish a list of revision questions to be answered prior to turning in the assignment. (Appendix p. 390)

Revision Checklist for Expository Writing

<u>First Paragraph</u>	Did you clearly <u>state the topic?</u>	Yes	No
	Did you include three or four <u>ideas/examples?</u>	Yes	No
	Did you capture the reader's attention and make the reader want to read further?	Yes	No
	Did you end with a <u>transition sentence</u> that connected the following paragraph?	Yes	No
<u>Following Paragraphs</u>	Did you write a <u>beginning sentence</u> that stated the main idea of each paragraph?	Yes	No
	Did you include <u>facts and examples</u> to support the main idea?	Yes	No
	Did you include a few <u>quotes</u> from authorities?	Yes	No
	Did you <u>reference</u> the quotes?	Yes	No
	Did you include some <u>illustrations</u> to explain main ideas and details?	Yes	No
	Did you <u>sequence the ideas</u> so they made sense and related to each other?	Yes	No
	Were there any words or sentences that did not need to be included?	Yes	No
	Did you use a <u>variety of words</u> rather than the same words over and over again?	Yes	No
	Did you use <u>adjectives</u> and <u>adverbs</u>?	Yes	No
	Did you <u>summarize</u> at the end of each paragraph?	Yes	No
<u>Concluding Paragraph</u>	Did you <u>rephrase the main idea</u> in words different from those used in the first paragraph?	Yes	No
	Did you <u>summarize</u> important ideas presented?	Yes	No
	Did you end with a <u>concluding statement</u>?	Yes	No

** If you circled "No" to any of the above questions, revise that part before turning in your paper.

Figure 19.6. Revision Checklist for Expository Writing

- Suggest tape recording the composition and then listening to it while reading the words.

- Provide <u>positive</u> corrective feedback noting strengths, weaknesses, sentences that are unclear or unnecessary, and missing ideas.

- Teach cognitive strategies for editing the mechanics of writing (spelling, grammar, capitalization, punctuation).
  - 🐾 *Assign editing one type of error at a time.*
  - Provide the elementary student with a visual proofreading strategy. Tape the strategy to the desk.

  Example for a first grade student:

  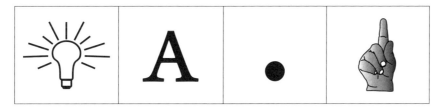

  Figure 19.7. Written Expression Editing Strip (15)

  - Light Bulb: Have I conveyed the whole idea (written it in a complete sentence)?
  - Capital A: Have I capitalized the appropriate letters?
  - Period: Have I punctuated correctly?
  - Pointing Finger: Have I put the appropriate spacing between words? (The width of a finger is usually sufficient for manuscript writing.)

  - Teach the student how to use cognitive strategies to edit ("police") mechanical errors.

    Example: **COPS** (16)

    (**C**) Capitalization   Title
    Beginning of each sentence
    Word "I"
    Proper names of people and places

    (**O**) Overall Appearance Neatness
    Legibility
    Spacing

    - 🐾 *If written on the computer, these factors usually become unimportant. (17) Substitute the following:*

      (**O**) Organization

Narrative	Expository
Beginning	Introduction
Middle	Paragraph(s) with Main Idea(s)/Details
End	Transitions
	Conclusion

      (**P**) Punctuation   End of each sentence
      Question/quotation marks
      Commas/colons/semicolons
      Apostrophes for contractions and possessives
      Periods after initials and abbreviations

      (**S**) Spelling

Section IV

- Provide a <u>proofreading checklist</u> for the student with strong visualization skills who has difficulty retrieving and holding in working memory the COPS strategy. (Appendix p. 391)

Proofreading Checklist

Did you <u>capitalize</u> the:

<u>Title</u>?	Yes	No
<u>First word</u> in each sentence?	Yes	No
Word "<u>I</u>"?	Yes	No
Proper <u>names</u> of people and places?	Yes	No

Did you put a <u>period</u> at the end of each sentence?	Yes	No
Did you put <u>question marks</u> at the end of each question?	Yes	No
Did you put <u>quotation marks</u> around people's words?	Yes	No
Did you put <u>commas</u> in a sequence of people, places, things?	Yes	No
Did you use <u>apostrophes</u> for contractions and possessives?	Yes	No
Did you check your <u>spelling</u>?	Yes	No
Did you use <u>complete sentences</u>?	Yes	No
Did you make the <u>subjects and verbs agree</u> with each other (singular/plural)?	Yes	No
Were the <u>verb tenses</u> consistent throughout the paper?	Yes	No
Could you <u>read</u> the essay aloud <u>without stumbling</u> over words?	Yes	No
Was your <u>handwriting legible</u>?	Yes	No
Did you provide enough <u>space between</u> the words?	Yes	No
Did you make the overall appearance of the <u>paper neat</u>?	Yes	No

** If you circled "No" to any of the above questions, correct that part before turning in your paper.

Figure 19.8. Proofreading Checklist – Checklist to assist with editing

- Permit the use of a computer word processing program to check spelling, punctuation, and syntax.

- Allow a personal editor (parent, teacher, or other adult) to offer revision and editing suggestions.

- Point out and discuss the type of errors that the student consistently makes (e.g., forgetting to punctuate, omitting words) to increase awareness when writing and editing.

Chapter 19

MEMORY PROBLEMS

Review interventions for Memory Problems in Chapter 14.

SHORT-TERM MEMORY PROBLEMS

Difficulty with Working Memory

Written expression requires the simultaneous integration of many cognitive skills and places a <u>heavy</u> demand on working memory. While maintaining ideas in short-term memory, the student must be able to shift back and forth between the tasks of remembering the text structure, selecting specific vocabulary words, spelling words correctly, utilizing age-appropriate grammar, and recalling capitalization and punctuation rules. An inability to fluently handle these tasks produces fatigue, frustration, and avoidance of writing.

The following behaviors serve as general indicators. The student will not exhibit every characteristic listed. These behaviors may also be indicative of other problems.

> Producing simplistic, concrete writing
> Having difficulty generating ideas to write
> Forgetting textual organization/sequence of ideas generated
> Repeating ideas previously stated
> Being unable to analyze different ideas to be used in writing
> Having difficulty retrieving specific vocabulary words to use
> Spelling words correctly on spelling tests, but having difficulty spelling accurately when writing
> Forgetting the rules of grammar
> Knowing capitalization and punctuation rules, but being unable to apply rules when writing
> Being able to express ideas orally, but having difficulty expressing thoughts in writing
> Including ideas vaguely related to the topic and inconsistent with intent/structure of the text

Research has demonstrated that inefficient working memory significantly impacts written expression. (18)

Interventions

- Remember that the capacity of working memory is affected by the <u>amount</u>, <u>type</u>, and <u>complexity</u> that written expression demands. (p. 36)

  ○ Reduce the amount of writing required.

  ○ Divide the writing assignment into its component parts (brainstorming, planning/organizing, writing first draft, revising/editing, rereading/writing final paper). Assign one segment for each writing lesson. (p. 212)

  ○ Focus on the generation of ideas on the first draft. Stress content and avoid requiring accurate spelling, punctuation, and grammar. Encourage the use of narrative and expository text structures and their corresponding graphic organizers to help maintain the flow of ideas.

  ○ Place the correct spelling of key words on the desk if the student frequently has to stop and think about the spelling of words.

  ○ Teach, encourage, and allow utilization of a <u>computer</u> with a good word processing program. Computer use circumvents not only the need to write quickly and legibly but the demand to maintain in working memory the sequence of ideas, spacing and organization of words on the page, proper spelling of words, recall of capitalization and punctuation rules, and monitoring and editing of errors.

Section IV

LONG-TERM MEMORY PROBLEMS

Difficulty Retrieving (Recalling)

The following behaviors serve as general indicators. The student will not exhibit every characteristic listed. These behaviors may also be indicative of other problems.

- Producing only a few factual ideas about a familiar topic
- Having difficulty accessing known vocabulary words to use
- Being unable to recall spelling/grammar/capitalization/punctuation rules
- Forgetting the skills needed to proofread and detect errors

Interventions

- Be aware that inefficient working memory makes the retrieval of information from long-term memory stores difficult.

    - Recognize that writing tasks that require the student to access information without the assistance of cues (bits of information) to stimulate recall are difficult for the student with retrieval problems.

    - Provide a template of the narrative or expository text structure and the steps needed to write the composition.

    - Recommend using a graphic organizer to aid recall of the information to be presented.

    - Provide a revision and proofreading checklist. (Appendix pp. 389–391)

- Allow and encourage the use of a spelling list with the basic sight vocabulary and frequently misspelled words. (Appendix p. 378)

- Stress content on the first draft and omit the requirement to access age-appropriate vocabulary words and accurate spelling, grammar, and capitalization and punctuation rules.

CHAPTER 20

MATH COMPUTATIONS

Difficulty with computational mathematics is the second most common academic problem associated with clinic-referred students with **ADHD**. Research suggests that approximately 20%-40% of students with **ADHD** (1, 2) compared to a 5%-14% of school age students (3, 4) have math learning disabilities (MLD). 5%-10% of students with **TS** (5, 6) meet MLD criteria. Problems are associated with a variety of deficits including impaired graphomotor (handwriting) skills, difficulty mastering math facts/procedures at an automatic level, slow speed of processing and performing calculations, difficulty using and sequencing cognitive strategies, inefficient and ineffective working memory, trouble quickly and consistently retrieving facts from long-term memory, making careless errors, and/or neglecting to edit and correct mistakes.

General Recommendations

Review Classroom and Individual Student Interventions in Chapters 8 and 9.

- Modify math assignments if the student has graphomotor impairment. (7)

    - *Many students with **ADHD**, **TS**, or **OCD** have neurologically-based graphomotor (handwriting) problems which may interfere with the ability to write legibly, align numbers and decimals, and space properly between problems. (p. 68) (8, 9, 10)*

  - Understand that the impulsivity associated with **ADHD** often results in rapid, unplanned writing that impacts the legibility of math papers.

  - Be flexible when **TS** hand or arm tics interfere with handwriting.

  - Remain sensitive to **OCD** compulsions to write and rewrite numbers or repeatedly erase until there is a hole in the paper.

  - Recognize that when handwriting is slow and laborious, the need to finish the work within a specified time frame affects both legibility and accuracy. Thus, it is essential to waive time limits on math assignments.

  - Reduce the number of math problems required on the work sheet, test, or homework assignment to a level which accommodates handwriting problems. For example, have the student complete every other problem, alternate rows, work selected problems, or finish half the assignment instead of the whole assignment.

  - Do not require the copying of math problems out of a book or off the board before answering them. This eliminates the excessive time, stress, and frustration produced by the copying task.

    - Always provide prepared or duplicated copies of the math assignment.

    - Obtain permission to photocopy or make enlargements of math book pages.

  - Avoid asking for math papers to be recopied. Muscle soreness and fatigue may cause handwriting to deteriorate and produce stress and inappropriate behavior.

Section IV

- Implement modifications if the student has trouble organizing math problems on a page and/or aligning and maintaining columns.
  - Reduce the number of problems on the page. Fold the paper into four or eight sections and place each problem in a separate section.
  - Suggest working on lined paper that has been rotated 90 degrees so the lines become columns.
  - Provide grid or graph paper with squares of the appropriate size to allow the student to write one numeral or sign in each box.
    - 🐾 *Art supply stores carry graph paper of varying sizes. Computer programs such as MS Excel can create appropriate sized graph paper to accommodate size of student's handwriting.*
  - Enlarge worksheets and tests to provide adequate space to work problems and line up digits.
  - Provide a cognitive cue card to prompt the student to space accurately between problems.
- Illustrate abstract concepts and procedures with concrete objects and real-life applications.
  - Provide many different kinds of manipulatives (blocks, beans, buttons, rods) to visually represent problems.
  - Use everyday situations to demonstrate concepts (e.g., cut 3 pizzas into 1/4, 1/6, and 1/8 pieces to show the size difference between 1/4, 1/6, and 1/8).
  - Suggest that the parents reinforce math concepts at home (e.g., cooking, earning an allowance, saving money to purchase a coveted item).
- Avoid teaching unnecessary concepts and rules that confuse the student and interfere with mastery of the concept being learned.
- Teach one skill at a time. Math is a sequential learning process. The student cannot progress to the next level until the current skill has been mastered.
  - 🐾 <u>*Mastery*</u> *is considered to be* <u>*nine out of ten*</u> *problems correct over an extended period of time.*
- Use graphic organizers to present operations visually. Suggest drawing operations and explaining them before solving problems.
- Ask the student to reteach an operation to a teacher, parent, or peer to ensure that the procedure has been understood.
- Create a <u>math folder</u> or notebook.
  - Provide the following:
    - addition and multiplication fact sheets. (Appendix pp. 392–393)
    - problem solving strategies.
    - examples of completed calculation problems.
  - Color coordinate the cover of the math book and math notebook.
  - Suggest referring to the notebook when the math facts or steps of the operations are forgotten.

Chapter 20

> **Tics/obsessions/compulsions, underarousal/slow processing speed, inattention/impulsivity/hyperactivity, executive dysfunction, and/or memory problems frequently interfere with ability to produce accurate math calculations.**

UNDEROUSAL/SLOW COGNITIVE PROCESSING SPEED

Review interventions for Underarousal and Slow Processing Speed in Chapter 10.

The following behaviors serve as general indicators. The student will not exhibit every characteristic listed. These behaviors may also be indicative of other problems.

- Performing math calculations slowly
- Being slow to learn/recall/retrieve math facts/operations
- Having difficulty sustaining focused attention on assignments
- Lacking persistence when completing seatwork
- Possessing age-appropriate math skills, but being unable to finish assignments/tests in allotted time

Processing speed impacts mastery of the basic number facts and procedures and, therefore, efficient and accurate calculations. (11, 12) Studies have shown that slow speed of processing tends to be associated with **ADHD, Inattentive type.** (13)

Interventions

- Check to make sure math facts have been mastered. When the math facts have not been automatized, the student performs more slowly and less accurately.

- Be aware that completing math assignments is very tiring and frustrating for the student who processes slowly.

- Evaluate the appropriateness of the math assignment and modify the length and requirements until the student can be successful.

- Permit the use of a calculator.

    - *Accuracy and fluency of the basic number facts are essential for the acquisition of higher level math skills. Calculators bypass difficulty learning the math facts at an automatic level and allow the student to focus on problem solving. The student still has to choose the numbers and operations that must be used.*

- Waive time limits or provide sufficient time for the math assignments to be completed.

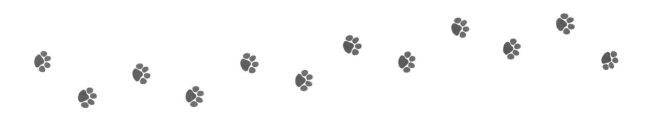

Section IV

INATTENTION/IMPULSIVITY/HYPERACTIVITY

Attention is fundamental to the acquisition of mathematical skills. (11, 14, 15) The student must be able to focus and sustain attention and return to the task after attentional shifts. Inattention interferes with the mastery of basic math facts and computational procedures.

The following behaviors serve as general indicators. The student will not exhibit every characteristic listed. These behaviors may also be indicative of other problems.

> Appearing to exert little effort
> Starting math assignment before learning directions/on the wrong page
> Being restless/distractible during math assignment
> Rushing impulsively through assignment/not stopping to use strategy
> Having difficulty concentrating long enough to complete problems
> Wanting to only do part of the classwork/homework
> Losing place/skipping steps in math procedures
> Misreading/failing to notice change in operational signs
> Omitting decimals/dollar and percentage signs from answers
> Needing reminders to persist on math assignment
> Having trouble performing mental calculations
> Having difficulty tracking math problems across page
> Overlooking spatial cues to assist in aligning numbers
> Making careless errors
> Being unable to finish math tests/homework
> Exhibiting variable performance from one day to the next
> Becoming frustrated/anxious/upset when encountering difficult problems

Students with **ADHD-Predominately Inattentive type** have an increased risk for impaired computational skills. (13)

Interventions

Review interventions for Inattention, Impulsivity, and Hyperactivity in Chapter 12.

- Modify the manner in which directions are delivered. (p. 99)

    🐾 *Understanding the <u>directions</u> is a prerequisite for completing math assignments correctly.*

- Always provide math assignments at the appropriate instructional level. (p. 64)

- Encourage the student to <u>read a problem aloud</u> before solving any mathematical operation. This will reduce the likelihood that visual details in the problem will be overlooked.

- Use a <u>highlighter</u> with visible ink to direct attention to calculation signs and slow impulsive work completion.

    ○ Color code signs when mixing operations (e.g., addition operation sign coded red, subtraction sign coded yellow). Use the same color on all math assignments.

    ○ Suggest tracing the operational sign with a highlighter before working the calculation.

- Recommend subvocalizing the steps of a problem while solving it.

- Provide a <u>completed example</u> of a math problem for use when teaching a new skill.

- Intervene if the student is having difficulty <u>tracking</u> math problems on the page. (7)
  - 🐾 **TS** *eye tics and head movements or the* **OCD** *need to reread, rewrite, and count numbers may cause tracking problems.*
  - Suggest using a finger to assist tracking.
  - Use graph paper.
  - Have a scribe write down the answers to the math problems.
  - Permit use of a computer if tracking problems do not interfere with its use.
- Design math assignments that result in a sense of accomplishment.
  - Give instructions that are clear and concise.
  - Reduce the number of problems and require accuracy.
  - Use several small groups of problems if more practice is needed.
  - Provide movement breaks between sets of problems.
- Diminish the stress and anxiety that is often associated with math.
  - Help the anxious student understand that the need to never make mistakes leads to excessive worry which interferes with the ability to perform well and causes one to stop trying.
  - Emphasize that mistakes are an important part of learning.
  - Confront negative cognitions ("I can't do these multiplication problems. They are too hard!"). Ask "What did you do the last time we had this type of problem? I recall that you worked every one of them correctly."
  - Encourage the use of positive self-statements ("I can do this! I tried hard the last time and was successful. I will work a few problems and check the answers.").
- Teach the student how to appropriately ask for help. (p. 126)

EXECUTIVE DYSFUNCTION

Review interventions for Executive Dysfunction in Chapter 13.

IMPAIRED PROBLEM SOLVING

- Provide a template of a problem solving strategy such as "**GET A CLUE**" or "**PLAN**" to assist with math calculations. Be sure the strategy includes steps for goal setting, planning (generating ideas, solutions; analyzing proposed ideas, solutions; prioritizing; organizing; sequencing; managing time), initiating, evaluating, and editing. (Appendix pp. 374–375)
- Model and demonstrate how to use <u>problem solving strategies</u>. (p. 108)

Section IV

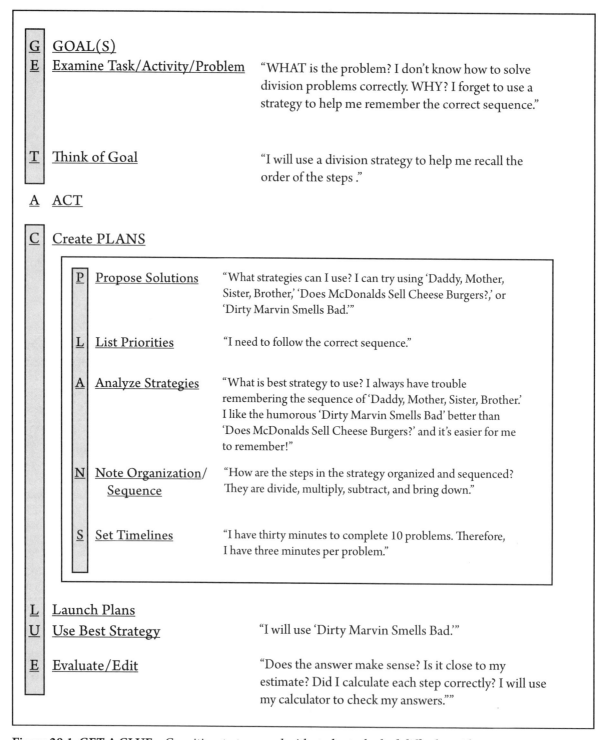

Figure 20.1. GET A CLUE – Cognitive strategy used with student who had difficulty with computation

Some students may not be able to follow the complexity of this strategy unless taught in incremental steps that must be mastered before continuing to the next step. Other students may need to learn a more simplified version "**PLAN**." If so, use "**GET A CLUE**" as a structure for discussing and teaching ways to solve tasks, activities, and problem situations.

P	Propose Goal	"I need to use a strategy to solve division problems correctly."
L	List and Analyze Strategies	"What strategies can I use? I might try: 'Daddy, Mother, Sister, Brother,' 'Does McDonalds Sell Cheese Burgers?,' or 'Dirty Marvin Smells Bad.' I always have trouble remembering the sequence of 'Daddy, Mother, Sister, Brother.' I like the humorous 'Dirty Marvin Smells Bad' better than 'Does McDonalds Sell Cheese Burgers?' and it's easier to remember!"
A	Apply Best Strategy	"I will use 'Dirty Marvin Smells Bad.'"
N	Notice Errors and Edit	"Does the answer make sense? Is it close to my estimate? Did I calculate each step correctly? I will use my calculator to check my answers."

Figure 20.2. PLAN – Cognitive strategy used with student who had difficulty with computation

Difficulty Setting Goals

The following behaviors serve as general indicators. The student will not exhibit every characteristic listed. These behaviors may also be indicative of other problems.

Being unaware of a problem with math calculation
Overlooking need to set goal to achieve mastery of math facts/procedures
Having difficulty thinking of strategies to carry out goal

Interventions

- Discuss the importance of mastering the math facts and procedures at an automatic level.
- Help the student self-evaluate mastery of the math facts and operations, identify strengths and weaknesses, and determine which skills need improvement.
- Teach, prompt, cue the student to stop and set goals.
- Provide assistance until goals can be set independently.

Difficulty Planning

Difficulty Proposing and Analyzing Ideas/Solutions/Strategies

The following behaviors serve as general indicators. The student will not exhibit every characteristic listed. These behaviors may also be indicative of other problems.

Lacking skills to generate/brainstorm solutions/strategies to solve math problems
Using trial-and-error approach to achieving goals
Needing help to analyze proposed strategy to carry out goal

Interventions

- Provide assistance in generating as many practical ideas as possible (e.g., choose strategy that can be easily recalled, use a math facts chart, use a cue card to help remember the sequence of steps in an operation).

Section IV

- Discuss both the positive and negative outcomes and consequences of each solution or strategy.
- Choose the best strategy.

Difficulty Prioritizing

The following behaviors serve as general indicators. The student will not exhibit every characteristic listed. These behaviors may also be indicative of other problems.

>Being annoyed at having to do math assignments
>Having trouble seeing reason to learn math facts and concepts
>Saying "Do I really need to do math when I grow up?"
>Missing the value of practice toward mastery
>Thinking practice work is boring/refusing to practice

Interventions

- Design problems that apply to mathematical procedures used in everyday situations (e.g., addition, subtraction, multiplication, and division operations are needed when shopping, saving enough money to buy a CD, going to a movie, or paying the bill when out on a date; fractions are required when cooking or filling the car with gas; percentages needed to compute sales tax or determine the cost of discounted items).

- Explain the meaning of the saying "No pain, no gain." In order to succeed, one has to do things that are considered frustrating and "BORING." Point out how others use math in their lives.

- Stress the advantages of learning math and its relationship to a good job.

- Demonstrate how math is a sequential process that builds on the mastery of previous steps (e.g., math is like building a tall sand castle – the first layer must be strongly built before the second layer can be added).

- Explain how automatic skills require no effort.

Difficulty Organizing/Sequencing

The following behaviors serve as general indicators. The student will not exhibit every characteristic listed. These behaviors may also be indicative of other problems.

>Appearing confused
>Becoming overwhelmed by large assignments
>Being unable to break down assignments into manageable steps
>Having trouble generating/using organizational strategies
>Using developmentally immature strategies (counting on fingers)
>Lacking skills to break down/order steps for completing multi-step problems
>Being unable to learn the sequence of the different operations
>Having trouble following steps needed to solve a math problem
>Working math problems in the wrong order
>Omitting part of a sequence
>Being unable to maintain conversion sequences
>Having difficulty working algebraic equations

Interventions

- Teach organizational and sequencing strategies to enhance mastery of the basic math facts and operations.

  - 🐾 *The student who has difficulty mastering the math facts learns more readily when taught organizational strategies which enhance learning. (16, 17)*

  - Make sure that the cognitive cue is meaningful to the student. For example, a common strategy used to remember the sequence of long division is, "Daddy, Mother, Sister, Brother" for divide, multiply, subtract, bring down. This strategy is more difficult for many students, especially those with sequencing problems, to recall than the humorous sentence, "Dirty Marvin Smells Bad." (p. 233) Suggest using the mnemonic "Kids Hate Doing Most Dirty Chores Mom" to cue the sequence "kilometer, hectometer, decameter, meter, decimeter, centimeter, millimeter" when teaching the conversion of one metric measure to the next.

  - Provide clear, explicit instructions. Point out <u>when</u> and <u>where</u> to use the strategy.

  - Model or demonstrate <u>how</u> to use the math strategy. Use an LCD projector with Power Point, an interactive whiteboard, or another multi-media aid. Describe the steps of the strategy.

  - Supply a cue card that indicates how to apply the strategy. The visual reminder lessens the demands placed on working memory.
    - Tape the cue card to the desktop or place inside the student's notebook as appropriate.
    - Discreetly touch the cue card to prompt its use.

  - Keep a sample of the strategy on the board.

  - Allow the student to quietly recite the strategy aloud while solving the math problem. Using self-directed speech will focus attention on the organization of the strategy.

  - Provide many practice lessons. Offer positive corrective feedback.

  - Encourage working independently without a visual cue when the strategy has been mastered.

  - Review and reteach the math strategy as needed.

  - Have the student add the strategy to the "trick" book or math notebook. (pp. 64, 222)

  - Remind the student to consult the book when a strategy that has previously been taught is forgotten.

- Determine whether <u>multi-step directions</u> are being followed correctly.

  - Be sure the math vocabulary words are understood before giving directions.

  - Give oral math instructions one step at a time. Say, "Take out your math book." (pause) "Turn to page 10." (pause) "Do the first problem."

- Have the student make and use a flow chart (map) of the steps of an operation and explain them before solving the problem.

Section IV

- Provide a list of the steps of the operation.
  - Color code the steps. For example, when calculating a multi-digit multiplication problem requiring regrouping (carrying), use a different color for each digit in the multiplier.

- Use concrete objects to help the student remember a sequence. For example, if the student is having difficulty remembering place value, demonstrate the ones place with pennies, the tens place with dimes, and the hundreds place with dollars.

- Provide sensory cues. Using the previous example, ask the student to put together 5 dollars, 8 dimes, and 6 pennies for 586 (use of visual and tactile cues).

- Ensure that a correct sequence is being followed before allowing classwork to proceed.

Difficulty Managing Time

The following behaviors serve as general indicators. The student will not exhibit every characteristic listed. These behaviors may also be indicative of other problems.

> Underestimating amount of time needed to complete math assignment ("My homework will only take 10 minutes!")
> Not scheduling enough time to think about/decide upon strategies for solving problems/completing classwork/checking for errors/correcting
> Starting assignment at last minute
> Needing extra time to finish assignment
> Becoming angry that there is not enough time to finish assignment/test

- Review interventions for Time Management. (pp. 119-121)

INFLEXIBILITY

The following behaviors serve as general indicators. The student will not exhibit every characteristic listed. These behaviors may also be indicative of other problems.

> Having difficulty alternating between math operations (addition to subtraction)
> Being able to calculate only one type of math problem at a time
> Continuing to use same approach to solving a problem when it repeatedly has produced mistakes
> Having trouble stopping/changing to a new activity (insisting on completing math assignment before engaging in different task)

Inflexibility interferes with problem solving that requires multiple steps or operations (e.g., multiplication problems that involve both multiplying and adding; division problems that require dividing, multiplying, subtracting). Difficulty in mentally changing to a new strategy, although the strategy being used has proven ineffective, impacts mathematical performance. (18)

Interventions

- Teach one procedure at a time until it has been mastered before providing worksheets with multiple operations.

- Have the student work the first two or three problems. Make sure the student is using the correct procedure.

- <u>Highlight</u> or color code calculation signs when mixing operations (e.g., addition operation sign coded red, subtraction sign coded yellow). Use the same color on all math assignments.

Chapter 20

INITIATION/EXECUTION DIFFICULTIES

The following behaviors serve as general indicators. The student will not exhibit every characteristic listed. These behaviors may also be indicative of other problems.

Appearing to lack energy/be uninterested in doing math assignment
Being slow to start/finish if assignment viewed as dull/tedious/"BORING"
Procrastinating/starting assignment at last minute
Needing reminders to begin/keep working

Interventions

- Work with the student until the first problem is completed.

- Teach the student how to appropriately ask for help. (p. 126)

- Positively reinforce task initiation.

IMPAIRED SELF-MONITORING/USE OF FEEDBACK/SELF-CORRECTION

The following behaviors serve as general indicators. The student will not exhibit every characteristic listed. These behaviors may also be indicative of other problems.

Being unaware of losing focus and concentration
Making careless errors
Being unable to calculate and edit at the same time
Omitting decimals/dollar and percentage signs in answers
Lacking skills to estimate/determine whether obtained answer is correct
Overlooking need to use strategies to check answers
Being unable to change problem-solving approach when answer is incorrect

Interventions

- Suggest working a problem and checking its accuracy. If the answer is incorrect, ask the student to explain how it was solved. The student frequently is able to identify the error.

- Reduce the number of problems to provide ample time for editing.

- Provide a cognitive cue card as a visual reminder to check the assignment. (Appendix p. 394)

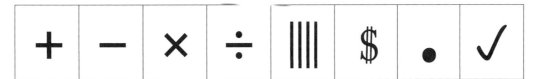

Figure 20.3. Math Editing Cue (19)

- <u>Operational signs</u>: check for correct operation (add, subtract, multiply, or divide).

- <u>Columns</u>: check for alignment of numbers into columns.

- <u>Dollar sign</u>: check for omission and appropriate placement.

- <u>Decimal point</u>: review placement and omissions.

- <u>Check mark</u>: check accuracy with a calculator.

Section IV

- Distinguish between lack of knowledge and editing errors before reteaching math concepts.
- Task analyze error patterns. Make modifications as needed. (20)

  🐾 *Calculation errors may be due to miscopying numbers, misaligning numbers in columns, and poorly spacing numbers on the page. However they more often result from poor mastery or retrieval of the math facts and operations.*

  o <u>Difficulty copying problems correctly</u>
    - Provide a work sheet.
    - Recopy problems for the student.
    - Obtain permission and make a photocopy enlargement of textbook page.
    - Reduce the number of problems on a page.
    - Recommend the use of a bookmark to maintain the place on the page.
    - Provide a "window" to reveal only one problem at a time.
    - Encourage verbal rehearsal (saying the number while copying it).

  o <u>Difficulty lining up and spacing numbers</u>
    - Use graph paper
    - Copy problems in a lattice.
    - Turn lined paper sideways.

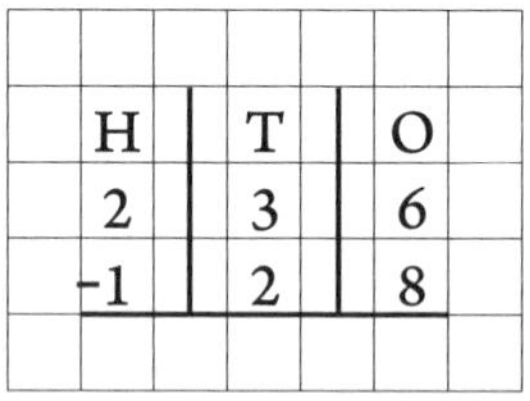

H	T	O
2	3	6
-1	2	8

Figure 20.4. Use of Graph Paper

  o <u>Difficulty using correct operational signs</u>
    - Color code signs.
    - Work one type of operation before changing to another.

  o <u>Difficulty mastering number facts</u>
    - Identify error patterns:

      Examples: Forgetting which facts?
      Missing answers by one number? (student may be counting)
      Wild guessing?
      Switching operations?

    - Teach strategies that are helpful for learning the facts. (21)

      Examples: When solving subtraction problems, count up from the smallest number to the largest number. (9 – 4 = ?) is 5, 6, 7, 8, 9 – the answer is 5.
      When multiplying by 9, the numbers in the answer always add up to 9 (e.g., 2 x 9 = 18, 3 x 9 = 27, 4 x 9 = 36).

    - Make a cue card that lists the student's most common errors.
    - Check facts orally using visual cue cards (e.g., flash cards).
    - Check procedure if knowledge of the facts is accurate and fluent.

- Difficulty regrouping (carrying) in addition/multiplication
    - Check understanding of place value and reteach if necessary.
    - Reteach procedure with manipulatives such as place value blocks.
    - Teach the student that an answer which is greater than 9 should be written at the side of the problem before deciding the appropriate number to carry.

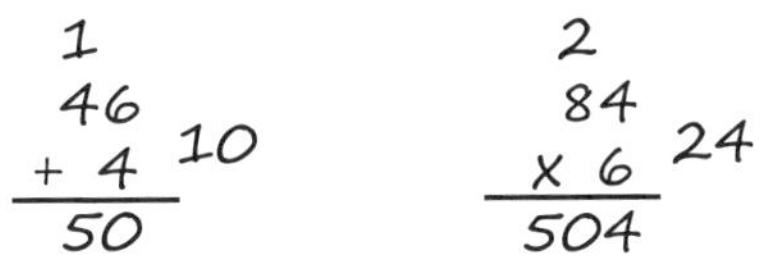

$$\begin{array}{r} 1 \\ 46 \\ +\ 4 \\ \hline 50 \end{array}\ 10 \qquad \begin{array}{r} 2 \\ 84 \\ \times\ 6 \\ \hline 504 \end{array}\ 24$$

Figure 20.5. Multiplication Carrying Strategy

For example, instead of saying, "Put down the 4 and carry the 2," say, "twenty-four." Have the student simultaneously write it and say it, starting with the tens place.

- Difficulty regrouping (borrowing) in subtraction
    - Check understanding of place value and reteach if necessary.
    - Play a game with $1, $10, and $100 bills. Appoint the student to be the banker. Make a withdrawal from the bank. Ask the student to make change. For example: If there is $356 in the bank account and a withdrawal of $137 is requested, the student will need to exchange a $10 bill for ten ones to make it possible. Encourage meaningful self-talk: "Is the big number on top? No, so I have to go next door and borrow a bundle of 10." Do NOT ask, "Can I take 7 from 6?" A student with sequencing problems may reverse the numbers.
    - Teach a cognitive strategy (e.g., the four **B**'s (**BBBB**) – **B**igger **B**ottom? **B**etter **B**orrow!) (21)
- Forgetting the sequence of division
    - Teach cognitive cues:

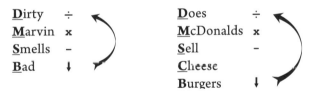

Figure 20.6. Long Division Cognitive Strategies (22) (source unknown)

The symbols are reminders to "**D**ivide, **M**ultiply, **S**ubtract, **B**ring down" or "**D**ivide, **M**ultiply, **S**ubtract, **C**heck, **B**ring down."

- Provide the student with a laminated cue card so that the steps can be checked off as they are completed. Use a pen or crayon that can be erased after the problem is solved. (Appendix p. 395)

Section IV

- ○ Difficulty keeping division problems aligned
  - Use graph paper.
  - Beginning at the greatest place value, have the student underline until reaching a number which can be divided and mark the place for the first number in the quotient:

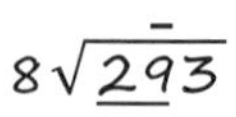

$$8\overline{)\underline{293}}^{\text{-}}$$

Figure 20.7. Alignment of Division Problem

Say, "8 cannot go into 2. But it can go into 29. So the first digit must go over the 9. Therefore, the quotient will have two digits, because beginning at the starting point which is 9, the quotient must have one digit over every following number in the dividend."

- Teach <u>estimation</u> by having the student round the numbers in problems to the closest whole value (e.g., 4723 + 2142 = ?; 5000 + 2000 = 7000). Ask the student to determine whether the answer seems reasonable.

- Provide immediate and specific feedback. Avoid waiting until all the problems have been solved to identify successes and errors.

  🐾 *Be sure to begin with a positive comment about the student's work, thinking process, or effort.*

- Teach strategies for checking answers. For example, to check a subtraction answer, have the student add the answer to the number being subtracted. To check a division answer, suggest multiplying the answer by the number being divided into the total.

- <u>Provide a self-editing checklist.</u> (Appendix p. 396)

Math Editing Checklist for Computations		
Did you <u>copy</u> the problem correctly?	Yes	No
Did you <u>line up and space</u> the numbers properly?	Yes	No
Did you <u>estimate</u> the answer?	Yes	No
Did you use the correct <u>operation</u>?	Yes	No
Did you remember the <u>math facts</u> correctly?	Yes	No
Did you miss the answer by one number?	Yes	No
Did you guess at the answer?	Yes	No
Did you regroup (<u>carry</u>) in addition/multiplication problems?	Yes	No
Was the answer more than 9?	Yes	No
Did you regroup (<u>borrow</u>) in subtraction problems?	Yes	No
Was the top number smaller than the bottom number?	Yes	No
Did you remember the <u>sequence of division</u> problems correctly?	Yes	No
Did you keep the division problems lined up correctly?	Yes	No
Is your <u>handwriting legible</u>?	Yes	No
** If you circled "No" to any of the above questions, correct that part before turning in your paper.		

Figure 20.8. Math Editing Checklist for Computation

- Permit the use of a calculator to check the accuracy of the answers as each individual problem is completed. If the answer is incorrect, point out the type of error and request that the problem be reworked.

- Suggest using a personal editor (teacher, parent, peer) to locate errors. A positive way to signal errors is to mark the problems that are <u>correct</u>. Ask the student to rework those that are not marked.

MEMORY PROBLEMS

Review interventions for Memory Problems in Chapter 14.

SHORT-TERM MEMORY PROBLEMS

Difficulty with Working Memory

Computation places high demands on working memory. The student must be able to hold in mind the type of problem to be solved while selecting a strategy to use, following the steps of the strategy, recalling relevant math facts, and executing the operation.

The following behaviors serve as general indicators. The student will not exhibit every characteristic listed. These behaviors may also be indicative of other problems.

> Rushing through assignments in order to not forget what one is doing
> Computing mental arithmetic problems incorrectly
> Having trouble recalling facts while calculating
> Losing place in middle of math problem due to difficulty remembering correct procedure
>   (carrying/borrowing/multiplying/dividing/using algebraic formula)
> Becoming overwhelmed when task has several parts or steps
> Being unable to remember math problems when copying from board or book

Research indicates that students with deficient math skills often have working memory problems. (18, 23, 24) When the basic number facts have not been mastered at an automatic level, the amount of mental workspace available for problem solving is reduced. (p. 36)

Interventions

- Increase <u>automaticity</u> of math facts so that fewer demands are placed on the processing space.

- Intervene if the student is having difficulty remembering how to perform an operation.

    Suggest that the student:

    - use a flow chart (map) of the operation.

    - use a cognitive or visual cue card.

    - color code the steps of operations before solving them. Use the same colors in the same sequence each time a procedure is followed.

    - subvocalize the steps of the procedure.

- Encourage and allow the use of a calculator if the student is slow accessing facts while solving problems.

Section IV

- Be aware that working memory problems result not only from trouble maintaining several pieces of information in the mind during processing (following steps of a math operation) but also from difficulty automatically <u>retrieving</u> information from long-term memory (recalling math facts/procedures) to use during processing.

LONG-TERM MEMORY PROBLEMS

Difficulty Encoding/Consolidating (Learning)

The following behaviors serve as general indicators. The student will not exhibit every characteristic listed. These behaviors may also be indicative of other problems.

> Having difficulty mastering math facts/procedures
> Using rote memory rather than strategies to learn facts/operations
> Using a slow, inefficient counting strategy (fingers)
> Having trouble recalling strategies to assist learning
> Learning new math skill one day and forgetting it the next day
> Requiring repeated reteaching of facts/procedures

Research indicates that students with **ADHD** often have difficulty mastering the basic number facts at an automatic level. (25)

Interventions

- Discourage rote memorization of the math facts.

    - 🐾 *Rote memorization of information is difficult for many students. Memorizing abstract, inherently boring and uninteresting material such as math facts and procedures requires sustained attention and intact sequential and working memory. Students who use rote memory to encode information may not be able to master the facts, apply concepts, or retrieve the materials efficiently.*

- Systematically introduce and repeat new math facts and concepts so that errors are <u>minimized</u>. "Errorless learning" has been found to be more effective than "trial-and-error" learning. (26, 27) Preventing errors during the learning process and practice sessions will keep the student from repeating and, thereby, encoding incorrect information.

    - 🐾 *Students with **ADHD** often do not learn from their mistakes due to inattention and inefficient working memory. Those with **OCD** may have difficulty unlearning errors that have become "stuck" in their minds.*

    - Avoid using a trial-and-error approach if the student has difficulty remembering and learning math facts and procedures from mistakes and feedback.

    - Teach concepts at a concrete level before introducing abstract ones.

    - Use prompts to ensure correct responding. Gradually remove cues as the information is mastered.

        - Give correct answers until the facts or operations have been learned.
        - Demonstrate a step or operation and ask the student to imitate it until it can be completed without modeling.
        - Provide a cue card listing the steps of an operation.

- Do not expect mastery immediately after introducing new material. (7)
  - Provide adequate repetition and review to ensure overlearning and mastery. Repetition is necessary to overcome the effects of forgetting.
  - Offer numerous opportunities to verbalize and/or demonstrate recently acquired skills.
  - Require mastery before moving on to the next skill.
    - 🐾 *Mastery is defined as knowing the information <u>90</u> percent of the time over an extended period.*
- Request a demonstration or explanation of new concepts and procedures.
- Use "backward chaining" (source unknown) to imprint math facts and teach multi-step skills. Initially, show the entire math fact or the steps in a math operation. Remove the last part of the sequence and ask the student to recall it. Delete one cue at each successive lesson. (7)
  - 🐾 *Gradual removal of cues reduces the chance for errors.*

  Example: If the student is having difficulty learning "7 X 9 = 63," write the problem on a board, in shaving cream spread on a Formica surface or desktop, on a white board with a dry erase marker, on a transparency with an overhead marker, or on a window with an erasable marker. Erase the last digit. Have the student write the "3" and say the whole problem. When the student is successful, erase the last two digits. Have the student rewrite the "63" and say the problem. Have the student say the problem during each step. Once mastered, recheck each week.

- Stimulate learning in the encoding phase. The student with **ADHD** frequently considers finishing math papers, completing workbook pages, and copying and solving problems from the board as "boring" tasks.
  - Ask the student to demonstrate a concept with the use of manipulatives (e.g., 5 X 5 = 25: five stacks with five wooden cubes each = 25 cubes).
  - Use flash cards to assist with the memorization of math facts and operations. Flash cards combine both auditory and visual modalities.
  - Increase understanding of math operations by having the student draw pictures or diagrams.
  - Suggest creating problems to be solved by other students.
  - Encourage use of computer programs to reinforce and consolidate math facts. Games provide drill and immediate reinforcement without being "BORING."
  - Play number games with cards.

- Use strategies to facilitate the acquisition of the basic number facts.
  - 🐾 *The student who uses strategies is able to solve problems more accurately and efficiently. (16, 17)*
  - Combine as many different sensory modalities as possible (verbal, visual, motor, tactile).
  - Encourage the use of manipulatives.
  - Build on known facts (if 5 + 5 = 10, add 1; therefore, 5 + 6 = 11).
  - Use a vertical number line.
  - Recommend visualizing math facts with the answers.

Section IV

- - Relate subtraction and division facts to appropriate addition and multiplication facts (e.g., To solve 15 – 9 = ?, ask what number added to 9 is 15? To solve 45 ÷ 9 = __, ask what number times 9 equals 45?).
  - Provide addition and multiplication facts charts. (Appendix pp. 392–393)
- Practice and review several math facts each day throughout the school year.
- Do not drill math facts for speed. Timed tests are stressful.
- Assist the encoding of <u>computational procedures</u>.
  - Demonstrate meaning with concrete materials and manipulatives.
  - Design problems that apply to everyday situations (e.g., making change, renting videos, purchasing tickets to sporting or musical events, measuring when cooking, paying at a toll booth).
  - Combine as many sensory modalities as possible (verbal, visual, motor, tactile).
  - Teach cognitive strategies that enhance encoding.
  - Encourage the verbalization of the steps of a math operation.
    - Suggest explaining the process to a classmate who needs assistance.
    - Tape record the student describing the steps of a math operation. Play back the tape before allowing the student to solve the problem.
  - Suggest drawing a picture or diagram of the problem.
  - Have the student make up problems related to concepts being learned.
  - Do not permit poor mastery of facts to delay or hamper success with math concepts and applications. Recommend using a calculator.

Difficulty Retrieving (Recalling)

Mastery of basic math skills is achieved when all of the facts and operations can be quickly and efficiently retrieved from long-term memory without errors. Automatic retrieval facilitates the acquisition of more complex skills.

The following behaviors serve as general indicators. The student will not exhibit every characteristic listed. These behaviors may also be indicative of other problems.

Being unable to quickly recall math facts/operations accurately
Completing math assignments slowly
Understanding/learning concepts when individually taught, but unable to recall them when calculating
Forgetting math facts/procedures learned yesterday
Making what appear to be "careless errors" that are actually retrieval errors
Forgetting cognitive strategies that assist retrieval
Needing frequent reteaching of rules/procedures

Interventions

- Determine whether an inability to solve a math problem is due to difficulty mastering the math facts or lack of understanding of the computational procedure.
- Provide extra time if the student is slow retrieving math facts.

- Encourage and allow the use of cognitive cue cards when completing assignments and taking tests.

- Permit use of a calculator.

- Suggest consulting computational procedures and work samples that were placed in the strategy ("trick") book. (p. 64)

- Recommend reviewing cognitive strategies just before completing an assignment or taking a test to enhance retrieval. Suggest writing them on the back of the assignment or test paper before working the first problem.

CHAPTER 21

MATH REASONING

Learning problems in the area of math reasoning are not as common for students with **ADHD** as those in math calculation. However, mastery and automatic retrieval of the basic number facts and understanding of the procedural aspects of computation are fundamental to higher level math skills and impact the ability to solve math word problems.

 Math reasoning includes conceptual understanding of time, money, measurement, estimation, data interpretation, algebra, geometry, etc. The recommendations in this section of the handbook are limited to skills needed to solve word problems.

The ability to solve word problems requires intact attention, executive functions, and memory. Furthermore, reading and language skills, reasoning, nonverbal problem solving skills, and speed of processing affect competence. (1)

General Recommendations

Review Classroom and Individual Student Interventions in Chapters 8 and 9.

- Evaluate not only attention, executive functions, and memory but also the individual components of word problems: reading level, math vocabulary, type of problem (concrete/abstract), placement of the question (beginning, middle, end), amount of relevant and irrelevant details and numbers, difficulty of the calculation (single or multiple operations), speed and accuracy needed for calculation, and mathematical concepts (money, measurement, distance, time).

- Actively engage the student in mathematical problem solving rather than passively assigning a problem and then monitoring its completion.
  - Incorporate novel and interesting instructional activities.
  - Personalize problems with student's name.
  - Suggest solving problems with another student.

- Construct word problems that are neither too abstract nor hypothetical.
  - Design problems relating to real-life situations.
  - Use concrete objects to illustrate abstract concepts and procedures.
    - Provide many different kinds of manipulatives (blocks, beans, buttons, rods) to help the student visualize problems.
    - Use pictures to illustrate the problem presented.

- Avoid teaching unnecessary concepts and rules that interfere with mastery of the concept being learned.

- Teach the meaning of math cue words (e.g., "more," "fewer," "all together," "in addition to," "total," "sum," "greater than," "less than," "how many," "difference").
  - Prepare a list of the cue words, their corresponding meanings, and calculation signs. (Appendix p. 397).

241

Section IV

- Check to make sure the student knows how to perform a calculation before assigning word problems requiring the operation.

- Construct one-step word problems. When mastered, gradually present more complex problems involving multiple operations.

- Ask the student to read a word problem without having to actually work the problem and explain which operations will be needed.

- Permit the use of calculators. Calculators bypass computational deficits and improve the ability to focus on the numbers and operations that should be used.

- Add the following to the math folder or notebook: (p. 222)
  - list of math cue words with their corresponding symbols. (Appendix p. 397)
  - word problem solving strategy. (Appendix p. 398)
  - examples of completed word problems.

- Suggest referring to the notebook when the basic facts, steps of an operation, or word problem solving strategies are forgotten.

- Recommend individualized remedial instruction in mathematics from an educational specialist as needed.

- Stress acquisition of functional math skills for the student with a serious math learning disability (e.g., basic arithmetic skills, fractions, decimals, percent, money, measurement, time).

> Tics/obsessions/compulsions, underarousal/slow processing speed, inattention/impulsivity/hyperactivity, executive dysfunction, and/or memory problems frequently interfere with math reasoning and the ability to solve word problems.

UNDERAROUSAL/SLOW COGNITIVE PROCESSING SPEED

Review interventions for Underarousal and Slow Processing Speed in Chapter 10.

The following behaviors serve as general indicators. The student will not exhibit every characteristic listed. These behaviors may also be indicative of other problems.

Solving word problems slowly
Being slow to recall math facts/operations
Having difficulty sustaining focused attention on assignment
Lacking persistence when completing seatwork
Possessing age-appropriate math skills, but being unable to finish assignments and tests in allotted time

Chapter 21

Research indicates that students with **ADHD** often have a slower computational speed which compromises the ability to solve word problems quickly and accurately. (2, 3) Slow speed of processing is associated with inattentive behaviors and is prominent among students with **ADHD, Inattentive type.** (4)

- Check to make sure the basic math facts have been mastered. When the number facts have not been automatized, the student will be unable to solve word problems quickly and accurately.

- Evaluate the length and requirements of the assignments. Modify them until the student can be successful.

- Eliminate time limits or provide ample time for the problems to be completed.

INATTENTION/IMPULSIVITY/HYPERACTIVITY

Review interventions for Inattention, Impulsivity, and Hyperactivity in Chapter 12.

The following behaviors serve as general indicators. The student will not exhibit every characteristic listed. These behaviors may also be indicative of other problems.

Being off-task
Daydreaming/looking around/staring into space
Being bored/lacking interest in solving word problems
Needing constant redirection
Starting math assignment without listening to directions
Rushing impulsively through math assignment
Being too impulsive to stop and use known strategy
Misunderstanding question being asked
Overlooking details
Mixing up details while solving problems
Having difficulty tracking words
Being unable to perform mental calculations
Losing place in middle of math procedures
Having trouble attending to lengthy word problems
Skipping math problems/parts of problems
Lacking ability to solve problems independently
Making copying errors
Missing mistakes
Exhibiting inconsistencies when solving word problems (answering first few problems correctly, missing one or two, then solving a few more correctly; correctly answering more difficult problems, then missing easier ones)
Becoming frustrated/anxious/upset when encountering difficult problems

Inattention and off-task behaviors compromise the ability to efficiently solve word problems. (1, 4)

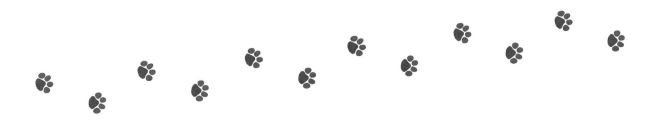

Section IV

Interventions

- Design math assignments for success.
- Direct attention to important details.

  Suggest that the student:

  - use <u>highlighters</u> with visible ink to color code words indicating different operations when the problem requires mixed operations (e.g., addition words coded red, subtraction words coded yellow). Use the same colors on all math problems.
  - underline or circle cue words with colored pencils or markers.

- Suggest <u>reading the word problem</u> aloud before solving it.
- This will focus attention and increase the likelihood that important details are identified.
- Provide a completed example of a math problem for use when teaching a new skill.
- Ask the student to <u>subvocalize</u> the steps of the problem while solving it to reduce impulsivity.
- Intervene if the student is having difficulty <u>tracking</u> (5)(e.g., losing place, skipping lines, and omitting or repeating words when reading problem aloud). (p. 169)

  - Suggest using finger to track.
  - Offer a bookmark, ruler, paper strip, or index card to remain on the line.

- Provide feedback after several problems are completed. Mark only problems that are correct.
- Diminish the stress and anxiety associated with math. (pp. 79–81)
- Teach the student how to appropriately <u>ask for help</u>. (p. 126)

EXECUTIVE DYSFUNCTION

Review interventions for Executive Dysfunction in Chapter 13.

IMPAIRED PROBLEM SOLVING

- Provide a template of a <u>problem solving strategy</u> such as "**GET A CLUE**" or "**PLAN**" to use when faced with complex word problems to be solved. Be sure the strategy includes steps for goal setting, planning (generating ideas, solutions; analyzing proposed ideas, solutions; prioritizing; organizing; sequencing; managing time), initiating, evaluating, and editing. (Appendix pp. 374–375)
- Model and demonstrate how to use <u>problem solving strategies</u>. (p. 108)

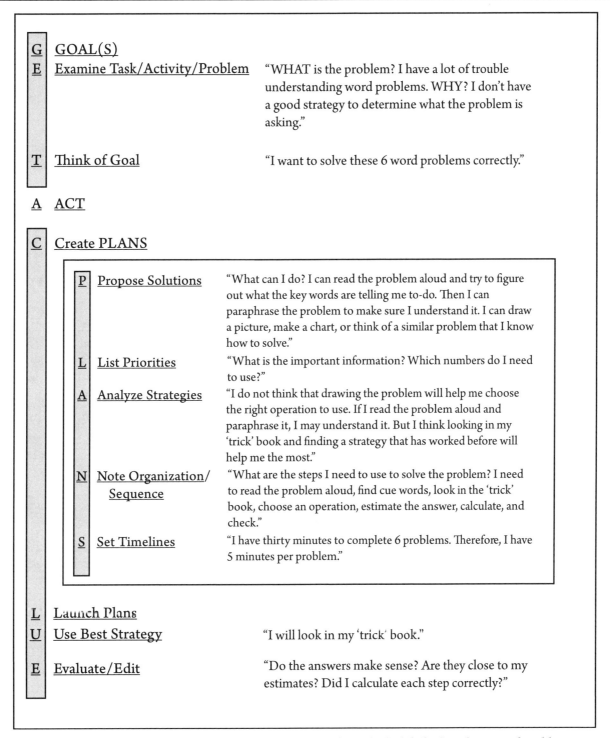

Figure 21.1. GET A CLUE – Cognitive strategy used with student who had difficulty solving word problems

Some students may not be able to follow the complexity of this strategy unless taught in incremental steps that must be mastered before continuing to the next step. Other students may need to learn a more simplified version "**PLAN**." If so, use "**GET A CLUE**" as a structure for discussing and teaching ways to solve tasks, activities, and problem situations.

Section IV

P	<u>Propose Goal</u>	"I need to solve 6 word problems correctly."
L	<u>List and Analyze Strategies</u>	"What can I do? I can read the problem aloud and try to figure out what the key words are telling me to do. Then I can paraphrase the problem to make sure I understand it. I can draw a picture, make a chart, or look in my 'trick' book for a similar problem. I do not think that drawing the problem will help me choose the right operation to use. If I read the problem aloud and try to paraphrase it, I may understand it."
A	<u>Apply Best Strategy</u>	"I will look in my 'trick' book and find a strategy that helped me with this type of problem."
N	<u>Notice Errors and Edit</u>	"Does the answer make sense? Is it close to my estimate? Did I calculate each step correctly? I will use my calculator to check my answers."

Figure 21.2. PLAN – Cognitive strategy used with student who had difficulty solving word problems

Difficulty Setting Goals

The following behaviors serve as general indicators. The student will not exhibit every characteristic listed. These behaviors may also be indicative of other problems.

Being unaware that there is a problem that needs to be solved
Overlooking need to set goal to better understand/solve word problems

Interventions

- Discuss skills required to solve word problems.
- Help the student self-evaluate mastery of those skills, identify strengths and weaknesses, and determine which ones need improvement.
- Teach, prompt, and cue the student to stop and set goals.
- Provide assistance until goals can be set independently.

Difficulty Planning

Difficulty Proposing and Analyzing Ideas/Solutions/Strategies

The following behaviors serve as general indicators. The student will not exhibit every characteristic listed. These behaviors may also be indicative of other problems.

Lacking skills to generate/brainstorm ideas/solutions/strategies for solving word problems
Using trial-and-error approach to problem solving
Having trouble identifying the what, when, where, how, and why of the problem
Needing help to analyze proposed strategy to carry out goal

Interventions

- Provide assistance in generating as many practical ideas as possible (e.g., determine meaning of cue words, paraphrase problem and question, draw a picture).

- Discuss both the positive and negative outcomes and consequences of each idea.

- Choose the best strategy.

Difficulty Prioritizing

The following behaviors serve as general indicators. The student will not exhibit every characteristic listed. These behaviors may also be indicative of other problems.

> Having difficulty deciding what is the most relevant information
> Focusing on less important information details

Students with **ADHD-I** are able to solve problems that present essential information but have difficulty when the problem includes nonessential information. Attending to irrelevant words and numbers results in procedural errors. (3, 6)

Interventions

- Introduce word problems containing irrelevant information after the student has mastered those containing only relevant details.

- Teach strategies that help the student discriminate between relevant and irrelevant information.

    Suggest that the student:

    ○ highlight, underline, or circle cue words and important numbers.

    ○ cross out nonessential details.

    ○ illustrate important information with a picture or diagram.

    ○ paraphrase the problem and question being asked. Include relevant key words and numbers.

Difficulty Organizing/Sequencing

The following behaviors serve as general indicators. The student will not exhibit every characteristic listed. These behaviors may also be indicative of other problems.

> Appearing confused
> Having trouble generating organized approach for solving word problems
> Lacking the skills to order the steps for solving word problems
> Skipping steps in the sequence of an operation
> Using all of steps of a procedure but in the incorrect order
> Being unable to maintain conversion sequences

Section IV

Interventions

- Teach an organized, step-by-step strategy for solving word problems.

    - *The strategy must include steps for understanding the word problems, developing plans to solve the problems, and generating the correct solutions.*

    Ask the student to "**READY THE PLANE for MATH'S FOUR C's.**"

    READY

    - <u>Read</u> problem aloud to focus attention on what is being asked and to ensure that no information is overlooked.
    - <u>Examine cue words</u> and key phrases.
    - <u>Ask the question</u> using different words.
    - <u>Draw</u> a picture, diagram, flow chart, or table.
    - **<u>You</u> are ready for take-off**.

    PLANE

    - <u>Propose</u> (brainstorm) possible solutions.
    - <u>Locate important</u> information and cross out irrelevant information.
    - <u>Analyze</u> advantages and disadvantages of proposed solutions.
    - <u>Name</u> the operation(s) to use.
    - <u>Estimate</u> answer.

    FOUR C's

    - <u>Calculate</u>.
    - <u>Compare</u> with estimate.
    - <u>Check</u> answer.
    - <u>Correct</u>, if necessary.

- Supply a cue card that indicates how to apply the strategy. The visual reminder will minimize the demands placed on working memory to remember it. (Appendix p. 398)

    - Have the strategy added to the "trick" book (p. 64) and math notebook. (p. 222)
    - Remind the student to consult the book when the strategy cannot be recalled

- Teach <u>self-questioning</u> as a means of guiding understanding and processing of word problems.
    - Explain self-questioning and how it helps solve word problems.
    - Model and demonstrate how to use self-questioning.
    - Help the student generate questions such as:
        - Have I <u>read</u> all of the words in the problem?
        - What are the <u>cue words</u>? What are they telling me to do?
        - What is the <u>question</u> being asked? What am I looking for?
        - Can I <u>draw</u> a picture/diagram/flow chart to illustrate the problem?
        - Which <u>operation</u>(s) can I use to answer the question?
        - What are the <u>advantages</u> and <u>disadvantages</u> of each procedure?
        - What is the <u>best solution</u>?
    - Prepare a list of the student's self-generated questions to serve as a guide to the cognitive processing of word problems.
    - Provide practice lessons for the use of the questions.
    - Place a list of the questions in the student's strategy ("trick") book or math notebook. Suggest referring to the list when the questions are not recalled.

Difficulty Managing Time

The following behaviors serve as general indicators. The student will not exhibit every characteristic listed. These behaviors may also be indicative of other problems.

Underestimating amount of time needed to complete assignment ("My math assignment will only take 10 minutes!" when actually it should take 30 minutes)
Not scheduling enough time to think about/decide upon strategies for solving problems/ completing classwork/checking for errors/self-correcting
Starting math assignments at last minute
Needing extra time to finish assignment
Becoming angry when there is not enough time to finish assignments/tests

- Review interventions for Time Management. (pp. 119-121)

INFLEXIBILITY

The following behaviors serve as general indicators. The student will not exhibit every characteristic listed. These behaviors may also be indicative of other problems.

Being able to calculate only one type of word problem at a time
Having difficulty switching between math operations (e.g., addition to subtraction) when problems require mixed operations
Continuing to use same approach to solving a word problem when it repeatedly has produced mistakes
Having trouble stopping and changing to new activity (insisting on completing math assignment before engaging in different task)

Difficulty mentally switching to a new strategy when the strategy being used has proven ineffective impacts mathematical performance and interferes with the student's ability to solve problems that require multiple operations or steps. (7)

Section IV

Interventions

- Assign word problems requiring only one type of operation. Wait until it has been mastered before providing problems that combine different operations.

- Have the student work the first two or three problems. Make sure the problems are understood and the correct procedures are being followed.

INITIATION/EXECUTION DIFFICULTIES

The following behaviors serve as general indicators. The student will not exhibit every characteristic listed. These behaviors may also be indicative of other problems.

> Appearing to lack energy/be uninterested in doing math assignment
> Being slow to get started/to finish if assignment viewed as dull/tedious/"BORING"
> Procrastinating/starting assignment at last minute
> Needing reminders to begin/complete working

Interventions

- Determine performance capability. Often the teacher is unaware that the student is not willing to admit that the math assignment is too difficult. This is particularly evident in middle and high school classes that demand independent work.

- Work with the student until one or two problems are completed.

- Teach the student how to appropriately <u>ask for help</u>. (p. 126)

IMPAIRED SELF-MONITORING/USE OF FEEDBACK/SELF-CORRECTION

The following behaviors serve as general indicators. The student will not exhibit every characteristic listed. These behaviors may also be indicative of other problems.

> Being unaware of losing focus and concentration
> Making careless errors
> Being unable to calculate and edit at the same time
> Omitting decimals/dollar and percentage signs in answers
> Overlooking need to stop and use strategies to check answers
> Lacking skills to estimate and know when answer might be incorrect
> Using same problem-solving approach even when answer is incorrect

Interventions

- Reduce the number of problems to provide ample time for editing.

- Suggest estimating the answer (e.g., rounding the numbers in the problem to the closest whole value (e.g., $4723 + 2142 = ? \rightarrow 5000 + 2000 = 7000$)) and comparing the estimate to the answer.

- Have the student work the first problem and check its accuracy. If the problem is incorrect, ask the student to explain how it was solved. The student is often able to identify the steps used to arrive at the answer and self-correct.

- Provide the student with visual strengths a template of "**READY THE PLANE for MATH'S FOUR C's**" as a visual reminder to check the completion of each step of the strategy. (Appendix p. 398)

- Furnish the student with verbal strengths a self-editing checklist. (Appendix p. 399)

Math Editing Checklist for Word Problems

Did you <u>read</u> the problem aloud?	Yes No
Did you locate the <u>cue words</u>?	Yes No
Did you ask for <u>unknown words</u> to be explained?	Yes No
Did you <u>paraphrase</u> the problem/question?	Yes No
Did you locate the <u>relevant</u> information?	Yes No
Did you cross out the <u>irrelevant</u> information?	Yes No
Did you make a <u>drawing</u>, diagram, or chart?	Yes No
Did you decide on the <u>correct operation(s)</u>?	Yes No
Did you <u>estimate</u> the answer?	Yes No
Did you <u>calculate</u> the answer?	Yes No
Did you <u>compare</u> the answer with the estimate?	Yes No
Did you <u>reread</u> the problem?	Yes No
Did you <u>check</u> the answer?	Yes No
Did you <u>correct</u> the answer when needed?	Yes No
Is your <u>handwriting legible</u>?	Yes No

** If you circled "No" to any of the above questions, correct that part before turning in your paper.

Figure 21.3 Math Editing Checklist for Word Problems

- Record and task analyze all of the student's errors. Provide immediate feedback with the student regarding both successes and errors.

- Distinguish between difficulty understanding the problem and editing errors before reteaching procedures for solving word problems.

- Provide a <u>calculator</u> for the student to check the accuracy of the answer as each problem is completed. If the answer is incorrect, ask the student to reread the problem, determine if the appropriate operation(s) was used, and rework the problem.

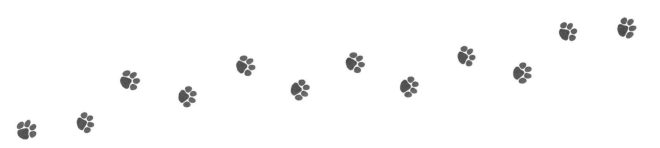

Section IV

MEMORY PROBLEMS

Review interventions for Memory Problems in Chapter 14.

SHORT-TERM MEMORY PROBLEMS

Difficulty with Working Memory

Students must hold "online" the question to be answered and numbers presented, while at the same time ignore irrelevant information, determine the appropriate procedure(s), retrieve number facts and steps of the operation(s), and compute the answer. If any of these tasks have not been mastered, the capacity of the cognitive processing space is compromised. (p. 36)

The following behaviors serve as general indicators. The student will not exhibit every characteristic listed. These behaviors may also be indicative of other problems.

- Using trial-and-error approaches when solving math problems rather than strategies
- Rushing through assignments in order to not forget what one is doing
- Allowing irrelevant information to enter processing
- Making errors when computing mentally
- Being unable to recall facts from long-term memory while trying to solve word problems
- Exhibiting procedural errors
- Losing place in the middle of a math problem due to difficulty remembering the correct procedure (carrying, borrowing, multiplying, dividing, using algebraic formula)
- Having difficulty recalling steps of operations while solving problems
- Becoming overwhelmed when the task has several parts or steps

Students who have difficulty solving word problems often have working memory problems. (8, 9)

Interventions

- Remember that the capacity of working memory is affected by the <u>amount</u>, <u>type</u>, and <u>complexity</u> of the information that must be processed simultaneously. (p. 36)
    - Distribute periods demanding extended concentration so that the student is not required to hold in working memory a large amount of information. Schedule several short sessions with breaks between tasks rather than scheduling one long session.
    - Extend time limits.
    - Limit the number of word problems that must be solved.
    - Avoid lengthy sentences with complex structure.
    - Omit nonessential information.
    - Include specific math cue words.
    - Place the question to be answered at the end of the problem.
- Increase amount and complexity as success is achieved.
- Provide a visual cue card indicating how to apply a strategy. The visual reminder reduces the demands placed on working memory. The cue card might be taped to the desk or placed in the math notebook as a reminder to use the strategy.

Chapter 21

- Implement modifications when the student is having difficulty remembering the correct procedures.

    Suggest that the student:

    o subvocalize the steps of the procedures.

    o make a flow chart ("map") of the operations.

    o color code the steps of the operations. Use the same colors in the same sequence each time procedures are performed.

    o use cognitive or visual cues to remember calculation sequences.

- Encourage and allow the use of a <u>calculator</u> if the student is having difficulty retrieving facts from long-term memory while solving problems. The calculator will free up workspace and permit the student to allocate more capacity to the processing of word problems.

LONG-TERM MEMORY PROBLEMS

Difficulty Encoding/Consolidating (Learning)

The following behaviors serve as general indicators. The student will not exhibit every characteristic listed. These behaviors may also be indicative of other problems.

Having difficulty learning abstract math vocabulary
Using math vocabulary words incorrectly
Forgetting procedures for solving word problems
Having trouble encoding and remembering abstract concepts

Interventions

- Create auditory, visual, motor, and/or tactile cues to help encode the meaning of abstract math concepts.

    o Greater Than/Less Than (5)

    The abstract math concepts of "greater than" and "less than" are sometimes difficult for the student to learn. If the student is having difficulty learning these concepts, use "higher than" and "lower than." Have two students stand on numbered stairs, starting with zero on the landing. The students can visually observe that the student standing on step 9 is "higher" than the student standing on step 1. Conversely, the student standing on step 1 is "lower" than the student on step 9.

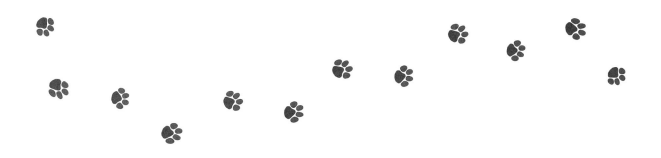

Section IV

- Liquid Measure: The Hand Trick (10)

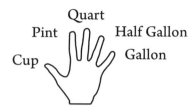

Figure 21.4. The Hand Trick – Visual cognitive strategy for converting liquid measures

The thumb represents cups, the index finger represents pints, the middle finger represents quarts, the ring finger represents half-gallons, and the little finger represents gallons. Starting with the thumb, two of each finger's liquid measurement unit equals one of the next finger's unit. For example, two cups equal one pint, two pints equal one quart, two quarts equal one half-gallon, and two half-gallons equal one gallon. This example brings meaning to an abstract sequential definition by using a cognitive cue linked with a tactile cue.

- Graphs: Slope

In algebra, when graphing, one of the characteristics of a line is the slope. Four kinds of slopes exist: positive, negative, zero, no. The values of these slopes are arbitrary. Up is positive, and so is right. Therefore, up and right (and down and left) are positive. Up and left (and down and right) are negative slopes. Zero slope is a flat line, and no slope is a vertical line.

Draw a stick figure skier on the right slope facing down the hill and skiing on the line. This is a positive and fun skiing experience. Then draw a line to the left with the skier going down hill backwards! This is not fun - it is a negative, dangerous skiing experience! Draw a flat line with the skier facing forward. This a "zero" slope just like the speed of the skier - zero miles per hour. Draw a vertical with the skier not skiing, but falling down the mountain. This line has no slope. (11)

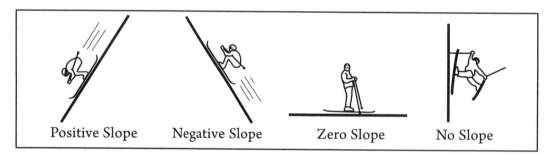

Figure 21.5. Slope – Visual cognitive strategy depicting different slopes

- Create cognitive stories to explain the meaning of math vocabulary words.

  - Isosceles Triangle

    Many algebra and geometry terms are Greek or Latin in origin. For example, a polynomial is an algebraic expression for "many names." A triangle literally means a figure with "three angles." Remembering the names of the different triangles often requires the use of a cognitive strategy. An isosceles triangle is a figure with three sides, two of which are congruent (equal in length). The prefix iso- means "same." The sceles part is derived from the root skelos, which means "leg." So the word isosceles means "same legs." The legs of most human beings form an isosceles triangle. To demonstrate this, ask the student to stand with the legs straight and spread apart. The legs form the two congruent "legs" of the triangle, and the floor becomes the third side of the isosceles triangle. (11)

Chapter 21

- Use backward chaining (source unknown) to imprint math words when the student must spell them correctly for a math test. (5)

  - "Celsius"

    If the student is having difficulty learning "Celsius," write the word on a board, in shaving cream on a Formica surface or desktop, with a dry erase marker on a white board, with an overhead marker on a transparency, or with an erasable marker on a window. Erase the last letter. Have the student write the "s" and say "Celsius." When the student is successful, erase the last two letters. Have the student rewrite the "u" and "s" and say the words. Continue erasing backwards until the student has learned the word. Recheck each week.

- Construct and provide a chart that links math vocabulary to math operations and symbols. (Appendix p. 397)

- Use computer programs to provide instructional practice in solving word problems.

Difficulty Retrieving (Recalling)

The following behaviors serve as general indicators. The student will not exhibit every characteristic listed. These behaviors may also be indicative of other problems.

> Being unable to recall math facts/operations
> Completing math assignments slowly
> Understanding/learning concepts when individually taught, but being unable to use them in word problems requiring multiple procedures
> Forgetting today math facts/procedures learned yesterday
> Making what appears to be "careless errors" when actually related to retrieval problems
> Forgetting cognitive strategies that assist recall
> Having difficulty recalling answers to questions requiring mastery of facts/procedures on cumulative tests (e.g., midterms, final exams).
> Needing frequent reteaching of rules/procedures/algorithms

Dysfluent retrieval increases the demands placed on working memory so that the processing of the word problem is inefficient.

Interventions

- Determine whether the inability to solve word problems is due to difficulty retrieving the math facts and operations or misunderstanding the problem.

- Provide extra time if the student is slow accessing facts.

- Encourage and allow the use of math fact charts and cognitive cue cards.

- Do not allow poor mastery of facts to delay or hamper success with math concepts and applications. Permit the student to use a <u>calculator</u>. The student must understand the word problem and select the proper operations and numbers to be used.

Section V
Study Skills

CHAPTER 22
NOTETAKING

Notetaking is a necessary skill for late elementary, middle, and high school students.

General Recommendations

Review Classroom and Individual Student Interventions in Chapters 8 and 9 and Listening Comprehension Interventions in Chapter 16.

- Be aware that research has consistently shown that students with **ADHD**, **TS**, and/or **OCD** often have neurologically-based graphomotor (handwriting) impairment associated with visual-motor integration problems. (p. 68) (1, 2, 3, 4, 5) Graphomotor difficulties interfere with the ability to take notes. Furthermore, inattention, impulsivity, poor planning (prioritizing, organizing/sequencing), and a lack of self-monitoring significantly impact handwriting. **TS** hand and arm tics and **OCD** compulsions to write, erase, and rewrite may limit the student's ability to keep pace with oral lessons and notetaking.

    🐾 *82% of students with **ADHD-C** and 57% of those with **ADHD-I** have been identified as having penmanship problems. (1)*

- Implement strategies to circumvent the handwriting problems associated with notetaking. (p. 68)

    ○ Designate a peer or "buddy" who is a good notetaker to share notes.

    ○ Have a classmate photocopy the notes or use lined NCR (Non Carbon Replica) paper.

    ○ Furnish a partially completed outline instead of expecting the student to write a complete set of notes.

    ○ Provide a copy of the teacher's notes or lesson plans.

- Permit the use of a laptop computer to take notes.

- Discourage the tape recording of lessons as a bypass strategy. The amount of time that must be spent outside of class listening to the lecture again is too overwhelming. Typing the notes is too frustrating.

    🐾 *An alternative might be the use of a tape recorder that syncs to a computer which then prints the lesson.*

- Be sure to ask a classmate to photocopy and share the notes if the student is absent and misses a lesson.

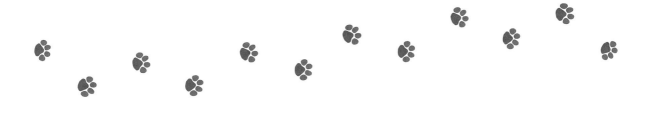

Section V

> Tics/obsessions/compulsions/underarousal/slow processing speed, inattention/impulsivity/hyperactivity, executive dysfunction, and/or memory problems frequently interfere with the ability to take notes.

UNDERAROUSAL/SLOW COGNITIVE PROCESSING SPEED

Review interventions for Underarousal and Slow Processing Speed in Chapter 10.

The following behaviors serve as general indicators. The student will not exhibit every characteristic listed. These behaviors may also be indicative of other problems.

    Lacking persistence
    Struggling to grasp/understand/follow lessons
    Becoming overwhelmed when confronted with complex information
    Having difficulty keeping up with lectures and taking notes
    Asking frequently for information to be repeated

Research suggests that students with **ADHD** have processing speed deficits. (2, 6, 7) A "sluggish cognitive tempo" (SCT) or slow speed of processing characterizes one-fourth to one-half of students with **ADHD, Inattentive type**. (8, 9, 10, 11, 12) Cognitive slowing may also be associated with **TS** and **OCD**. (13, 14, 15)

Interventions

- Recognize that the student's arousal level fluctuates throughout the school day and from one day to the next. Deregulated arousal may influence the ability to take notes.

- Schedule lessons requiring notetaking during the student's optimal arousal time.

- Present material at a slower-than-normal rate or pause at intervals. Fast-paced instruction makes it difficult to understand, process, and record the material.

- Pause frequently to allow time between statements for information to be processed and noted.

- Repeat, rephrase, and summarize material periodically.

- Divide lessons into smaller segments. Provide a movement break or change the activity between segments.

- Supply teacher-prepared mind maps to be filled in during lessons.

- Be alert to signs of misunderstanding and confusion.

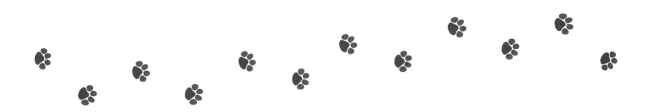

Chapter 22

INATTENTION/IMPULSIVITY/HYPERACTIVITY

Review interventions for Inattention/Impulsivity/Hyperactivity in Chapter 12.

Difficulty Focusing and Sustaining Attention

The following behaviors serve as general indicators. The student will not exhibit every characteristic listed. These behaviors may also be indicative of other problems.

> Becoming distracted
> Daydreaming/staring into space
> Fiddling/doodling during notetaking
> Getting up from desk repeatedly
> Becoming quickly bored/disinterested in taking notes
> Needing constant reminders to keep taking notes

Interventions

- Recognize that the student who is having difficulty focusing and sustaining attention will need more assistance and structure with notetaking than other students.

- Remember that the attentional and working memory problems of the student with **ADHD** may make it difficult to hold information in mind long enough to process and record it.

- Determine whether the inability to sustain attention when taking notes is modality-specific (verbal or visual) or content-specific (e.g., reading, writing, math, literature, science, history).

- Include many visual cues (e.g., highlighting, bullets, circles, letters, numbered sequences).

- Repeat information frequently to allow for lapses in attention.

- Permit questions to be asked during the lesson.

- Use cue words or filler sentences to attract attention before imparting important information (e.g., "Listen," "Ready," "What I'm going to say next is important."

- Instruct the student to pay attention and "listen" for key information such as who, what, when, where, how, and why.

- Periodically pause and request that the information be paraphrased or summarized.

EXECUTIVE DYSFUNCTION

Review interventions for Executive Dysfunction in Chapter 13.

Difficulty Prioritizing

The following behaviors serve as general indicators. The student will not exhibit every characteristic listed. These behaviors may also be indicative of other problems.

> Noting minor details and not including main ideas
> Recording irrelevant information
> Trying to take verbatim notes

Section V

Interventions

- Preview information prior to starting lessons.

  ○ Stress what will be most important about the material to be presented (answers to questions, main ideas, related facts).

  ○ Cue listening for who, what, when, where, how, and why.

  ○ Prepare a list of questions assessing key concepts that will be asked after the lesson. Have the student record the answers.

- Make sure the student has a strategy for identifying main ideas and important details.

  ○ Emphasize listening for cue words and phrases that signal key concepts and essential facts (e.g., "The main point is_____." "This is important _____." "Remember _____." "There are three important ideas _____." "In summary, _____." "You will need to know this for the test _____.").

  ○ Indicate that important information is often repeated.

  ○ Stress listening carefully to information that is presented in alphabetical or numerical order.

  ○ Hand out copies of the charts, definitions, graphs, tables, or formulas that are written on the board, overhead transparency, or computer generated slide.

- Omit information that is unnecessary for understanding.

- Exclude repetitious information.

- Summarize key ideas frequently.

- Supply a lettered or numbered outline or graphic organizer indicating main ideas. Ask the student to add important details.

Difficulty Organizing/Sequencing

The following behaviors serve as general indicators. The student will not exhibit every characteristic listed. These behaviors may also be indicative of other problems.

Producing disorganized, illegible notes
Taking notes that are difficult to understand
Putting the wrong information into the notes

The key to good notetaking is organization. Students with **ADHD** frequently are disorganized in their approach to notetaking.

Interventions

- Recommend that the parents purchase an 8 ½" x 11" <u>loose-leaf notebook</u> with sufficient lined pages for notetaking.

  ○ Divide the notebook into tabbed sections, one color-coded section for each course. Be sure to use the same color coding for all materials associated with a specific academic subject.

  ○ Demonstrate how supplemental materials can be filed, information inserted and deleted, and pages re-sequenced.

- Consider using a modified <u>Cornell Notetaking Technique</u>. (16) (Appendix p. 400)

Suggest that the student:

- put name, date, page number, and topic being discussed at the top of the page.
  - 🐾 *Notes often get disorganized, torn out, or misplaced. By dating and numbering the pages, they can be put back in the correct order.*
- fold or draw a vertical line 2 ½ inches from the left side of the paper.
- record in the large <u>right-hand column</u> words and phrases that express main ideas and important details. Do not try to write every word that is spoken.
- take notes on only the front of the paper so that the pages can be placed side by side when studying.
- skip lines to emphasize changes in ideas/topics and insert additional information.
- leave blank spaces with question marks when information is missed.
- learn and use strategies to increase notetaking speed. (Appendix p. 401)
  - abbreviate words (e.g., "&" for "and," "@" for "at," "w/" for "with," "etc." for "etcetera").
  - shorten words by eliminating the final letters (e.g., "imp" for "important," "info" for "information," "min" for "minimum," "max" for "maximum").
  - omit vowels and keep only enough consonants for word recognition (e.g., "bkgd" for "background," "wrt" for "write," "yrs" for "years," "vs" for "versus").
- following the lesson, reduce the notes to key words and phrases and record them in the <u>left-hand column</u>.
- keep the lessons in reverse chronological order (latest first, oldest last).

- Teach and provide practice notetaking.
  - Deliver short, organized lectures that cover familiar topics.
  - Emphasize key concepts and prompt the student to write them down.
  - Use a variety of visual aids.
  - Following the lecture, review notes and compare with a completed model.

INITIATION/EXECUTION DIFFICULTIES

The following behaviors serve as general indicators. The student will not exhibit every characteristic listed. These behaviors may also be indicative of other problems.

Appearing hypoactive/lacking energy/uninterested when required to take notes
Not knowing where/when to start taking notes
Fiddling with items in notebook/desk when needing to take notes
Avoiding taking notes, even when knowing failure to do so will result in negative consequences
Needing reminders to start/continue taking notes

Section V

Interventions

- Divide oral lessons into short, manageable segments. The student may become discouraged and frustrated when required to take notes during a long lecture and then be unable to overcome the inertia caused by feeling overwhelmed. Gradually increase the length and difficulty of the lesson as the student demonstrates success.

- Assist completion of the first one or two notes to make sure the student knows how to take notes.

MEMORY PROBLEMS

Review interventions for Memory Problems in Chapter 14.

SHORT-TERM MEMORY PROBLEMS

Difficulty with Working Memory

The following behaviors serve as general indicators. The student will not exhibit every characteristic listed. These behaviors may also be indicative of other problems.

Having difficulty listening to new/complex verbal material while taking satisfactory notes
Appearing confused during oral lessons
Becoming frustrated/overwhelmed when confronted with notetaking
Asking excessive number of questions
Needing repetition of phrases/sentences/instructions/information
Losing information heard at beginning of teacher's explanation/lesson while listening to rest of it
Being unable to paraphrase/summarize verbally presented information

Research suggests that students with **ADHD** have difficulty with listening comprehension tasks that require working memory, even though their ability to understand incoming information is normally developed. (17) Students must simultaneously pay close attention, remember the material, summarize accurately, write quickly in an organized and legible form, and continue to process the ongoing lecture.

Interventions

- Determine the student's auditory memory span. Do not present information in excess of the verbal memory span as the student may have difficulty maintaining it in working memory.

    The ability to process information in working memory decreases significantly when the student is trying to process more than the memory span can retain. Notetaking becomes impossible.

- Assign a chapter in the textbook for homework before it is taught in class. This familiarizes the student with the key points and terms that will be presented during the lesson.

    Suggest that the student:

    ○ review the vocabulary to be used during the lesson.

    ○ highlight the main ideas and details.

    ○ think about and connect the information to what is already known about the subject.

    ○ generate questions as the material is read.

- Stress reviewing notes from the previous lessons during homework sessions.
- Design well-organized lessons that are easy to understand and follow.
- Present ideas and explanations related to the text. Omit extraneous information.
- Slow down the rate of presentation to allow time for writing.
- Pause and ask students in the class to summarize the material. This provides more time for processing the information, writing, and/or and checking the accuracy of the notes.
- Write key concepts on the board, an overhead transparency, or an interactive whiteboard.
    - Use different colored pens or pencils to highlight or underline important points.
    - Frame main points with circles, squares, rectangles, and/or ovals.
- Modify <u>notetaking requirements</u> if the student has working memory problems.
    - Use <u>alternate forms</u> of notetaking.
        - Supply teacher-prepared mind maps or outlines identifying main ideas and related subtopics. Provide space for filling in facts, definitions, etc.
        - Furnish fill-in-the blank teacher-created notes or lists of details to be completed with the key concepts.
        - Furnish a graphic organizer to be completed during the lesson.
        - Provide incomplete charts, graphs, diagrams, and illustrations.
- Use strategies that enhance the workspace available in working memory. (p. 36)
- Provide a few minutes after the lesson for the student to read over the notes and fill in the information that was missed, make sure the notes are understandable, and correct illegible handwriting.

    Suggest that the student:
    - ask for further clarification from the teacher or reread the text if the notes are unclear.
    - borrow notes from another student to clarify missing information or illegible writing.

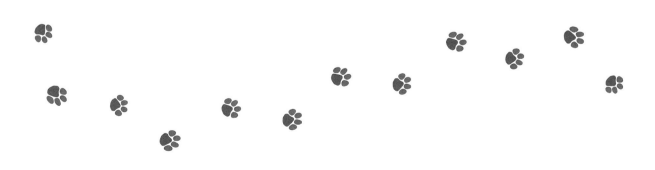

Section V

LONG-TERM MEMORY PROBLEMS

Difficulty Encoding/Consolidating (Learning)

The following behaviors serve as general indicators. The student will not exhibit every characteristic listed. These behaviors may also be indicative of other problems.

    Needing additional instruction to learn information in notes
    Forgetting today the material that was recalled yesterday

Interventions

- Recommend reviewing notes immediately following a lesson to mitigate a rapid loss of information. (p. 143)

    > *The more time that elapses without reinforcement, the more the information is forgotten. A quick review helps ensure that learning is permanent. Studying the material at a later time requires relearning, not just reviewing. (18, 19)*

- Teach strategies to encode information in the notes.

    Suggest that the student:

    - star major points or highlight/underline important concepts and facts with different colored pens or pencils.
    - summarize or restate in a few words the most salient information presented (key concepts, related facts, and conclusion).
    - cover up the right-hand column and use the left side to <u>rehearse aloud</u> the content of the lecture.
    - formulate questions that might be asked on a test and write them in the left-hand column.
    - reorganize or outline the notes.
    - create visual organizers.
        - organize the information into a mind map, written list, table, chart, or diagram. Most of the information will be encoded by the time the graphic organizer is completed.
        - draw pictures that illustrate important information.
    - transcribe the notes onto a word processor.
    - quickly review the notes before starting homework.
    - review the notes before the following lesson.
    - use the same procedure during the week prior to and just before a test.

CHAPTER 23

HOMEWORK

All students are required to complete homework as they progress through school. Homework is assigned to provide opportunities to help students develop good study habits, review what has been taught in class, practice skills and strategies, and use resources to find information about topics being studied in class. Students who spend more time on regularly assigned, meaningful homework improve their school performance, earn higher grades, and score better on standardized tests.

Students with **ADHD**, **TS**, and/or **OCD** frequently have difficulty completing homework. Underarousal/slow processing speed, inattention/impulsivity/hyperactivity, executive dysfunction, and working memory problems impact the students' ability to record homework assignments, to organize and to take home the necessary materials, to estimate the time required to complete tasks, to initiate, to focus and sustain attention until task completion, to self-monitor, edit, and/or to turn in assignments.

 *Many students with executive dysfunction (**EDF**) do not think about or plan for the future and, therefore, do not realize the value of doing homework.*

General Recommendations

Review Classroom and Individual Student Interventions in Chapters 8 and 9.

- Determine <u>why</u> a student is having difficulty with homework. Discuss the problem with both the student and parents.

  Consider the following questions:

  ○ Are the assignments at the appropriate instructional level? (p. 64)

  ○ Has the student mastered skills needed to work on assignments?

  ○ How is the homework assigned?

  ○ Are the assignments being recorded accurately?

  ○ How does the student keep track of the assignments?

  ○ How are the assignments taken home?

  ○ Are the necessary books and materials carried home?

  ○ What is the home study environment?

  ○ Does the student understand how to do the assignments?

  ○ Is the student able to organize homework assignments?

  ○ Is the homework started in a timely manner?

  ○ Are parental supervision and assistance required?

  ○ Is the homework completed with acceptable accuracy? If not, why?

  ○ Are the assignments finished within a reasonable time frame? If not, why?

  ○ How does the student keep track of the completed assignments?

Section V

- How is the homework returned to school?
- Does the student remember to turn in the homework?
- What is the method for collecting the homework?
- Is timely feedback provided?
- Does the student receive positive/negative reinforcement?
- What strategies have been tried to improve homework completion?
- Were they successful? If not, why?
- Does the student understand the benefits of doing homework?

- Ask the parents to complete the Homework Survey. (1) (Appendix p. 406)
- Assign homework that can be completed with a <u>minimum amount of stress</u>. (2)

  🐾 *Family stress levels increase during homework time and as the dinner and bedtime hours approach. Homework frequently interferes with family routines and leads to family battles and "storms." (pp. 81-95)*

  - Offer alternative activities for homework assignments (e.g., play computer games that reinforce the acquisition of basic sight vocabulary words, math facts, spelling words, history and science facts; make collages or posters; prepare Power Point presentations, demonstrations, oral reports).
  - Refrain from giving repetitive busywork.
  - <u>Never</u> assign extra homework as a punishment strategy.
  - Do not send unfinished class assignments home. The student who cannot complete classwork at school will be unable to finish it at home because of a decrease in physical and cognitive energy associated with the disorder(s).
  - Recommend that the parents avoid power struggles over homework.
  - Use after-school study groups or study periods to complete homework if the student is arguing with parents about homework assignments.

- Permit homework to be turned in late and receive credit if the symptoms associated with **ADHD, TS,** and/or **OCD** interfere with work completion.

  🐾 *Be sure all homework is completed, even if it is late, to instill good study habits.*

- Assign homework that can be <u>completed independently</u>. (2)

  🐾 *Parents should <u>not</u> have to teach the skills needed to complete assignments.*

  - Assign homework from the beginning of the school year to establish a homework routine.
  - Create interesting, motivating homework (e.g., write a different ending to a story; teach an adult a newly learned skill; interview an adult about the topic being studied; play an educational computer game; create a bulletin board).

- Find the level at which homework can be completed successfully.
  - Always give homework at the <u>independent</u> level (90 percent of the material is understood). (p. 64)
  - Assign homework as a means of <u>practicing</u> previously taught material.
  - Adjust homework requirements if the assignment is inappropriate (e.g., photocopy math problems, assign every other question/problem, permit use of the computer for writing tasks).
  - Question the effect of the homework on the family dynamics.
    - 🐾 *Homework that is too difficult or takes too long to complete often causes severe disruption in the family.*
- Set aside time during the day to provide assistance when homework cannot be completed independently.
- Discuss <u>homework expectations</u> with the parents. Explain:
  - how frequently homework will be assigned.
  - the type of homework that will be given.
  - how long each homework assignment should take.
  - expected parental involvement (e.g., provide assistance, carefully check the work and insist on corrections, make sure that the work is completed and turned in on time).
    - 🐾 *Parents should <u>assist</u> the student only when needed.*
  - how homework assignments will be graded.
- Scan homework papers which need to be completed into the student's computer. Permit the completed homework to be returned via the Internet.
- Create a homework website which the student and parents can access.

> **Tics/obsessions/compulsions, underarousal/slow processing speed, inattention/impulsivity/hyperactivity, executive dysfunction, and/or memory problems frequently interfere with the ability to do/complete homework.**

UNDERAROUSAL/SLOW COGNITIVE PROCESSING SPEED

Review interventions for Underarousal and Slow Processing Speed in Chapter 10.

The following behaviors serve as general indicators. The student will not exhibit every characteristic listed. These behaviors may also be indicative of other problems.

Having difficulty sustaining focused attention
Lacking persistence
Reading/writing/solving math problems slowly
Needing additional time to finish homework
Responding slowly when being quizzed by the parents for tests

Section V

Interventions

- Take into consideration the physical and emotional consequences of having **ADHD**, **TS**, and/or **OCD** and the impact on the ability to quickly and efficiently complete homework. By the end of the day, the student is often tired and cognitively exhausted.

    - 🐾 *Inattention, distractibility, hyperactivity, tics, obsessions, and compulsions frequently increase as the day progresses.*

    - Be flexible and modify assignments when the neurological problems associated with the disorder(s) make it difficult to finish homework.

- Coordinate homework with the other teachers to ensure that unreasonable amounts of work are not assigned (e.g., report/project due at the same time, more than one test/quiz scheduled on the same day).

- Determine the level at which homework can be completed within reasonable time limits. (2)

    - Write down how long the assignment is expected to take.

        - 🐾 *Teachers often underestimate how long it takes students with slow processing speed to complete homework.*

    - Ask the parents to keep a daily record for the first six weeks and note the <u>actual time</u> needed to finish the homework.

        - 🐾 *Students and parents often do not communicate with teachers that homework takes an excessive amount of time to complete.*

    - Analyze whether the type and amount of assigned work was realistic.

    - Modify the requirements and the length of homework assignments. Lengthy, complex assignments frequently lead to frustration and agitation.

        - Assign shorter tasks requiring accuracy and quality of response.

        - Separate a long-term assignment into small segments that appear as independent assignments.

        - Gradually increase the length and difficulty of the homework as the assignments are successfully completed.

        - Recommend dividing study periods into several short sessions with breaks between tasks.

        - Do not assign the student with **OCD** any homework assignment that cannot be finished within a reasonable time frame. The student may have a compulsive need to finish all homework, even if it requires staying up past bedtime. Being unable to change tasks often increases anxiety and precipitates inappropriate behaviors.

- Provide practice and rehearsal of cognitive and academic skills until mastered. When information is automatized, speed of processing increases.

- Suggest using a word processor, calculator, or tape recorder.

Chapter 23

INATTENTION/IMPULSIVITY/HYPERACTIVITY

Review interventions for Inattention/Impulsivity/Hyperactivity in Chapter 12.

Difficulty Focusing and Sustaining Attention

The following behaviors serve as general indicators. The student will not exhibit every characteristic listed. These behaviors may also be indicative of other problems.

- Becoming distracted
- Daydreaming/staring into space
- Fiddling/doodling
- Shifting position/getting up from desk repeatedly
- Needing constant reminders to keep working
- Having difficulty working independently
- Becoming quickly bored/disinterested in homework
- Being unable to complete homework
- Neglecting to use internalized speech to control behavior
- Beginning assignments without reading directions
- Impulsively starting homework before planning/organizing
- Rushing through assignments
- Making careless errors due to impulsivity
- Having low tolerance for frustration/responding with irritability/anger
- Lacking skills to deal with negative emotions regarding homework
- Giving up/quitting when confronted with difficult homework

Interventions

- Be aware that the ability to attend and concentrate deteriorates as the day progresses and as the end of the school year approaches. Adjust homework assignments accordingly.

- Recognize that the student who is having difficulty focusing and sustaining attention will need more assistance and structure at home than other students.

- Assign tasks that keep the student active while studying (e.g., underlining, highlighting, drawing diagrams, reading aloud, taking notes).

- Vary homework assignments. The student with **ADHD** often becomes inattentive when confronted with dull, boring, repetitive homework. The stimulation of new, different, and interesting assignments, which offer more satisfaction and immediate reward, helps maintain attention.

    - Utilize games and hands-on projects.

    - Pair the student with a classmate who has a special interest in the subject being studied.

    - Provide magazine articles with color photographs to be read for homework.

    - Assign watching a video related to the topic and writing questions to ask the other students the following day.

    - Give homework that requires the use of the computer as the student with **ADHD** often attends more readily to the computer screen.

Section V

- Recommend using <u>cognitive strategies</u> to assist on-task behavior.

  - Suggest quietly reciting or thinking aloud while completing assignments. Using self-directed speech will help the student focus on the homework and remain on task.

  - Provide visual cues that indicate the steps needed to complete an assignment.

  - Recommend taping a visual cue to the study desk or inside the notebook as a reminder to pay attention and finish the homework.

- Encourage the parents to provide frequent opportunities for <u>physical movement</u> to decrease the restlessness and overactivity associated with **ADHD**. (2)

  - 🐾 *The student with **ADHD** and/or **TS** has great difficulty following rules that restrict movement.*

  Suggest that the parents:

  - <u>ignore minor motor movements</u> which release hyperactivity and increase attention. Minor motor movements include drumming fingers, doodling, fiddling with objects, or moving papers on the desk.

    - 🐾 *When the student must sit and read an assignment, permit gum chewing, eating, or fiddling with a small, squeezable object to increase attention to task.*

  - allow standing, shaking legs, kneeling, or repositioning self in chair while completing homework assignments.

  - schedule frequent, short movement breaks. Periodically have the student stand up, reach for the sky, stretch or shake arms and shoulders, press hands together, touch toes, twist waist, or do chair push ups.

- Recommend using a <u>timer</u> or clock set for the amount of time needed to focus on and complete a task (e.g., every 5 to 15 minutes, depending on the student's attention span).

  - 🐾 *Set a timer that ticks to cue attention to task unless it is too distracting.*

- Encourage the parents to restrict the use of electronics (e.g., emailing, instant messaging, talking on telephone, text messaging) until all assignments are completed.

- Modify homework if the lesson is <u>impulsively</u> completed and contains many mistakes.

  - Assign shorter tasks with accuracy being the criterion.

  - Encourage the use of self-talk. Self-directed speech is a means of slowing down responding and reducing impulsivity.

- Adjust assignments if parents report that the student becomes <u>frustrated</u> during homework sessions.

  - 🐾 *Students with **ADHD**, **TS**, and/or **OCD** often become discouraged and frustrated when confronted with long, complex assignments. No learning can occur when the student is upset.*

  - Minimize negative reactions to frustration by always making sure that the assigned homework is at the <u>independent level</u> (<u>90</u> percent of the material is understood). (p. 64)

  - Assign short tasks that can easily be completed. Gradually increase length and difficulty of homework as success is demonstrated.

- Reduce parental expectations for perfection. An expectation for perfect work may be unrealistic and increase frustration and stress.

- Suggest taking a break or stopping homework for that evening if the student becomes agitated. However, if the homework must be stopped, it should be finished at a later time so the student does not think that homework can be avoided.

- Ask the parents to write a note explaining the situation and requesting a conference to discuss the problem.

• Provide in-school reinforcers for completing and turning in homework. For example, the elementary student might be given stickers, allowed to be first in line, draw, pass out and collect papers, have extra time to use the computer, or take care of the classroom pet. The middle school student might be permitted to engage in an activity of personal choice, to use a learning center, to work on an art project, to watch a video, or to receive a "no homework" pass. The high school student might use an area of interest or expertise to tutor a peer, work on a project in a preferred medium, do a task for the teacher to earn extra credit, or to use electronics.

- Discuss in advance with the student homework expectations and together select an appropriate reward.

    • Make sure that the assignment can realistically be completed.

> **Motivational programs make the possible possible; they do not make the impossible possible.**
> Greene, R. W. (2001). International Symposium on TS and Other Neurodevelopmental Disorders. Tourette Syndrome Foundation of Canada. Toronto, Canada

    • Interview the student or observe the student's choice of activities to determine which one might be proposed as a reward.

- Change rewards frequently if the student tends to become quickly satiated with the reinforcers.

    Variety and novelty are potent reinforcers. However, some students are satisfied with rewards such as the use of electronic devises and infrequently need the reward changed.

- Accompany the reward with an enthusiastic, clearly stated comment regarding homework completion (e.g., "I understand that you started your work as soon as you got home and remained on task. Look what happened. You finished all your homework!").

- Evaluate the efficacy of the reinforcer used.

    • Was the failure to complete or turn in the homework the result of an ineffective reward?

    • Was the reward considered positive and meaningful to the student?

        What is motivating for one student may not be for another student.

    • Had the student become bored with the reinforcer?

    • Was there too long of a delay between completing or turning in the homework and the reinforcer?

Section V

- Teach the parents how to <u>positively reinforce appropriate homework behaviors</u> (e.g., writing down the homework in the assignment book, bringing home the necessary materials, starting and persisting on work without reminders, completing assignments in the designated time, finishing homework as independently as possible, self-monitoring, editing, remembering to turn in homework).

    Recommend that the parents:

    - <u>ignore</u> off-task behavior. Paying attention to off-task behavior increases the likelihood that the student will continue the off-task behavior. The simultaneous use of reinforcing the positive and ignoring the negative improves behavior. (2)

    - use a log as a means of providing an accurate record if weekend privileges are being rewarded.

    - use a contract for the older student that essentially conveys a "no work, no play" message. Include positive reinforcers and rewards according to the student's interests. The following contract might be written for the student who likes electronics, driving, and going out with friends.

Behaviors	Positive Reinforcers
Materials taken home for the week	Movie/game rental for the weekend
Homework recorded correctly for the week	Credit toward purchase of electronics
Monday's homework completed	Use of electronics for 2 hours
Tuesday's homework completed	Use of electronics for 2 hours
Wednesday's homework completed	Use of electronics for 2 hours
Thursday's homework completed	Use of electronics for 2 hours
Friday's homework completed	Use of electronics for 2 hours
Homework in bookbag by door without cue for the week	Stay up one hour later Saturday
No homework arguments for the week	Permission to go out Saturday night
No homework reminders needed for the week	Gas credit
Homework started right after school for the week	Choice of weekend activity
Homework completed/turned in for the week	Car keys available for weekend night

Figure 23.1. Example of Homework Contract

- Indicate that it is necessary to set firm and consistent consequences for not completing homework that is within the student's capabilities (e.g., being unable to go outside and play with friends or losing telephone, computer, television, CD player privileges for the rest of the evening).

Chapter 23

- Recommend that the parents intervene if the student becomes overwhelmed.

  🐾 *Sometime **ADHD** medication has worn off during homework time and can make cognitive tasks quite difficult.*

  Suggest that the parents:

  - associate anxiety and anger with distress or lacking skills.
  - provide a movement break before trying again.
  - offer a protein snack to increase arousal and improve attention.

- Teach the parents how to intercede when <u>acting-out behavior</u> interferes with the rest of the family. (pp. 94-95)

EXECUTIVE DYSFUNCTION

Review interventions for Executive Dysfunction in Chapter 13.

IMPAIRED PROBLEM SOLVING

(Tasks/Activities/Situations)

- Provide a template of a problem solving strategy such as "**GET A CLUE**" or "**PLAN**" to enhance the ability to do homework. Be sure the strategy includes steps for goal setting, planning (generating ideas, solutions; analyzing proposed ideas, solutions; prioritizing; organizing; sequencing; managing time), initiating, completing, and editing. (Appendix pp. 374–375)

- Model and demonstrate how to use <u>problem solving strategies</u>. (p. 108)

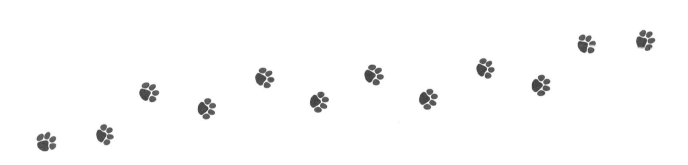

Section V

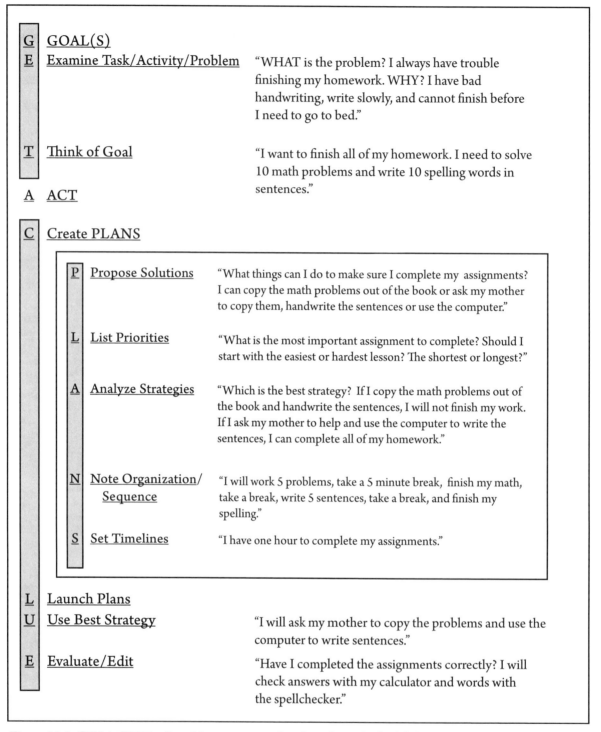

Figure 23.2. GET A CLUE – Cognitive strategy used with student who had difficulty completing homework

Some students may not be able to follow the complexity of this strategy unless taught in incremental steps that must be mastered before continuing to the next step. Other students may need to learn a more simplified version "**PLAN.**" If so, use "**GET A CLUE**" as a structure for discussing and teaching ways to solve tasks, activities, and problem situations.

P	<u>Propose Goal</u>	"I want to develop a plan to complete my homework. I need to solve 10 math problems and write 10 spelling words in sentences."
L	<u>List and Analyze Strategies</u>	"What things can I do to make sure I complete my homework? I can copy the math problems out of the book or ask my mother to copy them, handwrite the sentences or write them on the computer. If I copy the math problems out of the book and handwrite the sentences, I will not finish my homework. If I ask my mother to copy the math problems and I use the computer to write the sentences, I think I can complete all of my work."
A	<u>Apply Best Strategy</u>	"I will ask my mother to copy the problems and I will use the computer."
N	<u>Notice Errors and Edit</u>	"Have I solved the math problems correctly? I will check the answers with my calculator. Oh! I need to redo this one! Have I spelled the words correctly? They are all correct."

Figure 23.3. PLAN – Cognitive strategy used with student who had difficulty completing homework

Difficulty Setting Goals

The following behaviors serve as general indicators. The student will not exhibit every characteristic listed. These behaviors may also be indicative of other problems.

Using trial-and-error approach to completing homework
Overlooking the need to set goals for completing homework effectively and efficiently
Being unable to generate solutions to homework problems

Interventions

- Teach the use of the strategy for setting goals.

- Have the student self-evaluate the skills required to complete homework successfully, identify strengths and weaknesses, and determine the skills which need improvement.

- Recommend that the parents help the student set goals before beginning homework.

- Provide the parents with templates of "**GET A CLUE**," "**PLAN**," or another homework strategy for setting goals. (Appendix pp. 374–375)

Difficulty Planning

Difficulty Proposing and Analyzing Ideas/Solutions/Strategies

The following behaviors serve as general indicators. The student will not exhibit every characteristic listed. These behaviors may also be indicative of other problems.

Lacking skills to generate/brainstorm ideas/solutions/strategies for solving homework problems
Using trial-and-error approach to problem solving
Having trouble identifying the who, what, when, where, how, and why of the problem
Needing help to analyze proposed strategies to carry out goal

Section V

Interventions

- Provide assistance in generating as many practical ideas as possible (e.g., "I will make a 'To Do' list and put it in my daily, weekly, and monthly calendars, ask an adult to copy assignments before completing them, use the computer and email lesson to teacher.").

- Discuss both the positive and negative outcomes and consequences of each idea.

- Choose the best strategy.

Difficulty Prioritizing

The following behaviors serve as general indicators. The student will not exhibit every characteristic listed. These behaviors may also be indicative of other problems.

Misjudging significance of homework assignments
Spending too much time on unimportant activities
Being unclear as to why homework should be considered a priority
Having difficulty determining most important reading/math/writing assignment to be completed
Struggling to decide what material to study for tests

Interventions

- Discuss the value of homework.

    - Explain that completing homework increases learning and produces good grades.

    - Show how school achievement and good grades help the student get "great adult toys" (e.g., car, computer, large screen TV).

- Teach the student how to prepare homework "To Do Lists" that prioritize, organize, and consolidate all of the essential tasks that need to be carried out each day, week, and month. (p. 121)

    🐾 *A "To Do List" will help reduce the demands placed on working memory to remember several different assignments.*

Ask the parents to help the student:

- list all the homework assignments that must be completed for that day, week, and month.

- separate important tasks and activities from time-consuming unimportant ones.

    🐾 *Check to see if priorities are correct.*

- divide difficult tasks and assignments into several smaller ones and add them to the list.

- include due dates and steps for completing long-term assignments and studying for tests.

- highlight steps for completing book reports in one color, test dates in another color, etc.

- list special events such as athletic games, club meetings, holidays, birthdays, family events, etc.

- rank order and number the sequence in which the tasks should be completed. Students differ in their preferences. Some prefer beginning with the most difficult or tedious assignment. Others choose to start with an easy assignment, complete a more difficult task, and end with another easy assignment.

- rewrite the list in priority order.

Difficulty Organizing/Sequencing

The following behaviors serve as general indicators. The student will not exhibit every characteristic listed. These behaviors may also be indicative of other problems.

> Overlooking need to use assignment book
> Neglecting to take home needed books/materials
> Becoming overwhelmed by large homework assignments and unable to break assignments into manageable segments
> Finding it impossible to sequence homework tasks
> Using a disorganized approach to completing homework
> Having difficulty organizing materials/belongings/backpacks
> Forgetting to return books/materials to school

Interventions

- Be aware that organizational skills tend to be better developed in a classroom that provides structure and routine regarding homework assignments.

- Require the use of an assignment book.

- Use the <u>assignment book</u> as a communication log with the parents. (2)

    - 🐾 *Email or fax comments when the use of the assignment book is unsuccessful.*

    ○ Initial that the homework was copied correctly.

    ○ Ask the parents to initial that the homework was completed. This will prevent unfair accusations if the work was misplaced between home and school.

    ○ Keep an accurate record in the log if weekend privileges are being awarded for homework completion. A Friday summary report can determine what rewards a student can earn (e.g., watching television, using the computer, staying up late, driving, receiving extra allowance).

- Establish a <u>classroom procedure for assigning homework</u>.

    ○ Post <u>written</u> homework assignments in the same location every day.

        - 🐾 *Avoid giving oral directions as students leave class.*

    ○ Set a specific time for writing down assignments and gathering materials. Follow the same schedule every day.

        - 🐾 *Schedule enough time to copy homework assignments accurately.*

- Intervene if the student is having difficulty <u>recording homework assignments</u> accurately.

    - 🐾 *Always provide <u>written</u> instructions if the student has a handwriting problem or ask a "buddy" to copy the directions on lined NCR (Non Carbon Replica) paper to be placed in the student's assignment book.*

    ○ Give the student a copy of the homework assignments.

    ○ Suggest tape recording homework assignments.

    ○ Post homework assignments on the school or class website.

    ○ Provide the names and phone numbers of two or three classmates who are willing to discuss the assignments with the student.

Section V

- Recommend using the Internet to obtain information regarding assignments from other classmates.
- Email parents regarding homework assignments, what is expected from the student, due dates, etc.
- Ask the parents to provide self-addressed and stamped envelopes to have the class syllabus, deadlines, and instructions for long-term assignments mailed home.

• Help the student remember to <u>take the needed materials home</u>. (2)

- Suggest keeping an extra set of books at home.
- Recommend that the parents supply the study area with necessary materials (paper, pencils, pens, highlighters, paper clips, stapler, scissors, tape, glue, ruler, calculator, dictionary, thesaurus) to eliminate the need to look for the items to put in the bookbag.
- Provide time throughout the day for organizing books and materials needed for the homework assignments.
- Color coordinate textbooks, folders, and assignment sheets so that it is easier to find materials (e.g., yellow math book cover, yellow math notebook, yellow assignment sheet).
- Have a separate, color-coded folder for permission slips and teacher-parent communications.
- Insist that the assignment book and homework folders containing the work sheets be placed in the <u>front</u> of the notebook.
- Allow the student to leave class two to three minutes early. The extra time will enable the student to go to the locker to calmly pack the school bag without the distraction of other students. This will increase the likelihood that the necessary items do go home.
- Have an aide or resource teacher monitor whether the homework instructions are correctly recorded in the assignment notebook and check the book bag to make sure the needed books and materials are included.
- Conduct a weekly cleanup of the folders, notebook, and bookbag.

• Suggest that the parents have a large container into which the student can put all school materials upon arriving home so messages from the teacher, permission slips, library cards, and other school communications will not be overlooked.

• Recommend creating a <u>study environment</u> that allows the student to concentrate and is conducive to work completion.

Suggest that the parents:

- designate a quiet study area that is free of distractions such as televisions, video games, CD players, and telephones.
  - insist that all family members engage in quiet activities during homework time. This is particularly important if the student lives in a small, noisy household.
  - permit the student to select and to listen to music to block out the noises that are distracting in the home. However, if the privilege is abused (decline in grades, failure to complete homework), the privilege is lost.
    - *The student should not listen to music on the radio as the intermittent interruptions may be distracting.*

- allow the student to choose the location for doing the homework (desk, bed, kitchen or dining room table, floor). If the work is not finished, all assignments must be completed in a specified location. After a period of time, permit the student to try again. (2)
- take into consideration the student's sensory preferences when choosing the study place. (2)

    Does the student:

    - study better with familiar music masking background noises?
    - prefer soft lighting to bright lighting, or incandescent lighting to florescent lighting?
    - prefer a cool room to a warm room?
    - prefer a soft or hard chair, one that rocks or swivels?
    - prefer rocking to sitting?
    - prefer walking while reading?
    - need to snack while studying?

- Recommend designating a <u>specific time</u> every day to study and do homework. (2)

    Suggest that the parents:

    - require homework be completed before dinner. Often the student and parents are too tired to handle the demands of the homework routine later in the evening.

        When after-school activities interfere with doing homework, start homework as soon as possible. If activities prevent homework completion, review priorities and adjust schedule for success.

    - provide enough time (about 30 minutes) to have a snack, relax, and release energy and tics before starting homework, but not enough time to get distracted or involved in another activity that might prevent shifting focus to the homework (e.g., playing with friends, watching TV, playing a video game, IM-instant messaging).

        It is often difficult for the student to engage in an interesting activity and then stop and think about homework. If the student wants more time, there must be an agreement to stop immediately when called or the privilege will be denied in the future.

    - set a <u>required amount of time for studying</u> whether or not homework has been assigned so that studying becomes a regular routine. If the student does not have any homework or finishes the work before the designated time, the student can read for pleasure, review for tests, work on an upcoming project, or complete practice lessons. A set time will negate rushing through homework to watch TV, play a video game, or talk on the telephone.

        The amount of time the student should spend doing homework depends on the student's grade level. The National Education Association (NEA) recommends that students in kindergarten through the second grade have 10 to 20 minutes of homework each night. Students in grades 3 to 6 should be assigned 30 to 60 minutes of homework. The amount assigned to middle and high school students should vary depending on the subject and the course requirements (answering questions, solving math problems on a daily basis, or writing reports and research papers). (3)

Section V

- Encourage the parents to help <u>structure and organize the completion of homework</u> assignments.

  Suggest that the parents:

  - offer assistance in listing and prioritizing (p. 278) all tasks that need to be completed during the homework period (e.g., solving a specified number of math problems, answering history questions, completing a step needed to write a report or complete a long-term project, studying for a science test later in the week).
  - help separate longer assignments into subtasks.
  - make sure that breaks are scheduled between tasks.
    - 🐾 *Schedule more frequent breaks for more difficult assignments.*

- Recommend providing a structure that ensures that completed <u>assignments are returned</u> to school.

  Suggest that the parents:

  - <u>always</u> keep the school bag by the door through which the student leaves in the morning.
  - check to make sure that the completed assignments have been placed in the color-coded homework folder in the front of the notebook.
  - provide reminders to put the notebook in the school bag.
  - have the student scan homework papers and submit them on the Internet when possible.
    - 🐾 *The ability to email homework assignments to the teacher increases homework completion and negates the loss of homework between home and school.*

- Establish a classroom routine for <u>collecting homework</u>.

  - Designate a location in the classroom for the homework to be placed.
  - Use color-coded folders to hold completed assignments.
  - Routinely remind <u>all</u> students at the beginning of class to turn in their assignments.
  - Discreetly cue the student to place the homework in the specified area. Gradually decrease cues as success is experienced.
  - Check completed assignments and return them as soon as possible so the student and parents can see if the work was completed satisfactorily. Make positive, corrective comments.
    - 🐾 *Returning corrected assignments and tests <u>promptly</u> reinforces learning.*
  - Contact parents when two or three assignments have not been turned in. This will help the student keep up with the homework and not become hopelessly behind. (2)

Difficulty Managing Time

The following behaviors serve as general indicators. The student will not exhibit every characteristic listed. These behaviors may also be indicative of other problems.

> Having trouble organizing homework schedule and using calendar/planner
> Being unable to create a timeline to complete long-term assignments
> Lacking time estimation skills
> Starting homework/long-term assignments at the last minute
> Having difficulty allocating time to study for tests

Interventions

- Provide instruction in time <u>estimation</u> for the completion of homework assignments. (p. 120)

- Suggest that the student transfer the "To Do List" (p. 121) to the daily, weekly, and monthly planners/calendars, <u>estimating</u> and <u>allocating</u> the time it will take to complete the tasks. Schedule accordingly.

    - schedule the hardest, least liked tasks early in the study session to reduce the tendency to procrastinate.

        - 🐾 *The most difficult subject should <u>not</u> be left until last because the student may concentrate on the easier assignments and not have enough cognitive energy to finish the more difficult one.*

    - plan activities with breaks between tasks.

        - 🐾 *More difficult tasks require more frequent breaks.*

    - post the "To Do List" and calendars on the wall in front of the study desk to jog the memory.

    - cross off homework assignments as they are completed to provide a sense of accomplishment.

INITIATION/EXECUTION DIFFICULTIES

The following behaviors serve as general indicators. The student will not exhibit every characteristic listed. These behaviors may also be indicative of other problems.

> Appearing hypoactive/lacking energy/uninterested in doing homework
> Seeming "lazy" or "unmotivated"
> Procrastinating/hesitating/avoiding beginning homework
> Needing constant reminders to sit down and get started
> Requiring repeated encouragement/direction

Interventions

- Always assign homework with which the student can experience success. Ensure that the homework is at the <u>independent</u> instructional level (<u>90</u> percent of the material is understood). (p. 64)

- Provide clearly defined, <u>written directions</u> so that the student understands the assignment and the parents can provide assistance, if needed. Instructions should include:

    - purpose of the assignment (e.g., practice newly learned skill, review notes, prepare for test).

    - specific directions for doing the homework.

    - estimate of time that should be spent on each assignment.

Section V

- description of the type of work expected (e.g., short answers, complete sentences, written or oral report, poster).
- list of the materials needed to complete the assignment.
- due date(s).
- grading criteria.

- Determine whether the student understands the instructions and feels capable of performing the homework assignment. (2)

    🐾 *Often the teacher and parents are unaware that the student is not willing to admit that the work is too difficult to perform. This is particularly evident in middle and high school classes that expect significant amounts of increasingly difficult homework assignments to be completed independently.*

    - Ask for the directions to be restated by the student before sending assignments home.

        🐾 *Avoid using this approach in front of peers.*

    - Have the student begin the homework assignment in class.
    - Check the accuracy of the first few answers.

- Allow the student to select between two or three different homework alternatives (e.g., using a computer program to reinforce learning an academic skill, listening to a book on tape, watching a TV program or video related to the topic being studied, preparing a demonstration or oral report). This will increase the likelihood that the student will work on and complete the homework.

    🐾 *Be sure the choices are of equal difficulty and require the same amount of work so that the student does not learn to opt for the least challenging assignment.*

- Suggest that parents help the student get started by discussing the different assignments that need to be completed.

- Recommend that the parents provide assistance with the first two or three problems to make sure the assignment is understood and can be completed successfully. (2)

- Stress the importance of reminding the student that the homework must be finished before being allowed to go outside and play with friends, watch TV, play electronic games, etc.

- Instruct the parents to offer an enthusiastic, clearly stated comment regarding the student's initiation to task and work completion ("I was impressed with the way you started and finished your homework without any reminders!"). (2)

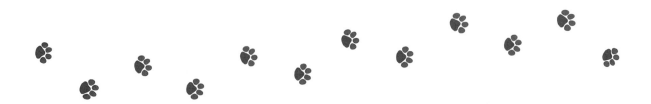

Chapter 23

IMPAIRED SELF-MONITORING/USE OF FEEDBACK/SELF-CORRECTION

The following behaviors serve as general indicators. The student will not exhibit every characteristic listed. These behaviors may also be indicative of other problems.

- Being unaware of losing focus and concentration
- Missing important details
- Making careless errors
- Neglecting to use strategies to monitor homework
- Continuing to work even though the materials are not understood
- Lacking skills to know how and when to self-correct
- Neglecting to stop and clarify thinking and then continue working
- Forgetting to use self-questioning to determine if understanding/completing assignment correctly
- Making same types of mistakes even though repeatedly shown correct way to solve problems

Interventions

- Assess the student's ability to self-monitor and self-correct homework by using materials at the <u>instructional</u> level (<u>70-85</u> percent of the material is familiar) so that some errors will be made.

- Suggest completing homework orally. Working aloud forces the student to slow down, listen to information, and self-correct.

- Teach the use of <u>self-questioning</u> to monitor assignments.

    ○ Help generate questions such as:

        • "What is the homework? Did I copy it correctly? Do I need to look on the class web site?"

        • "Do I know how to do it?"

        • "What does this word/phrase/sentence/problem/direction mean?"

        • "Does this make sense to me?"

        • "I don't understand my homework. What should I do? Should I ask someone to help me?"

        • "Have I finished all of my homework?"

        • "Have I made any mistakes?"

        • "Is there something different that I should do next time?"

        • "Did I put the work in my notebook? Is the notebook in my bookbag? Is my bookbag by the door?"

    ○ Prepare a list of the student's self-generated questions to serve as a visual guide.

    ○ Suggest placing the list of questions in the student's notebook.

- Recommend that the parents emphasize and cue the use of self-monitoring strategies that produced correct answers (e.g., "Be sure to read the instructions and underline important words before starting." or "Remember to work more slowly and use the cue card to follow the steps of the problem.").

- Review homework assignments with the student and analyze why answers were correct or incorrect (e.g., "I didn't read the directions." or "I was working too fast and forgot to use the cue card to solve the problem.").

285

Section V

- Remind the parents that the student will rarely complete homework without making mistakes. Suggest providing positive reinforcement for work effort and completion.

MEMORY PROBLEMS

Review interventions for Memory Problems in Chapter 14.

SHORT-TERM MEMORY PROBLEMS

Difficulty with Working Memory

The following behaviors serve as general indicators. The student will not exhibit every characteristic listed. These behaviors may also be indicative of other problems.

- Having trouble holding directions in memory when homework assignments are given orally
- Having difficulty remembering steps of tasks while executing them
- Rushing through assignments in order to not forget what one is in the process of completing
- Becoming overwhelmed when task has several parts or steps
- Using trial-and-error approaches rather than strategies
- Being unable to retrieve facts from long-term while completing assignments

Interventions

- Give the student <u>written</u> copies of homework assignments.
- Post written directions at the beginning of the class period to give the student with handwriting problems more time to record assignments.
- Use a homework "buddy," if needed, to write down assignments.
- Provide written directions that indicate the steps needed to complete assignments.
- Divide homework assignments into small segments.
- Recommend using a mind map or computer program to brainstorm ideas, organize, and/or recall the sequence for completing projects and solving problems.
- Suggest quietly thinking aloud while completing assignments.
- Using self-directed speech helps the student maintain information in working memory.
- Allow the use of a computer and calculator to circumvent the need to maintain information in working memory.
- Permit the parent to act as a scribe.

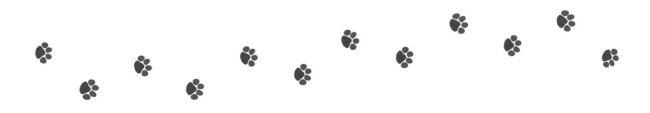

CHAPTER 24
TEST PREPARATION

- Explicitly <u>teach</u> study skills.

  - 🐾 *Do not assume that, when students say they are "studying," they know what studying means.*

- Give sufficient advance notice of tests to provide ample time to organize and prepare for tests.

- Create study guides which indicate the most important material to be learned.

- Point out information that is most likely to be asked on the test (specific facts, details, definitions; characters, places, events; comparison and contrast of ideas; predictions) so the student does not spend time studying content that will not be included.

- Identify the types of questions (multiple-choice, matching, true/false, fill-in-the-blank, short answer, essay).

- Review information for tests by having the students write questions for classmates to answer or write answers for which others must pose the questions.

- Indicate how the test will be graded and how much the test will count toward the final grade.

- Teach the student how to <u>allocate and manage time prior to test taking</u>.

  - 🐾 *Students with **ADHD** and executive dysfunction (**EDF**) typically procrastinate until the day before the test to begin studying.*

  Suggest that the student:

  - <u>always</u> write test dates in the assignment book and on the weekly and monthly calendars as they are assigned. (p. 120)
    - write reminders 1 week, 5 days, 3 days, and 1 day before tests.
    - highlight the review days and the test date.
  - determine the most important information to be learned.
  - decide how much time will be needed to encode the material.
  - divide study sessions into several small segments with breaks in between them. The beginning and ending of each segment is remembered better than the middle. Thus, there will be more opportunities to learn the information. (p. 139)
  - schedule most difficult material to be studied when the student is most alert.

- Recommend reviewing materials and class notes as part of daily and weekly study sessions. This avoids "cramming" the night before the test.

  - 🐾 *There is a rapid loss of information immediately following the lesson. The more time that elapses after learning without reinforcement, the more the information is forgotten. A quick review helps ensure that learning is permanent. Studying the material at a later time requires relearning, not just reviewing. (p. 143) (1)*

Section V

Suggest that the student:

- review the information 5-10 minutes after the lesson is completed and when memory is at its strongest.
- review 24 hours later after the material has been consolidated during sleep. (p. 74)
- review again after one week, one month, and six months.

  🐾 *Reinforcing learning at intervals negates the 80% decrease in memory over time.*

- Remind the student to study information emphasized in class (e.g., material that was repeated or written on the board or overhead; questions that were asked and discussed; clues that indicated importance "This is important to remember _____." "Listen carefully, _____." "This will be on the test _____.").

- Provide assistance in deciding what needs to be memorized and what can be reasoned out during the test.

- Discourage rote memorization.

  🐾 *Rote memorization of information is difficult for students with **ADHD**, **TS**, and/or **OCD**. Memorizing abstract, inherently uninteresting facts requires sustained attention and intact memory. Students who use rote memory to consolidate information into long-term memory will have considerable difficulty efficiently retrieving it on tests.*

- Teach effective <u>encoding strategies</u> based on the student's cognitive strengths. (2)

Suggest that the student with <u>verbal</u> strengths:

- <u>explain</u> difficult concepts to parents or friends without referring to the textbook or notes.
- form a <u>study group</u> with three or four peers to review the material and to reinforce learning.

  🐾 *A small group allows each member time to talk and ensures that the material is understood.*

  - choose classmates who are attentive, serious and knowledgeable about the topic, participate in class, ask important questions, and take good notes.
  - arrange several short meetings rather than only one the day before the test.
  - determine in advance the material to be discussed at each session.
  - suggest that each student prepare and present a specific section from the material, prepare and copy graphic organizers to share, and write and supply several questions.
  - review all the materials, class notes, old homework, and previous tests before the meetings.
  - think of questions to ask the other students.
  - brainstorm possible test questions and answers.
  - write outlines to proposed essay questions.
  - ask the teacher to clarify any areas of confusion.
  - conclude by reviewing the key concepts and important facts discussed.

- incorporate information to be learned into a story. The more ridiculous or silly the <u>story</u> the more likely it is to be recalled (e.g., story relating how Pierre from South Dakota fell in love with Helena from Montana as a means to learn those two state capitals).

- make <u>acronyms</u> by combining the first letter of each word to be encoded. For example, an <u>acronym</u> for recalling the names of the Great Lakes would be HOMES – Huron, Ontario, Michigan, Erie, Superior (source unknown).

- create <u>acrostics</u> by using the first letter of each word to be learned to make a sentence or rhyme. For example, an acrostic for memorizing the planets and their order is "<u>M</u>ost <u>V</u>olcanoes <u>E</u>rupt <u>M</u>aking <u>J</u>ust <u>S</u>uch <u>U</u>nusual <u>N</u>oises" for <u>M</u>ercury, <u>V</u>enus, <u>E</u>arth, <u>M</u>ars, <u>J</u>upiter, <u>S</u>aturn, <u>U</u>ranus, <u>N</u>eptune (source unknown). Make the acrostics humorous and absurd to ensure encoding.

- set new information to <u>music</u>. For example, it is a daunting task for a four-year-old child to learn the sequence of the twenty-six abstract letters of the alphabet. However, singing the "ABC" song or listening to *Schoolhouse Rock* recordings makes encoding of the sequence much easier.

Recommend that the student with <u>visual</u> strengths:

- complete a <u>graphic organizer</u>. (Appendix pp. 379–388)

- organize the information into a written <u>list, table, chart, or diagram</u>. This provides the same benefits as outlining in a more visual and nonsequential format. Furthermore, most of the information will be encoded by the time the organizer is completed.

- picture a <u>whiteboard</u> in the mind and draw pictures on it.

- create <u>images</u> of nonsensical or unusual pictures relating to the information.

- <u>draw</u> pictures to illustrate important points.

- use a <u>mind mapping strategy</u> to consolidate information. (p. 208)
    - emphasize various concepts and related facts by highlighting with different colors.
    - divide the diagram into several sections.
    - make meaningful shapes out of the diagram.

- utilize the "<u>Method of Loci</u>" strategy. (Ancient Rome)
    - visualize a familiar location such as the home and choose specific places (e.g., living room, dining room, family room, kitchen, hallway).
    - place the information to be remembered in the various rooms.
    - remember the information by walking through the rooms and recalling the items associated with each room.
    - use the same sequence of rooms each time that the strategy is applied.

- make <u>flash cards</u>. Using index cards, write vocabulary words, key concepts and facts, dates, questions, chemistry and physic elements, or formulas on one side and definitions, events, explanations, and answers on the other side.

    Flash cards are easily transported and can be studied throughout the day.

    - answer the questions aloud.
    - review the questions in random order.
    - concentrate on the answers that are difficult to remember.
    - study the flash cards with parents or friends.

Section V

- Recommend <u>self-testing</u>.

  Suggest that the student:

  - predict test questions from textbooks, class notes, cognitive maps, and charts.
    - turn main ideas and specific details into questions.
    - use headings and subheadings to construct questions.
  - outline the answers to the questions.
  - write the answers to the questions.
  - check study materials to correct or improve upon the responses.
  - practice math problems.
  - make a question and answer study recording.
    - record questions with sufficient pauses to answer them.
    - listen to a question, pause or turn off the tape.
    - answer the question.
    - listen to the correct response.

- Suggest reviewing cognitive strategies and graphic organizers a few minutes before taking the test.

- Offer the parents suggestions that will help the student prepare for tests.

  Ask the parents to:

  - create a study environment that is free from distractions. (p. 280)
  - encourage reviewing prior tests, lecture notes, study guides as part of the <u>daily</u> study periods.
  - make sure the student is well rested and has a healthy breakfast on the day of the test. If the student is tired and/or hungry, attention and thinking skills will be affected.
  - do not pressure the student to do well on tests.
  - avoid arguments and power struggles while the student is studying or getting ready for school on test days.

    🐾 *Excessive stress decreases learning and information retrieval.*

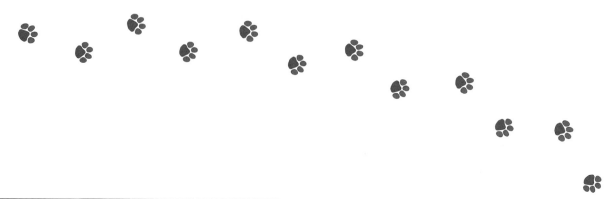

SECTION VI
TESTS

CHAPTER 25
TESTS

Tests are used to determine whether students have mastered academic skills and concepts. However, there are many factors other than a lack of achievement that influence test scores of students with **ADHD**, **TS**, and/or **OCD** (e.g., inattention, deregulated arousal levels, slow speed of processing, executive dysfunction, memory problems). Therefore, it is essential that accommodations be made to allow students to demonstrate knowledge without being penalized by their learning problems. The Individuals with Disabilities Education Act (IDEA) mandates that students with disabilities be provided accommodations based on their individual strengths and weaknesses. These accommodations must be documented in the students' Individual Education Plan (IEP)/504 Plan. Research suggests that the performance of students with disabilities is frequently improved with test accommodations. (1, 2, 3)

General Recommendations

- Be aware that excessive anxiety and stress regarding tests interfere with the student's ability to think clearly, recall information, and answer questions accurately.
    - Provide assurances that mistakes are normal and only indicate areas which need improvement.
- Analyze with the IEP/504 team the need for accommodations.
    - *Not all students need accommodations. Not all students with the same problems need the same accommodations. Students often need different accommodations in different academic areas.*
- Take into consideration the student's perception of the need for accommodations.
    - *Students who are allowed to take part in the decision-making process view accommodations positively and are willing and motivated to use them.*
- Determine, as appropriate, accommodations in the areas of setting/environment, timing/scheduling, presentation format, and response format.
- Document appropriate accommodations as part of the student's IEP/504 Plan. Specify the who, when, where, and how the accommodations will be implemented.
- Communicate accommodations to all test administrators.
- Teach the student how to use the accommodations in the classroom setting. Incorporate them into the student's daily curriculum and into teacher-prepared tests.
- Assess the student's perception of whether the accommodations helped. Modify as needed.
- Provide accommodations in the setting/environment in which the test is administered.
    - Create a quiet setting where the student feels comfortable and distractions are minimized.
    - Arrange seating near the test administrator so supervision and reminders to start working and remain on task can be provided.
        - *Students with **TS** and/or **OCD** may need to sit in the back of the room so they can concentrate on taking tests rather than suppressing tics or obsessions and compulsions.*
    - Administer tests in small group settings of 3-5 students.

Section VI

- Administer tests in the resource room or a separate location.
- Use a carrel or portable room divider.

- Modify the <u>timing/scheduling</u> of tests.
  - Schedule tests throughout the school year to reduce test-related anxiety and teach test-taking strategies.
    - 🐾 *Assign no more than one test each day.*
  - Give tests during the optimal arousal time. Many students with **ADHD**, **TS**, and/or **OCD** are not fully alert at the beginning of the day and experience a decline in energy and attention in the afternoon. When possible, schedule tests late morning or early afternoon.
  - Plan movement breaks during testing.
  - Divide tests into several parts and administer at different times.
    - 🐾 *This accommodation is important if the student with **OCD** becomes "stuck" on the need to make work "just so."*
  - Extend time limits or permit the test to be finished later in the day if time is expiring and the test is not completed.
  - Waive time limits. Timed tests often penalize the student with **ADHD**, **TS**, and/or **OCD** and do not accurately assess the amount of knowledge mastered. Note extra time on the test paper.
    - 🐾 *Test administrators often do not understand that the elimination of time constraints reduces anxiety and stress thereby allowing the test to be completed within time limits.*
  - Schedule extra time at the end of tests for checking answers.

- Take into consideration the <u>presentation format</u> of tests.
  - Modify the manner in which <u>test instructions</u> are delivered.
    - Always provide written directions.
    - Simplify the wording of the instructions.
    - Highlight or underline important words in directions.
    - Read the directions orally.
    - Repeat instructions, if necessary.
    - Ask for the directions to be restated before beginning the test. This will also help maintain the instructions in working memory until they can be followed.
      - 🐾 *Avoid using this approach in front of classmates.*
    - Have the student complete the first two problems and check for comprehension.
  - Design tests that accommodate <u>graphomotor problems</u>. (p. 68)
    - Give tests orally.
    - Do not require the student to copy questions or problems out of textbooks or off the board before answering them. This will eliminate the excessive time, stress, and frustration produced by the copying task.

- Provide teacher-prepared or duplicated copies of textbook tests.
- Ask an assistant/scribe to copy the questions or problems.
- Reduce the number of test items on a page.
- Provide extra space between test items.
- Leave ample workspace next to math problems.
- Increase the size of the space for the answer to be recorded.
- Write questions in a multiple-choice or true-false format. Eliminate fill-in-the-blank, short answer, and essay tests.
- Arrange multiple-choice test answers vertically. Place answer circles to the right of each possible answer.
- Assign letters to each of the possible answer choices when a student has difficulty on multiple-choice tests which require filling in bubbles. Allow the student to write or circle the letters.
- Avoid asking the student to recopy illegible test papers. Muscle soreness and fatigue can cause handwriting to deteriorate and produce stress and inappropriate behavior.
- Arrange for a demonstration of mastery (e.g., completion of a project, computer presentation, oral report).

- Modify the response format.
    - Give tests orally. Have aides, volunteers, or resource teachers read the questions and record word-for-word dictated answers. Allow the answers to be reviewed and edited by the student.
    - Permit moving or standing during test taking.
    - Permit essay questions to be answered in outline form.
    - Recommend recording answers on tape.
    - Suggest using a word processor with spelling and grammar checks.
    - Monitor placement of the student's answers on the test sheet.
    - Allow the use of a ruler or index card to assist tracking.
    - Accommodate retrieval problems.
        - *Fill-in-the-blank, short answer, and essay tests are especially difficult for the student who has difficulty accessing information stored in long-term memory.*
        - Provide word banks for fill-in-the-blank tests.
        - Give multiple-choice or true-false tests.
        - Assign open book tests.
        - Permit the use of cognitive cue cards/graphic organizers during testing.
        - Allow the use of a calculator or basic math facts charts. Calculators and charts bypass computational deficits, increase the ability to select the appropriate numbers and operations to be used, and help focus attention on problem solving.
            - *It is not possible to be successful using a calculator if the math concept is not understood.*

Section VI

NONSTANDARDIZED/TEACHER-PREPARED TESTS

- Avoid evaluating the student's achievement based on a single test at the end of a grading period. Cumulative tests require the organization and memorization of more material than the student can successfully handle.

- Use tests to analyze which skills need to be practiced or retaught.

- Evaluate improvement rather than compare the student's test performance to that of the other students.

  🐾 *Assess privately, not publicly.*

- Ask the students in the class to write the test questions.

- Balance test questions between understanding and factual recall.

- Limit the number of questions asked to ensure the quality and accuracy of the responses and to determine mastery of skills and knowledge.

- Assess content, not handwriting, punctuation, syntax, or spelling.

- Arrange math test items from easiest to most difficult.

- Adjust scoring criteria.

  ○ Suggest re-answering incorrect responses for a higher grade.

  ○ Allow tests to be retaken until passing grades are achieved.

  ○ Assign partial credit if the correct math procedure or formula was used, but the answer was wrong due to a calculation error.

  ○ Award points based on effort.

STANDARDIZED TESTS

Standardized tests are used to measure the students' achievement relative to same age and grade peers. These tests are always administered in a specified manner so that the individual student's scores can be compared with the scores of other students who took the test under the same conditions. Students with **ADHD, TS,** and/or **OCD** often have difficulty demonstrating their knowledge on standardized tests.

- Provide direct training and extensive practice in taking standardized tests.

- Design practice test booklets using a standardized format.

  ○ Provide a separate answer sheet.

  ○ Include increasingly more difficult paragraphs that contain unfamiliar words.

- Teach the student how to interpret different types of questions. The questions posed on standardized tests are often quite different than those asked on teacher-prepared tests (e.g., "The purpose for the last sentence in the article is to _____." "Which statement is NOT true?" "There is enough information in the story to show that _____." "What question does the first paragraph answer?" "The author uses the word corruption to mean _____.").

  ○ Search through outdated tests and note the type of questions.

Chapter 25

- Use these types of questions when making practice tests.
- Provide direct instruction for answering multiple-choice questions as standardized tests are constructed with multiple-choice formats. (p. 300)

- Construct <u>reading comprehension tests</u>.

  🐾 *Write questions that assess both factual recall and inferential reasoning.*

  Suggest that the student:

  - read the questions before reading the paragraphs.
    - paraphrase the questions.
    - compare paraphrased questions to the original questions.
  - read <u>all</u> of the paragraphs even if unknown words are encountered.
  - underline important points in the paragraphs.

- Design tests that evaluate <u>interpretation of tables and charts</u>.

  Suggest that the student:

  - avoid memorizing the material in the charts and tables.
  - scan the information to determine how the material is organized so that an answer can easily be located.
  - read a question and refer to the table or chart to locate the answer.

- Provide practice taking <u>math tests</u>. Be sure to include questions which assess estimation, rounding, money, measurement, and time.

  Suggest that the student:

  - observe and underline operational signs, decimals, etc.
  - read word problems carefully and underline important words and facts.

    🐾 *Check comprehension of the vocabulary of mathematics (e.g., sum, difference, product, quotient, greater than, less than).*

  - estimate answers.
  - work the problems on a separate sheet of paper.
  - look at all the choices and then choose the answer that exactly matches the calculation.
  - use the estimate to determine whether the calculations appear to be correct. (p. 234)

- Review all answers and ask how the answers were derived.

Section VI

- Intervene if the student is having difficulty reading the questions in the standardized test booklet and then using a separate answer sheet.
    - Have aides, volunteers, or resource teachers read the questions and record the answers dictated by the student.
    - Permit writing or circling the answers in the test booklet. Have an aide transfer the answers onto the computer sheet.
        - *The student with **ADHD** and/or **TS** may have difficulty filling in the circles on computerized test sheets due to poor fine motor control and inattention to visual details. If the answers are not completely filled in or marked in the wrong circle even though the answer is known, the answer will be scored incorrect. The student with **OCD** may need to compulsively fill the circles until they are perfect, thus affecting test completion.*
    - Suggest folding the test booklet so that only one page is visible.
    - Provide an index card to act as a placeholder on the page.
    - Monitor the student carefully during testing.
        - Make sure the student is on the correct page in the booklet and on the answer sheet when the last question on the page is answered and the page is turned over.
        - Be sure the numbers in the test booklet match those on the answer sheet.
- Encourage the student to use <u>all</u> of the allotted time to proofread, check, and edit answers.

Suggest that the student:

- attempt to answer the difficult questions that were skipped, if guessing is not penalized.
- try for partial credit by writing everything that is known about the question.
- reread troublesome questions and answers to make sure the questions were clearly interpreted and no mistakes were made.
- be the <u>last</u> student to turn in the test.
    - *The student with **ADHD** who is impulsive and hyperactive often has difficulty using extra time to check the answers. Divide a test into segments. Have the student check answers after finishing each section and provide a movement break. This will allow a more accurate assessment of the student's mastery of information.*

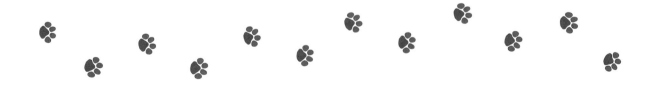

CHAPTER 26
TEST-TAKING STRATEGIES

Students with **ADHD**, **TS**, and/or **OCD** frequently do not acquire effective strategies spontaneously, tend to become very anxious during testing, and forget the academic skills that have been learned. Test-taking skills must be directly taught. (1, 2, 3, 4)

- Encourage the student to bring all the necessary materials, such as several pencils with erasers, paper, ruler, and a calculator.

- Have extra supplies available. These can be provided by the parents and stored by the teacher.

- Select a place without distractions so tics can be released. Suppressing tics interferes with concentration.

- Recommend jotting down all the information that might be forgotten (mnemonic strategies, formulas) immediately upon receiving the test.

- Instruct and practice previewing the whole test rather than impulsively starting to mark the test paper.

  Recommend that the student:

  ○ listen to or read all directions carefully.

  ○ scan the entire test first.

  ○ examine the test format (multiple-choice, true-false, matching, short answer, essay).

  ○ determine the number of points assigned to each question to avoid discovering an essay question that comprises one-third of the test grade with no time to complete it.

  ○ find out if there is a penalty for guessing. Avoid guessing if points for incorrect responses are subtracted from the final grade.

- Teach the student how to allocate enough time to answer each question.

  Suggest that the student:

  ○ divide the time according to the number of questions.

  ○ allow more time to answer essay questions and those worth the most points.

  ○ schedule time at the end to make sure answers or parts of answers have not been omitted and to complete unanswered questions.

- Recommend answering the easiest questions first and then the ones with the highest point value in order to earn as many points as possible.

  Suggest that the student:

  ○ mark or circle the numbers of the more difficult questions.

  ○ return to the unanswered questions after completing the test.

Section VI

- Teach strategies for answering <u>multiple-choice questions</u>.

  Suggest that the student:

  - cover up the choices, read the question, and try to answer it.
  - determine from the stem whether the question has one or more ("which two") correct choices.
  - read the stem with each choice before selecting the answer.
  - consider each of the choices as a true-false statement and select the statement that is true. (see strategies for true-false questions.)
  - recognize that positive choices are more likely to be correct than negative choices.
  - underline words in the questions that may help determine the correct choice.
  - cross out choices that are obviously incorrect.
  - eliminate choices that mean the same thing.
  - pay attention to all questions and answers that contain double negatives. Cross out negative words and then answer the question.
  - remember that, if the stem ends with "a," then the choice will begin with a consonant. If the stem ends with "an," the answer will begin with a vowel.
  - eliminate choices that are grammatically incorrect.
  - select "all of the above" if two or three choices are correct and "none of the above" if one choice is incorrect.
  - <u>guess</u>, if there is <u>no penalty</u>.
  - be reluctant to change an answer as the first guess is more likely to be correct. This is particularly true for students with **OCD**.

- Teach strategies for answering <u>true-false questions</u>.

  Suggest that the student:

  - assume that a statement is false if any part of it is false (e.g., name, date, fact).
  - assume that a statement is most likely <u>false</u> if it contains <u>absolute words</u> such as "everyone," "nobody," "every," "all," "best," "none," "only," "always," "never," or "definitely."
  - assume that the statement frequently is <u>true</u> when there are <u>qualifiers</u> including "often," "seldom," "some," "most," "many," "few," "generally," "frequently," "usually," "sometimes," or "probably."
  - mark a statement as true unless it is actually false as most true-false exams generally contain more "T" than "F" statements.
  - guess if there is no guessing penalty because there is a 50-50 chance of the answer being correct.

- Teach strategies for answering <u>matching tests</u>.

  Suggest that the student:

  - determine if there are an equal number of matches or whether a response might be used more than once.

- focus on only <u>one</u> column.
- match each item in that column to all items in the second column and select the appropriate match.
- match easier associations first.
- mark through each match as it is selected so that it is easier to locate the remaining items. However, do not cross out items if there is an unequal number of matches.

• Teach strategies for answering <u>fill-in-the-blank</u> or <u>short answer tests</u>.

Suggest that the student:

- read the question carefully as some questions have several parts to be answered.
- decide the type of response needed (e.g., person, place, date).
- highlight or underline key words in the questions.
- use grammatical clues as indicators of correct answers.
- write short answers which contain as much information as possible.
- guess, if there is no penalty for guessing, rather than leaving an answer blank. Partial credit may be awarded.

• Teach strategies for answering <u>essay questions</u>.

Suggest that the student:

- allocate more time to essay questions.
- read essay questions carefully and highlight or underline the different parts of the questions.
- underline or circle all instructional words.

  Be sure that student has learned the meaning of the different instructional words. A list of the words might be placed in the strategy ("trick") book and consulted when they are forgotten. (p. 64)

  • <u>analyze</u> – describe the whole, identify the parts, and explain the relationship between the parts and the whole.
  • <u>compare/contrast</u> – explain the similarities and differences between two or more concepts.
  • <u>define</u> – provide a clear, concise, and accurate definition.
  • <u>discuss</u> – write in-depth reasons, facts, details that demonstrate understanding.
  • <u>explain</u> – clarify the reasons or causes of something.
  • <u>illustrate</u> – draw a graphic organizer or picture to describe the major components of a concept.
  • <u>justify</u> – argue for or against one's statements or conclusions.
  • <u>outline</u> – outline the main ideas and details.
  • <u>relate</u> – explain the relationship between ideas.
  • <u>summarize</u> – succinctly paraphrase main ideas and details.

- ask for clarification if the directions are not understood.

Section VI

- note in the margins ideas and mnemonic strategies that relate to the answers.
- treat each essay question as a mini-report (e.g., brainstorm ideas; organize thoughts with a graphic organizer or outline; and write an introductory paragraph that directly answers the question, paragraphs that provide supporting ideas and details, and a concluding paragraph). (pp. 211-212)
- write legible and complete sentences and paragraphs.
- stop writing when the time allocated for the answer is over, leave some space, and begin the next essay question.
- complete answers or outline remaining information during the scheduled review time. Partial credit may be assigned for demonstrating knowledge of the material.

- Teach strategies for solving <u>tests requiring calculations</u> (e.g., math, chemistry, physics). Suggest that student:

  - review strategies just prior to testing to enhance retrieval.
  - write in the margins or on the back of the test paper all the mnemonics, formulas, equations, and/or rules pertaining to the test before beginning to work the test problems.
  - highlight or underline calculation signs in computational problems.
  - highlight or underline words indicating different operations in word problems.
  - estimate answers to determine whether the answer appears to be correct. (p. 234)
  - skip difficult problems and come back later if time permits.
  - leave space between answers to recheck or rework problems.
  - recheck all answers using a different strategy (e.g., adding down a column and then checking by adding up the column; dividing a problem and then multiplying the answer times the divisor).
  - write down all the steps in problems as partial credit might be awarded even if the answer is incorrect.

TEST REVIEW

- Review the graded test with the student and determine the reasons for the mistakes. (5) Were the mistakes caused by:

  - getting anxious when taking the test?
  - having to handwrite the answers?
  - not studying the appropriate material?
  - not using the correct study skills?
  - not spending enough time studying?
  - having difficulty with the format of the test (multiple-choice, fill-in-the-blank, matching, short answer, essay)?
  - not understanding or misinterpreting the questions or directions?
  - not paying attention to relevant details?

- not being able to recall or retrieve the information?
- not asking for help when the material was not understood?
- making careless mistakes?
- rushing through test and not checking answers?
- running out of time?

- Recommend saving the test for later review and cumulative tests.
- Recommend reworking errors to discover why the answers were incorrect.
- Suggest looking for answers to incorrect responses in the textbook, supplementary reading materials, class notes, lab work, and previous quizzes and tests. This will help the student prepare for future tests.
- Stress saving the tests to review for cumulative tests.

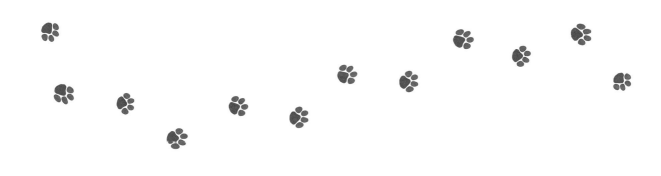

SECTION VII
SOCIAL COMPETENCE

CHARACTERISTICS OF POPULAR CHILDREN
They are often seen smiling and laughing.
They greet other children.
They extend invitations to other children.
They converse with other children.
They share with other children.
They compliment other children.
They have a good appearance.

Richard Lavoie. (2000). International Learning Disability Convention. Reno, NV

CHAPTER 27
SOCIAL SKILLS INTERVENTIONS

Students with **ADHD** are at high risk for a "social disability." (1) They often have difficulty initiating and sustaining conversations; communicating their own ideas, feelings, and needs; understanding and empathizing with others; expressing and interpreting verbal and nonverbal social cues; getting along with peers; negotiating, compromising, and resolving conflict situations; and/or forming and maintaining developmentally appropriate friendships. Comorbidity associated with ADHD presents a greater potential for social dysfunction than **ADHD-only**. Social skills do not spontaneously improve as a function of age. Rather, research suggests that social competence deteriorates as social interactions require increasingly more mature and complex behaviors during adolescence. (2, 3)

22% of boys and 15% of girls with **ADHD** in clinically referred samples were determined to be socially disabled. (1, 4)

Teachers rated as socially impaired:

53% of ADHD, Predominately Hyperactive/Impulsive type
59% of ADHD, Predominately Inattentive type
82% of ADHD, Combined type (5)

Behaviors associated with **ADHD** that adversely affect social functioning may include several of the following: (6)

ADHD-C	ADHD-I
Interacting aggressively	Being shy/passive/withdrawn
Displaying intense emotional reactions	Displaying few emotional reactions
Interrupting/intruding on others	Avoiding peer interactions
Trying to control/direct peers	Engaging in solitary play
Having problems sustaining attention	Having problems focusing attention
Responding impatiently/impulsively	Processing social interactions slowly
Misinterpreting social cues	Missing nonverbal social cues
Being insensitive to needs of others	Showing little interest in others
Neglecting to self-monitor/inhibit/shift behavior	Appearing lethargic/daydreamy/underaroused
Being overly competitive	Preferring noncompetitive activities

 ADHD-Hyperactive-Impulsive type has not been included in more recent studies comparing the behaviors associated with the disorders as the subtype is primarily found in preschool students and is often a precursor to ADHD-Combined type. (7)

Figure 27.1. Impact of ADHD on Social Functioning

Section VII

The social disabilities that the students with **ADHD** experience are considered to have different causes and outcomes.

ADHD-C students, who are intrusive and aggressive, are often rejected. They are considered by their peers to be unpopular and the "least liked" students in the classroom. Unable to handle the frustration of peer rejection, they frequently become angry and react aggressively. A cycle of aggression, rejection, and aggression is established. Although often possessing knowledge of appropriate social behavior, they are unable to use these skills due to their impulsivity and overarousal. This **"social performance deficit"** (8, 9) interferes with students' opportunities to have normal social relationships and practice prosocial behaviors. Being disliked and rejected leads to poor self-esteem and secondary psychological problems. Furthermore, a social disability in childhood may result in poor social outcome in adolescence, including increased peer rejection, association with friends who use alcohol and drugs, substance abuse, conduct disorder, delinquency, school failure, and school dropout. (10, 11, 12)

ADHD-I students, on the other hand, often have not mastered the necessary social skills and interact awkwardly and inappropriately. These students are rated by their classmates as shy, teased, and "left out." They have difficulty making and keeping friends, paying attention to and properly interpreting social cues, and communicating effectively. A **"social skills deficit"** or a deficit in social knowledge (13) promotes a cycle of social neglect, withdrawal, and isolation. (8, 9)

*Clinical and teaching experience suggests that the distinction between the subtypes of ADHD is not so clear. Some students with **ADHD-C** have not learned strategies (clues) that guide and direct behavior and help solve problems. Others do not perceive and interpret accurately verbal and nonverbal social signals (cues).*

Evidence indicates that students with **TS** may struggle with the development of age-appropriate peer relationships. A large population-based study found that 24% of students with tics and 39% of students with **TS** have more social problems than those without tics (15%). (14) While some students with **TS-only** have more trouble with peer relationships than their classmates and tend to be socially withdrawn, students with **TS plus ADHD** exhibit poorer social adjustment than students with **TS-only** and normally developing peers. It is the problems that accompany **ADHD** which interfere with social expression and understanding rather than the severity of the tics or the chronicity of the disorder. (15, 16, 17, 18).

OCD may likewise have a significant impact on social competence during childhood and adolescence. (19, 20, 21) The Obsessive-Compulsive Foundation notes: "Friendships and peer relationships are often stressful for those with OCD because they try very hard to conceal their rituals from peers. When the disorder is severe, this becomes impossible, and the child may be teased or ridiculed. Even when the OCD is not severe, it can affect friendships because of the amount of time spent preoccupied with obsessions and compulsions, or because friends react negatively to unusual OCD-related behaviors." (22) Approximately one-third of the students with OCD are reported to have difficulty establishing and maintaining friendships, engaging in peer activities, and experiencing positive peer interactions. (20, 23) Students with **OCD plus ADHD** experience many of the social problems associated with ADHD and are more impaired than those with **OCD-only**. (21, 24)

Chapter 27

> **Social behavior is, at least in part, a brain function just like memory and language ... Even though we typically think of these emotional, psychological, or moral capacities as learned, the existence of a social brain indicates that our social skills also have a partly biological basis.**
>
> John J. Ratey, M.D. (2001). <u>A User's Guide to the Brain</u>. New York, NY: Random House. (p.296)

General Recommendations

Review Classroom and Individual Student Interventions in Chapters 8 and 9.

- 🐾 *While medication is the most common intervention for* **ADHD**, *medication alone will not remediate a social deficit. The socially disabled student requires <u>direct</u>, <u>intense</u>, and <u>ongoing</u> treatment.*

- Ensure availability for learning and practicing social skills.
    - Determine whether the student is able to perform socially in all settings.
        - 🐾 *Unmedicated teenagers have an increased rate of risk-taking behaviors.* (p. 9)

- Assess the processing of social information through the auditory, visual, and tactile modalities. The student must be able to adequately process and express that which is seen and heard and then respond appropriately. The student who has auditory or visual problems cannot accurately attend to and interpret verbal or nonverbal social cues. The student who is hypersensitive to being touched by anyone and/or anything may react aggressively. The student with a heightened awareness of sounds may become agitated in social settings (e.g., cafeteria, playground, assemblies). (25)

- Determine the strengths and weaknesses of the student's social behavior by observing the student during peer interactions.

- Match interventions to the student's <u>individual</u> cognitive and social deficits. (26)
    - Integrate social skills lessons into the daily curriculum.
    - Design interventions that are based on the student's cognitive (learning) style (e.g., use discussions and role-playing when addressing the social problems of the highly verbal student; use visual materials and written scripts with the student who has strong visualization skills).
        - 🐾 *When planning social interventions, remember that many students with a "social disability" tend to be more <u>immature</u> than same age classmates.*
    - Explain and discuss the unspoken social rules that often are not directly taught, but most students intuitively understand and use (e.g., looking the other student in the eye and smiling, maintaining spatial boundaries, listening and not interrupting, making appropriate and relevant comments, taking turns, observing verbal and nonverbal social cues and then adapting behavior accordingly). (27)
    - Teach anger management and problem-solving strategies to the student with a "social performance deficit."

Section VII

- Engage the student with a "social skills deficit" in a social skills program (e.g., teach strategies for initiating and maintaining friendships, processing verbal and nonverbal social cues, communicating effectively). (6, 28)

- Divide social skills into successive steps.
  - Focus on only one social behavior at a time to enhance attention and responsiveness to intervention.
  - Do not progress to the next step until the previous skill has been mastered.

- Recognize that intense instruction, guidance, and assistance are required to teach social skills. They must be taught, reviewed, practiced, and reinforced in all settings.

- Be aware that research suggests that the expression of feelings and attitudes is primarily conveyed through <u>verbal and nonverbal social cues</u> rather than spoken words. (29)

  - 55% of the message is expressed by nonverbal cues (e.g., facial expressions, body language, gestures).
  - 38% of the meaning is projected by the tone of voice.
  - 7% of the communication is attributed to the words spoken.
    - 🐾 *These figures cannot be generalized to all communication situations. However, they underscore the importance of body language and tone of voice rather than the actual words spoken.*

- Teach and practice the <u>verbal expression of emotions</u>. (30)

  Suggest that the student:

  - act out different social situations using verbal social cues. <u>Exaggerate</u> to stress the feeling being conveyed.
  - practice talking with a normal tone, volume, and intensity.
  - tape record self talking and evaluate tone, volume, and intensity.
  - watch for a prearranged signal indicating improper tone, volume, intensity.
  - provide a script and rehearse effective verbal responses to the feelings of others. (31)
  - practice the difference between language used with classmates, same sex peers, teachers, principal, parents, and other adults.

- Teach and practice the <u>nonverbal expression of feelings</u>. (30)

  Suggest that the student:

  - role-play and <u>exaggerate</u> different social interactions and portray feelings with appropriate facial expressions and body positions.
  - play "Charades." Act out an emotion using a variety of nonverbal cues to express the feeling and ask the other students to interpret the feeling.

Chapter 27

- Create opportunities that promote a sense of belonging, provide the means to practice prosocial behaviors, and build confidence and self-esteem.
    - Determine peers with whom the student might prefer to interact and attempt to facilitate interactions.
    - Highlight and point out interests shared between students.
    - Have the students in the classroom talk with each other and discover what they have in common. (31)
    - Organize some classroom activities around the student's special interests and talents. If the student can share information about a topic, be the classroom artist, or act as the Internet investigator, the student may earn the respect of classmates.
    - Help the student decide which classmates are good friends to everyone (peers all students like). Discuss the qualities that make these classmates good friends. (31)
    - Appoint a "Classroom Captain for the Day." Have the students discuss and list the things that the captain should do to be a good leader.
        - Suggest playing "Watch Your Captain." (Classmates carefully watch and try to "do what the captain does." The next captain is the student who comes the closest to exhibiting prosocial behaviors.). (31)
    - Assign the student an appropriate classroom "job" (responsibility) or a "no-fail" leadership activity (e.g., office messenger, teacher's assistant, attendance keeper, class librarian). (31)
        - Reinforce the student when the task is completed.
            - *If the student has difficulty controlling behavior, reward effort.*
        - Pay particular attention to the withdrawn student. Make the student feel a part of the class by assigning a task that can be carried out successfully.

- Be sensitive to the <u>emotional needs of the student</u>.
    - Establish a policy of no bullying (e.g., teasing, name-calling, harassment, embarrassment, humiliation, intimidation). (pp. 54-57)
    - Model understanding, acceptance, and care for the student.
        - *The teacher's attitude is the most important factor in preventing negative interactions.*
    - Engage the support of the other students.
        - Educate peers about the symptoms of ADHD, TS, and OCD that impact social behaviors. (p. 53)
            - *Be sure to obtain permission from the student and parents before discussing the disorders.*
        - Assign willing peers with prosocial skills to be "buddies" (e.g., lunch buddy, free-time companion, project partner, or after-school friend). A peer buddy system promotes friendship, respect for individual differences, and prosocial interactions.
            - *Make sure the student is comfortable having a buddy assigned and that the buddy wants the job.*
    - Hold class meetings to discuss social issues. (p. 58)

Section VII

- Reduce competition between students.

- Establish <u>cooperative learning experiences</u> and group activities to optimize social interactions (e.g., work on a science experiment, write and publish a class newsletter, create a bulletin board or mural, complete an art project).

    - Assign the student to a group that will be accepting and exhibit prosocial behaviors.

    - Keep the size of the group small so that the student has many opportunities to interact and use communication skills.

    - Schedule the group activity at a time when the student is most likely to successfully interact with others.

    - Guide the group process (e.g., "Before selecting a topic, let's allow everyone a chance to offer an idea. Everyone will have a turn to speak but must respect each other's ideas.").

    - Predetermine roles (e.g., secretary, group artist, computer expert, research specialist, oral presenter). Capitalize on the student's interests and talents and select a task with which success can be experienced.

    - Review group rules before beginning an activity.

    - Monitor group interactions.

    - Frequently rearrange the composition of the groups to provide opportunities for interacting with different classmates.

- Encourage participation in extracurricular activities with peers who share similar interests (e.g., <u>structured</u> and <u>supervised</u> art, music, acting, chess, photography, computer clubs).

- Create opportunities for the student to support others such as giving computer instruction to a classmate with less advanced skills or helping younger students with reading, writing, math, and physical education. Allow the student to act as an aide and accompany elementary students on field trips. Mentoring helps improve not only academic competence but also social skills.

- Increase structure, support, supervision, and cueing during unstructured activities.

- Reinforce the student frequently in front of peers both inside and outside the classroom. If the student can experience a sense of accomplishment, it will improve the student's self-esteem and provide an incentive for prosocial behavior in the future.

- Recommend learning and practicing the social skills offered in this chapter of the handbook in a <u>socialization group</u>. (25)

    - *A social skills group is by far the most powerful setting for teaching appropriate social skills. The small group environment provides opportunities for the student to learn and practice social skills, receive positive feedback from peers, and apply behavior in other settings. Group participation must be <u>ongoing</u>, <u>not time limited</u>. Social skills training should be conducted by two experienced specialists who know how to teach practical strategies for remediating social deficits. The specialists should model and reinforce appropriate social skills during instructional times and assist the student who is struggling.*

- Read and discuss books/stories that reflect real-life social problems and outcomes. Books can help the student view situations from the perspective of others, develop empathy, and evaluate problem-solving strategies.
    - Match the story to the social skill being taught and reinforced.
    - Circumvent attentional and memory problems by choosing a story that can be read and discussed in one lesson.
    - Select a story with a simple, straightforward plot.
- Diminish the stress experienced by the student who has a <u>social anxiety disorder</u> and is worried about being embarrassed or humiliated in front of others. (Appendix p. 372)
    - Help the student understand that fearing embarrassment in front of peers causes the student to withdraw and avoid social activities.
        - Determine if circumstances at school or during social events are producing anxiety. (e.g., being embarrassed by the teacher, teased by peers)
        - Confront negative thoughts ("Nobody likes me. No one will ask me to play!"). Ask "What happened to make you think that?"
        - Encourage the use of positive self-statements ("I can ask to join a group of girls on the playground. If they act like they don't want to include me, I won't get upset and will find other friends.").
        - Provide reassurance by noting that similar situations were handled appropriately.
    - Provide assistance with peer interactions.
        - Design small group cooperative learning activities. (p. 59)
        - Permit sitting with familiar or preferred classmates.
        - Role-play different social scenarios.
            - *Always provide the student with a suitable conversational partner.*
    - Intervene if the student is anxious about being called on in class or reading aloud.
        - Schedule small group interactions in which the student can demonstrate special interests and talents in front of friendly peers.
        - Call on all students rather than focusing on the anxious student.
    - Design a gradual approach to giving demonstrations and presenting reports. (32)

    Suggest that the student:
    - select a topic of personal interest and familiarity.
    - incorporate visual aids, pictures, or diagrams to lessen the stress of forgetting due to anxiety.
    - observe how classmates introduce topics, where they look, how long they speak, what they do when mistakes are made, and how they conclude presentations. Discuss with teacher.
    - practice the presentation in advance with parents, siblings or trusted adults.
    - audiotape or videotape the presentation so classmates can listen to it.
    - choose a classmate to read the report.

Section VII

- take turns reading the paper with another student.
- practice making presentations in front of a small group of four or five compatible students.
- give presentations to class as anxiety is reduced.
  - 🐾 *Incorporate activities into the daily curriculum that require all students to speak in front of others in order to develop confidence in public speaking.*
- Positively reinforce all attempts to conquer social anxiety. Acknowledge that the student handled the stressful situation and was successful at doing something considered too difficult to do.

- Encourage parental involvement in promoting age-appropriate social skills.

Suggest that the parents:

- provide social exposure through clubs and activities outside of school (e.g., art, dance, chorus, band, drama, sewing, scouting, 4-H, Boys and Girls clubs, sports, religious groups).
- arrange social activities that provide successful experiences (e.g., having play dates in the home; going to a playground, pizza restaurant, movie, or concert; playing miniature golf; bowling).
  - schedule play dates on a regular basis.
  - invite only one friend at a time to provide ample opportunities to learn and practice social skills (e.g., taking turns, problem solving, negotiating).
  - permit the student to select a peer with similar interests. However, the other student should not have social difficulties.
    - 🐾 *Students who tend to be immature may need to interact with younger students.*
  - plan a short, structured, interactive activity (game, art project). Increase duration as the student is able to socialize successfully.
  - play games with the student prior to play dates so that the rules and strategies of games are understood. If the student typically tries to change the rules of games, indicate that the game will be discontinued if the rules are not followed.
  - remain in close proximity and be prepared to facilitate interactions. Intervene if the student becomes overly excited, irritable, or frustrated. Many times a word at the right time or another distracting activity can save a situation that is about to turn negative.
  - discourage solitary activities such as watching television, using the computer, and playing electronic games.
- Recommend that the student join a sport team to provide the opportunity to interact with peers and practice prosocial behaviors.
  - 🐾 *Sport activities are often topics of common interest among students and informally organized on the playground.*

Suggest that the parents:

- take into consideration the student's interests and ability level when choosing a sport. There are usually teams available that accommodate students with different skill levels.
  - 🐾 *The **ADHD-C** student may prefer more active and competitive sports (baseball, football, soccer, wrestling) if visual-motor problems do not interfere. The **ADHD-I** student may prefer more noncompetitive sports (swimming, horseback riding, hiking, martial arts).*

- make sure the sport activity is structured and has appropriate adult supervision.
- educate the instructor or coach about the symptoms associated with the disorder(s) so that the student will not be considered a "behavior problem." Explain the student's neurology rather than just hoping a problem will not arise. (31)
- interview the martial arts teacher and visit the studio before enrolling the student.
  - *Martial arts teach self-discipline and self-control and encourage individual achievement. They do not make the student aggressive. Some leaders pair making acceptable grades and respecting others with being promoted to a higher level.*
- interview the coach and assess the league to ensure that they are not too competitive, allow each member to play, and stress having a good time over winning.
- select a team that focuses on teaching and practicing the skills needed to play the sport and provides extra practice for splinter skills that interfere with success.
- determine whether good sportsmanship is taught as well as encouraged (e.g., taking turns, following the rules of the game, working together, knowing when it is appropriate to play aggressively, complimenting other players, winning is not the most important goal).
- be sure the coach offers positive reinforcement for trying and does not criticize or stress mistakes.
- allow the student to make the choice.
- practice with the student the skills needed to participate successfully (throw, catch, kick a ball; dribble a basketball).
- arrange for an assistant (e.g., older student, trusted relative, someone from the Big Brother program) to practice specific sport and game skills with the student and to provide social skills instruction.
  - *If the student has difficulty playing team sports, encourage participation in a sport that is based on individual rather than group performance (e.g., gymnastics, field and track, bicycling, tennis, golf, skating).*

Tics/obsessions/compulsions, underarousal/slow processing speed, inattention/impulsivity/hyperactivity, executive dysfunction, and/or memory problems frequently interfere with ability to interact socially.

UNDERAROUSAL/SLOW COGNITIVE PROCESSING SPEED

The following behaviors serve as general indicators. The student will not exhibit every characteristic listed. These behaviors may also be indicative of other problems.

Having difficulty sustaining focused attention during social conversations/interactions
Appearing not to listen
Being slow to understand/grasp social interactions
Being unable to quickly adapt to changing social situations
Failing to respond to peers who try to initiate conversations
Retrieving words/thoughts slowly in conversations
Responding with short, unclear statements
Needing additional time to respond in conversations/interactions
Hesitating to participate in conversations/social situations

Section VII

Processing speed affects the ability to quickly assimilate and integrate incoming social information. Research studies have shown that slow speed of processing is associated with inattentive behaviors and is common among students with **ADHD-I**, **TS**, and **OCD**. (33, 34, 35, 36, 37)

Interventions

Review interventions for Underarousal and Slow Processing Speed in Chapter 10.

- Teach awareness and educate those interacting with the student.
- Allow additional "thinking time."
- Limit the number of students with whom the student interacts.
- Teach appropriate delaying tactics.

    Suggest that the student:

    - ask peers to speak more slowly.
    - say "Give me a minute and let me think about that."

- Teach strategies for appearing to process and understand conversations.

    Suggest that the student:

    - nod in an affirmative way or say, "Hmm." "That's very interesting." "I agree."
    - ask for clarification.

- Instruct the student to <u>not</u> go first when playing games or sports to provide enough time to observe and understand the instructions and rules before needing to follow them and to process the interactions of the other students.

- Encourage the parents to schedule only one playmate/friend at a time to decrease the need to quickly process and respond to complex social interactions.

INATTENTION/IMPULSIVITY/HYPERACTIVITY

The following behaviors serve as general indicators. The student will not exhibit every characteristic listed. These behaviors may also be indicative of other problems.

Impact on Communications

Interjecting unconnected comments into conversations
Beginning conversations at awkward moments
Jumping from one topic of conversation to another
Having difficulty listening to/following conversations
Interrupting ongoing conversations inappropriately
Overlooking verbal and nonverbal social cues (tones of voice/meaning of words/facial expressions/body language/gestures)
Losing interest/becoming bored/walking away in middle of conversations
Talking excessively when not appropriate
Giving over detailed accounts/failing to notice signs of listener's disinterest/boredom
Having difficulty moderating tone of voice and language when upset/stressed – seeming disrespectful/rude/inconsiderate
Making socially inappropriate/embarrassing/rude comments without realizing/meaning them
Having trouble inhibiting aggressive/negative comments

Impact on Behavior

 Daydreaming/looking around/staring into space
 Being distracted by/preoccupied with one's own thought
 Being unable to wait turn to speak and then interrupting
 Intruding into games without being asked
 Becoming upset/complaining if not allowed to join games
 Trying to choose/control/direct games or change rules
 Grabbing things from other students
 Breaking the rules of a game/pointing out when peers break the rules
 Needing to win rather than just having a good time
 Failing to stop and consider consequences of behavior
 Having difficulty using internalized speech to control behavior/solve social problems
 Lacking skills to negotiate/compromise
 Constantly touching others when inappropriate
 Denying/placing blame for inappropriate behavior on others

Impact on Emotions

 Having a low tolerance for frustration/being easily irritated
 Having difficulty ignoring teasing and provocation
 Handling frustration in impulsive/intense/aggressive manner
 Overreacting in difficult social situations with anger/arguments/fights
 Reacting negatively when touched (tactile reactivity)
 Being unable to moderate emotions (too high/too low)
 Allowing feelings to control thoughts/actions
 Having trouble calming down

Prosocial behavior is the key factor in receiving peer acceptance. Students who are inattentive, impulsive, and/or hyperactive have been found in both clinic and community samples to have poor social functioning. (38, 39) They often have a very limited range of responses available. An effective intervention program must be multimodal and include, as needed, information processing skills (attention to and interpretation of social cues), social communication skills (pragmatic language skills), problem-solving skills, anger management training, and instruction and rehearsal of self-control techniques.

Interventions

Review interventions for Inattention, Impulsivity, and Hyperactivity in Chapter 12.

- Demonstrate and have the student mimic <u>appropriate</u> as well as <u>inappropriate</u> prosocial behaviors. Analyze and discuss the impact of those behaviors on others.

    - *Take into consideration the student's awareness of and ability to control behavior. Inattention and impulsivity are <u>neurologically-based</u> and an expectation for eliminating these behaviors is unrealistic.*

  ○ Repetitiously practice prosocial behaviors.

  ○ Provide written guidelines for acceptable and unacceptable behaviors based on the student's unique needs.

    - Place the guidelines in the student's strategy ("trick") book. (p. 64)

    - Review them frequently.

Section VII

- Teach and practice strategies for <u>focusing</u> and <u>sustaining attention</u> during conversational interactions.

    Suggest that the student:

    - stand one arm's length away from the other person.
    - look at and focus on the individual who is talking.
        - 🐾 *Making eye contact may produce anxiety and overarousal. Suggest looking in the area around the eyes (e.g., bridge of nose).*
    - <u>listen</u> carefully when the other person is speaking and interpret the underlying feelings being expressed by the <u>tone</u> (soft/shrill, gentle/harsh; friendly/distant; happy/sad); <u>loudness</u> (too loud/too soft); <u>speed</u> (too fast/too slow); and <u>intensity</u> of the voice.
    - carefully <u>examine</u> the facial features (smiles, frowns, glares) of the classmate and identify the feeling.
    - <u>observe</u> the body language and gestures in response to an interaction (looking away, turning the body around, looking at watch) and <u>interpret</u> the reaction.
    - make facial expressions and use body language that indicate listening and understanding (e.g., lean slightly forward, nod in an affirming manner, appear sincere when listening to a serious story, smile at jokes).
    - ask questions or paraphrase what was said so that the person knows that the comments were heard correctly.
        - 🐾 *Paraphrasing is an excellent way to teach the student how to listen and respond to the emotional content or message of the other student.*
    - comment on what the individual is saying and feeling or make a scripted response (e.g., "Hmmm." "Really." "Yeah." "Wow!" "I can tell you're excited." "I'm sorry that happened to you."). (31)

- Conference privately with the student to establish verbal and visual cues to indicate loss of focus.

    - Discuss <u>when</u> and <u>why</u> off-topic verbalizations occur.
        - Repeat what was said immediately prior to digressions.
        - Help the student identify the words or associations that occurred.
    - Suggest focusing on the primary stimuli (who, what, when, where, how, why) when telling a story, recounting a past experience, or describing the plot of a movie. (25)
    - Make a flow chart or mind map as the student speaks to illustrate inappropriate changes of topic.

- Teach conversational <u>turn-taking</u> routines to reduce impulsive interruptions. (25)

    - Assess the frequency of speaking and discuss privately with the student. Suggest limiting the number of times for talking.
    - Practice turn-taking in structured, teacher-directed lessons.

- Minimize problems with interrupting and waiting one's turn by assigning the student to a small group in which there are frequent opportunities to talk.
- Demonstrate concretely and visually how a conversation is like "playing tennis."
    - Throw a ball back and forth. Whoever has the ball is allowed to say something.
    - Limit the time the ball is held with an egg timer when practicing.
- Suggest pausing periodically to allow the other student to comment.
- Stress that, when another student is talking about a topic, it is important to ask two or three questions rather than changing the conversation to a subject of personal interest.
- Explain that students often do not want to talk with peers who try to dominate conversations.
    - Discuss the nonverbal cues classmates exhibit when they are annoyed (e.g., frowning, talking to others, making excuses to stop the conversation prematurely).
- Positively reinforce other students who demonstrate the appropriate turn-taking behavior. Always define the behavior ("I like the way John waited before taking his turn to speak.")
- Determine the interests of the quiet, withdrawn student and arrange topic-centered activities so the student has a chance to contribute. Ask the student a question or for an opinion.
    - *Notify the student in advance of the topic to be discussed.*

- Teach and practice strategies for inhibiting or controlling <u>impulsive comments</u>. Research suggests that the impulsivity of students with **ADHD** negatively influences communications. (40)

Suggest that the student:

- determine frequency of interrupting and discuss the impact this action has on other students.
- scan the environment to determine what is occurring before making any comments.
- practice the way to appropriately become a part of an ongoing conversation without interrupting.
    - observe whether the peer is talking to someone else.
    - notice if they are talking very softly and seem to be engaged in a private conversation. If so, postpone initiating a conversation.
    - determine if the conversation seems serious. If so, refrain from interfering.
    - check to see if the classmate is working intently on something and does not want to be disturbed.
    - ask the student if it is a good time to talk when unsure.
- understand that making inappropriate comments (e.g., "That is a stupid game! Who would want to play that!") is like going "PSSST" or spraying the classmate with insect repellent. (31)
    - *Using this concept teaches the student to recognize behaviors that attract or repel others.*
- wait for pauses in a conversation before speaking.
- inconspicuously place a hand over the mouth when wanting to comment while another student is talking.

Section VII

- recognize that making impulsive, negative comments is like making "Poison Stew." A tasty stew is made with fresh meat, carrots, peas, etc. However, when poison mushrooms are added, they spoil the whole pot. (41)

- Teach language that conveys <u>respect for others</u>.
  - Define respect and why it is important.
  - Demonstrate how to show support and concern for one's classmates.
  - Recommend asking about other students' feelings.
  - Stress the importance of making feeling comments that relate to the emotions being expressed.
  - Discuss the difference between appropriately sharing positive experiences with peers and boasting or bragging.
  - Model and practice <u>giving and accepting compliments</u>.

    Suggest that the student:
    - praise and make peers feel good with compliments.
    - tell classmates when they being helpful, kind, or smart. (25)
    - realize that it is common to feel uncomfortable when someone receives a compliment.
    - understand that the compliments are valid.
    - listen to peers without discounting what they are saying.
    - act out different responses to compliments.
    - rehearse scripts for offering and receiving compliments.
    - watch for a prearranged cue when compliments are required or are being rejected.
    - practice the proper way to thank a person.

- Explain the difference between assertive and aggressive language.
  - Role-play various interactions making both assertive and aggressive comments.
  - Discuss the feelings engendered.
  - Practice using assertive language.

- Implement strategies for <u>curbing impulsive, intrusive actions</u>.
  - Ignore impulsive behavior as much as possible. Address only those behaviors that disrupt and annoy other students (e.g., interrupting or intruding into ongoing games, grabbing objects from others).
  - Teach the student how to use a <u>self-talk strategy</u>. Self-directed speech reduces impulsivity, slows down responding, and provides time to objectively evaluate tasks and situations before reacting.
  - Explain to the student who interrupts and tries to control games and activities that others often become irritated and angry.
  - Supervise group activities and be sure the reticent student takes turns.
  - Tape a simple visual cue, such as a picture of the reward, to the desktop or inside the notebook to remind the student to stop and think before acting. (25)

- Positively reinforce behaviors that reflect appropriate impulse control.
- Compliment other students for self-regulating behaviors rather than continuously correcting the student.

- Arrange for classmates to <u>play cooperative, rule-based academic games</u>. Successfully playing games requires many social skills (e.g., following the rules of the game, taking turns, cooperating, handling competition, continuing to play even when losing, controlling angry feelings, assisting other players, complimenting the plays of other team members, losing gracefully, congratulating the winners, making positive comments after the game is finished).
  - Initially select a short game. Increase duration of game as success is experienced.
  - Choose a game that will not overarouse the student (frustrate, increase activity level) and make positive interactions difficult.
  - Limit the number of peers in the group.
  - Predetermine group membership rather than allowing the students to choose team members. Select compatible classmates.
  - Help the students negotiate/decide the order of the players.
  - Make certain beforehand that the student knows how to play the game, understands the rules, and has the skills to participate.
  - Pair the student with a prosocial "buddy" who knows the rules of the game and will be supportive.
  - Be sensitive to the tactilely defensive student who may respond negatively when touched. If a game or activity requires physical contact, make arrangements for the student to participate in an alternate manner.
  - De-emphasize winning. Remind the student that, regardless of the rules, the object of the game is to enjoy playing with friends.
  - Teach and rehearse good sportsmanship.
  - Supervise the playing of the game.
  - Discuss privately with the student the <u>positive</u> and negative behaviors exhibited during the game.
- Help the student <u>apologize</u> for inappropriate comments. (p. 95)

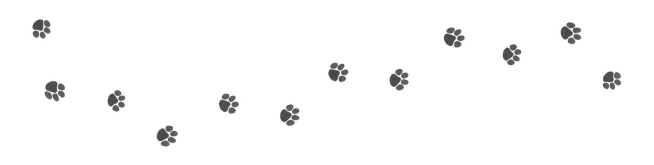

Section VII

EXECUTIVE DYSFUNCTION

Review interventions for Executive Dysfunction in Chapter 13.

Executive deficits can have a profound impact on social behaviors. Students with executive dysfunction are usually able to perform adequately in automatic and familiar social situations that require few executive skills. However, when they are confronted with more novel and complex social situations, they often engage in ineffective and inappropriate social interactions. Deficits in executive functions (problem solving, organization, and self-monitoring/self-correcting) account for many of the executive problems experienced by students with **ADHD**.

IMPAIRED PROBLEM SOLVING
(Tasks/Activities/Situations)

The following behaviors serve as general indicators. The student will not exhibit every characteristic listed. These behaviors may also be indicative of other problems.

Being unaware of communication/social problems that need to be solved
Being unable to solve new/unfamiliar/stressful social situations
Responding, "I don't know" when faced with an inquiry as to what to do

Interventions

- Provide a template of a <u>problem solving strategy</u> such as "**GET A CLUE**" or "**PLAN**" or another strategy to solve social problems. Be sure the strategy includes steps for goal setting, planning (generating ideas, solutions; analyzing proposed ideas, solutions; prioritizing; organizing; sequencing; managing time), initiating, and self-monitoring. (Appendix pp. 488-489)

- Model and demonstrate how to use the <u>problem solving strategy</u>. (p. 108)

Chapter 27

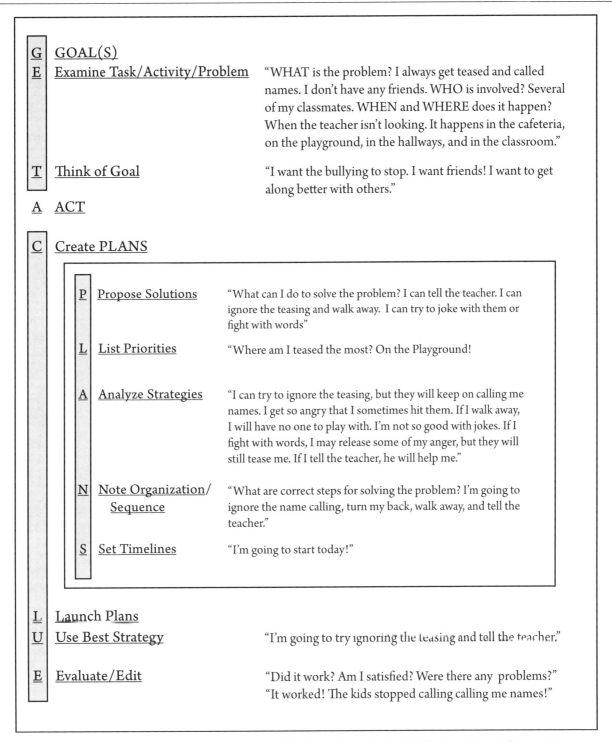

Figure 27.2. GET A CLUE – Cognitive strategy used with student who had difficulty with social interactions

Some students may not be able to follow the complexity of this strategy unless taught in incremental steps that must be mastered before continuing to the next step. Other students may need to learn a more simplified version "**PLAN.**" If so, use "**GET A CLUE**" as a structure for discussing and teaching ways to solve tasks, activities, and problem situations.

Section VII

P	Propose Goal	"I need to develop a plan to stop the other kids from bullying me by teasing me and calling me names."
L	List and Analyze Strategies	"What things can I do to solve the problem? I could ignore the teasing, I could walk away, or I could fight with words. When I try to ignore the teasing, they keep on calling me names. I sometimes get so angry I hit them. If I walk away, I will have no one to play with. If I fight with words, I may release some of my angry feelings and not hit them. If I ask the teacher to help me, I think he can stop the bullying."
A	Apply Best Strategy	"I will ask the teacher to help me."
N	Notice Errors and Edit	"Did it work? Am I satisfied? Were there any problems? It worked! The kids stopped!"

Figure 27.3. PLAN – Cognitive strategy used with student who had difficulty with social interactions

Difficulty Setting Goals

The following behaviors serve as general indicators. The student will not exhibit every characteristic listed. These behaviors may also be indicative of other problems.

Being unable to step back from present situation and think about future social needs
Having trouble identifying who, what, when, where, how, and why of problem situations
Having no concept of realistic, successful social goals

Interventions

- Define prosocial behaviors. Discuss when, where, how they are used and why they are critical to positive interactions.
- Have the student self-evaluate social strengths and weaknesses and determine which skills need improvement.
- Teach, prompt, and cue the student to stop and set goals.
- Provide assistance until goals can be set independently.

Difficulty Planning

Difficulty Proposing and Analyzing Ideas/Solutions/Strategies

The following behaviors serve as general indicators. The student will not exhibit every characteristic listed. These behaviors may also be indicative of other problems.

Overlooking need to conceptualize a step-by-step plan to achieve social goals
Lacking skills to generate/brainstorm ideas/solutions/strategies

Interventions

- Provide help in generating as many practical ideas as possible (e.g., wait for a turn rather than interrupting others when they are talking, ignore teasing rather than reacting aggressively, pay close attention to the body language of classmates).

- Discuss the positive and negative consequences of each idea.

- Use a cartooning format as a means to verbally and visually analyze problem social situations and set goals. (42)

    Suggest that the student:

    - discuss and draw the negative interaction on the right side of the paper.
    - working right to left, continue sketching previous interactions.
    - include conversation bubbles with the words that were spoken and idea bubbles containing the thoughts, feelings, or points of view.
    - discuss the who, what, when, where, how, and why of the interactions and identify the critical point when the incident turned negative.
    - propose and analyze strategies that might have avoided the problem.
    - set a new goal.
    - redraw the interaction from left to right using the goal to achieve a positive outcome.

- Practice problem solving using different social vignettes that the student often encounters.

- Show video tapes. Pause and brainstorm subsequent steps in the solution of the social problem.

- Suggest observing and then discussing how other classmates solve problematic social interactions.

Difficulty Prioritizing

The following behaviors serve as general indicators. The student will not exhibit every characteristic listed. These behaviors may also be indicative of other problems.

    Talking about topic inappropriate for context
    Assuming prior knowledge and not providing enough information
    Focusing on small details and not relating main idea
    Giving over detailed accounts and failing to notice signs of listener's disinterest/boredom
    Responding with irrelevant comments

Interventions

- Discuss strategies for adapting a conversation to the listener (e.g., talking with a classmate/teacher, parent/unknown adult, acquaintance/stranger).

- Review appropriate topics for different situations (playground/classroom/cafeteria/library/birthday party/movie theater). (25)

- Have the student role-play conversations with different people and in various contexts.

- Suggest keeping the conversation focused on the main topic and eliminating extraneous details.

Section VII

- Recommend limiting comments to who, what, when, where, how, and why.

- Explain the importance of using self-disclosure appropriately (personal problems are discussed with a close friend or family member, but not with an acquaintance or stranger). (25)

Difficulty Organizing/Sequencing

The following behaviors serve as general indicators. The student will not exhibit every characteristic listed. These behaviors may also be indicative of other problems.

> Having difficulty expressing self clearly and concisely
> Offering comments that are poorly organized and sequenced
> Seeming to "talk around" a subject and not getting to main idea, making it difficult to follow train of thought
> Interjecting disconnected/tangential thoughts
> Using ambiguous referents ("thing"/"stuff;" or "he"/"she" rather than names of objects/persons)
> Being unable to organize/generate comments to direct questioning

Students with **ADHD** often talk more than other students, but, when confronted with a situation in which responses must be generated and organized, they are likely to talk less and be more dysfluent. They tend to relate ideas in a disorganized and illogical sequence that makes comprehension by the listener difficult. (43, 44, 45)

Interventions

- Teach the student how to <u>organize communications</u> and provide enough information without giving overly detailed accounts.

    - *When relating stories or events, students with **ADHD** often go around and around in circles before getting to the point. At other times, they forget the main idea and interject tangential information. An inability to tell an organized, coherent story is frustrating for the listeners as well as the students who are trying to communicate.*

    ○ Distribute a who, what, when, where, how, and why outline and have the student practice using it to tell a story, to recount a past experience, or to describe the plot of a movie. Limit comments to the primary stimuli.

    ○ Use a mind mapping strategy to organize thoughts before relating an event or story.

    ○ Ask the student to record a personal experience on tape and then listen to the tape and evaluate the organization.

    ○ Have the student explain a simple board game to a classmate who does not know how to play.

    ○ Make a flow chart or mind map as the student speaks to illustrate inappropriate changes of topic.

    ○ Conference privately with the student to establish verbal and visual cues to indicate disorganization and rambling.

    ○ Suggest monitoring whether the other students are listening (looking at the speaker, leaning slightly forward, nodding, making relevant comments).

- Teach the student how to <u>sequence communications</u>.

    ○ Discuss and decide which information is primary, secondary, etc.

    ○ Stress the importance of using keywords to indicate a sequence.

- Ask the student to use "first," "next," and "last" and tell a peer about a movie (e.g., "Tell me what happened first." (pause) "Then what happened?" (pause) "What happened last?").
- Suggest using "first," "second," "third" to explain the rules of a game or sports activity to a classmate who is unfamiliar with the game.
- Listen for disorganized verbalizations. Say "I could not follow what happened."

○ Provide picture cues to help the student relate the sequence of a story or give directions. Rearrange the pictures and ask for them to be resequenced.

○ Suggest visualizing and explaining how to make something simple (e.g., peanut butter and jelly sandwich). Write down the sequence dictated by the student. Then have the student read and follow the directions to determine if they are properly sequenced. Increase the length and complexity as success is achieved.

INFLEXIBILITY

The following behaviors serve as general indicators. The student will not exhibit every characteristic listed. These behaviors may also be indicative of other problems.

Not knowing what to talk about
Being unable to change the topic of conversation/rambling on and on
Failing to adapt conversation to listener (peer/parent/teacher)
Having difficulty responding to different students during class discussions/group conversations
Having black-and-white points of view/intolerance for shades of gray
Having rigid/moralistic ideas of right and wrong ("moral policeman")
Being unable to listen to another point of view without imposing own
Not letting go of an argument, even if other student disagrees
Having trouble knowing when peer is joking/being sarcastic/using slang
Interpreting abstractness of idioms/metaphors literally
Being unable to change behavior when confronted with complex, unfamiliar social situations that require new/different responses
Becoming "stuck" on negative emotions (hurt/scared/angry feelings)

Interventions

- Increase recognition of when it is time to <u>change the topic</u> of conversation. (25)

  🐾 *A student with **OCD** may be unable to change topics.*

  ○ Suggest stopping and noting whether the other students have finished talking about one subject and have already moved on to another subject.

  ○ Have the student determine if the classmates are listening (e.g., looking at the speaker, nodding, adding comments).

  ○ Limit the student's comments on a topic to one per turn.

  ○ Teach transition words and phrases to form logical ties and relationships to new subjects.

  ○ Make statements that signal and stress a change in topic, such as "That reminds me of _____." or, more directly, "Now we are going to change the subject and talk about _____."

  ○ Prearrange a cue that alerts the student to being "stuck."

Section VII

- Teach the meanings of <u>figurative language</u> (phrases that contain images and do not mean what they say).

  - 🐾 *Some students interpret figures of speech literally and do not understand their meaning.*

  ○ Ask the student to brainstorm different figurative sayings.

    - A <u>simile</u> is a comparison using "like" and "as" (e.g., "like a bolt out of the blue," "as smooth as silk," "as quick as lightening").

    - A <u>metaphor</u> is a way to describe how two things that are not alike in most ways and similar in an important way without using "like" and "as" (e.g., "He was boiling mad." "He began to simmer down." "I was down in the dumps.").

    - A <u>hyperbole</u> is an exaggerated statement (e.g., "In order to finish my report, I need to burn the midnight oil." "I'd give my right arm to get a good grade in math." "I'd go out on a limb to help you.").

    - A <u>personification</u> gives human qualities to a non-living object (e.g., "A smiling moon looks down on me." "Stars dance in the night sky." "My dog read my mind.").

  ○ Make a list of figurative expressions and their actual meanings. Discuss what they mean. Begin with the more easily explained, humorous ones.

- Discuss the slang used by the student's peers (informal words and expressions that are not part of the standard language). For example, "awesome" for really great; "be real" for be serious, or "whatever" for not wanting to talk about something.

  - 🐾 *Remind the student to use peer slang only with friends and <u>not</u> with adults.*

- Teach the student how to recognize when a peer is joking and using humor.

  - 🐾 *Joking and humor rely on tone and inflection for effect. The student may focus on only the words and not process the verbal and nonverbal cues.*

- Read statements containing sarcasm (cutting remarks intended to ridicule and hurt the other person). Ask for an interpretation.

- Teach and practice <u>perspective-taking skills</u> (recognizing that others may have alternative points of view).

  - 🐾 *When a student understands the thoughts and feelings of other students, the student is better able to generate solutions to interpersonal problems. Misunderstandings often lead to social problems and peer rejection.*

Ask the student to:

○ listen carefully to what is being said (tone, loudness, intensity of voice; words).

  - paraphrase what was heard. This helps the student focus on the peer's words and feelings and understand the point of view.

○ observe nonverbal social cues (facial expressions, body language, gestures).

○ discuss <u>what</u> might have happened and <u>why</u> the other student might perceive the situation differently.

○ pose several alternative interpretations regarding the thoughts and feelings being expressed.

○ choose the most likely interpretation.

- request confirmation of the interpretation.
    - *If the student is unable to identify what the other person is thinking or feeling, teach the appropriate way to ask for clarification.*
- put one's self in the place of the other student and imagine how it would feel to be that person.
- role-play several different points of view. Exaggerate until the point of view is understood.
- make a scripted response when there is disagreement (e.g., "I can tell you love football. It isn't my favorite sport, but I know lots of kids who really enjoy it."). (31)
- provide examples showing how classmates might misinterpret situations (e.g., being bumped in the hallway or on the playground – accidental/intentional; being teased – joking/rejection).

• Teach and rehearse strategies for changing behavior when confronted with complex, unfamiliar social situations that require new or more adaptive responses.

Suggest that the student:

- pause and observe the interactions before responding.
- make facial expressions and body positions that show interest while adjusting to the situation.
- recognize when emotions are becoming intense and change to a more positive and calming activity.
- look for a prearranged cue from the teacher that indicates that a different response is required.
- learn a script for offering a polite comment (e.g., "Excuse me, I need to go now.") and making a "graceful exit" (p. 90) when a response is not forthcoming.

• Prepare the student for changes in social events. For example, if there is going to be a pep rally and a new format will be used (everyone wearing a certain color), make sure that the student knows what is different and is prepared for the event.

- *Being out of step when changes occur is embarrassing and may lead to overarousal and out-of-control behavior.*
- Discuss social situations in advance.
    - Review what will be happening (e.g., playing games, singing, dancing, watching a play or musical performance) and behavioral expectations.
    - Show photographs of peers who will be attending the event and review their names.
    - Consult social strategies placed in the strategy ("trick") book. (p. 64)
    - Practice previously learned scripts and social routines.
    - Suggest having trusted friends or adults remain nearby to provide prompts and/or facilitate interactions.

• Discuss the social customs of the new school if the student is changing schools or transitioning to a middle or high school, (e.g., where the students congregate before the school day starts/after lunch/at recess; social hierarchy; trends in clothing, hairstyles; popular music; slang used by peers). (27)

Section VII

INITIATION/EXECUTION DIFFICULTIES

The following behaviors serve as general indicators. The student will not exhibit every characteristic listed. These behaviors may also be indicative of other problems.

Having trouble initiating a verbal response (answering questions/starting conversations)
Being reluctant to speak in class
Looking bored and disinterested
Having difficulty asking peers questions
Avoiding making phone calls
Having difficulty initiating social interactions/social plans

Interventions

- Teach, model, and practice strategies for recognizing the <u>correct timing for approaching</u> another student to initiate a conversation.

    Suggest that the student:

    - pause and observe whether the classmate is engaged in a serious conversation with another student (standing or leaning close to each other, whispering or speaking softly) and should not be interrupted.

    - move toward the peer and observe the reaction.

    - retreat if the peer is frowning, not looking up, or moving away.

    - proceed if smiling, making eye-contact, or coming forward.

- Demonstrate and rehearse appropriate social <u>greeting skills</u>.

    Suggest that student:

    - stand up straight and smile.

    - make eye contact.

        - *Some neurologically challenged students become anxious looking into another person's eyes. If the student experiences anxiety trying to make eye contact, demonstrate how to give the appearance of making eye contact by looking at an area surrounding the eyes (forehead, nose).*

    - practice and follow a prearranged script.

        - say "Hi! How are you today?" or, if greeted first, respond "Fine, thank you, how are you?" (31)

        - introduce self.

        - wait and listen for the name of the other student. If there is no response, ask "What's your name?"

            - *Suggest using the other student's name as often as possible.*

    - identify the peer's response to the greeting (smiling, frowning, looking away). Modify the greeting, if necessary.

    - examine pictures of people greeting each other and analyze eye contact, social boundaries, and facial expressions.

- Teach strategies for <u>becoming a member of a group conversation</u>.

  Suggest that the student:

  - approach the group, make eye contact, and smile.
  - make friendly greetings and gestures.
  - wait and notice the topic about which everyone else is talking.
  - stop and think what else might be said about the topic.
  - avoid interrupting while someone is talking.
  - wait for a pause in the conversation and then offer a relevant comment.
  - refrain from changing the topic of conversation to one of personal interest.
  - choose another activity if the other students do not return eye contact, frown, or are unresponsive.

- Demonstrate and practice how to <u>introduce a friend</u>.

  Suggest that the student:

  - look at and greet the other student.
  - state the name of the student and then tell the name of the friend.
  - say something that might be of mutual interest.
  - repeat until everyone has been introduced when wanting to include a friend in a group.

- Discuss ideas for <u>initiating and maintaining a conversation</u>.

  Suggest that the student:

  - choose a topic of common interest.
    - *If the student has difficulty thinking of topics, assist preparation of a list of common interests (e.g., TV programs, movies, music, electronic games, sports, school activities and events, topics heard during lunch/on playground).*
  - make sure the conversation is interesting and animated.
  - allow the other student to frequently express ideas.
  - ask questions (e.g., who, what, when, where, how, why).
  - listen intently to the peer's responses.
  - determine if the peer is listening (e.g., looking at speaker, nodding, adding comments).

Section VII

- Teach strategies for <u>initiating social plans</u> with other students. Provide and rehearse scripts, if needed.

    Suggest that the student:

    ○ phone a classmate early in the week and say, using the practiced script, "Hello! This is _____. Would you like to come over to my house on Saturday? We can play with my new interactive electronic game! It is a lot of fun!"

    ○ plan in advance a social activity with a classmate while at school. Ask "Hey, _____, want to do something this weekend? We can get a pizza and then go to a movie."

- Recommend using the Internet to communicate. This reduces the effort and anxiety associated with initiating face-to-face conversations.

    🐾 *However, do not allow the computer to become a substitute for personal contact and <u>always monitor</u> the use of the Internet. (41)*

- Teach the student a script for terminating conversations (e.g., "I enjoyed talking to you, but I have to go now. See you later.").

IMPAIRED SELF-MONITORING/USE OF FEEDBACK/SELF-CORRECTION

The following behaviors serve as general indicators. The student will not exhibit every characteristic listed. These behaviors may also be indicative of other problems.

Lacking insight into one's own vocal/motor/emotional behavior
Misperceiving/not assessing the effect own behavior has on self/others
Having trouble modulating tone/volume/speed/intensity of voice
Not noticing off-topic digressions in social conversations
Failing to perceive that peers are not interested in topic
Saying wrong thing at wrong time
Failing to modify/adapt conversation to listener's needs/interests
Missing need to clarify comments when misunderstood
Neglecting to ask for clarification when one does not understand
Missing changing aspects of social situations
Having difficulty analyzing/interpreting own feelings/feelings of others
Having trouble interpreting feelings of others when they are speaking (angry/joking/serious)
Overlooking/misunderstanding/responding inappropriately to social feedback cues
    (body movements/gestures/facial expressions/tones of voice)
Being unaware of social boundaries/touching rules (standing too close/touching when inappropriate)
Being unable to learn from past mistakes
Failing to modify behavior based on either positive or negative feedback (repeatedly making same
    social blunders even when it repeatedly has not worked or when told the strategy was incorrect)
Appearing to not care when really "clueless" about feedback
Not knowing how to repair a relationship

The ability to self-monitor and self-correct in social situations requires awareness of one's own behavior, of the implication of that behavior on self and others, and of verbal and nonverbal social cues being exhibited by peers.

Interventions

- Improve the student's <u>understanding and awareness of feelings</u>.

  - 🐾 *Decreased awareness contributes to ineffective pragmatics (use of verbal and nonverbal communication skills) in social situations which in turn leads to rejection and social isolation.*

  ○ Teach and rehearse the use of <u>feeling words</u>. Streamline the myriad of feeling words and start with the four basic words – "mad," "sad," "glad," and "scared." Once these are mastered, introduce synonyms for the feeling words. (Appendix p. 402) (25)

    - 🐾 *Research suggests that "happy" is the easiest to identify, followed by "angry," "surprised," "sad," and "afraid." (46)*

  Suggest that the student practice:

  - identifying and labeling feelings portrayed in pictures and films.
  - using synonyms for feeling words after the basic words are mastered and can be generalized to other situations.

- Help the student learn to <u>identify feelings in self</u>.

  Encourage the student to:

  ○ understand that feelings are neither "good" nor "bad". What is important is how the student reacts to them.

  ○ recognize that feelings are in response to experiences.

  ○ discuss the body's reactions to those feelings (e.g., flushed face, racing heart, butterflies in the stomach).

  ○ determine the causes of those feelings.

  ○ discuss previous situations in which a particular feeling was experienced.

  ○ role-play various social situations. Identify and label the feelings generated.

    - 🐾 *<u>Exaggerate</u> feelings at first and then more indirectly until the feeling can be identified independently and the underlying cause can be stated.*

  ○ look into a mirror and make facial features associated with various emotions.

  ○ pose for photographs and use different body language to convey feelings.

  ○ create hypothetical scenarios and predict the feelings.

  ○ start sentences by saying "I feel _____."

  ○ realize that others often may experience different feelings to the same situations.

Section VII

- Develop understanding of the <u>feelings being expressed by others</u>.
  - Directly teach the interpretation of <u>verbal social cues</u>, especially the way something is said rather than what is said. Students with **ADHD** sometimes have difficulty identifying the tone of emotionally laden sentences. (47)

    Suggest that the student:
    - listen to the tone, loudness, and intensity of a voice and identify the feeling.
    - interpret hesitations, pauses, and silence.
    - note sounds like groans and sighs.
    - identify and state the feelings expressed by a classmate during an ongoing conversation.
    - listen to video tapes or television programs with the screen darkened and interpret the feelings based on the tone, loudness, and intensity of the conversations. (30)

  - Use a variety of teaching methods to promote awareness of feelings being projected through nonverbal social cues. Students with **ADHD** may misinterpret subtle <u>nonverbal social cues</u> or unspoken messages. Research suggests that many of these students have deficits in their ability to accurately interpret facial expressions. (47, 48, 49)

    Suggest that the student:
    - examine a series of cartoons and discuss the feelings being expressed by the face, interpersonal space, body stance, and/or gestures.
    - identify the feelings being expressed in photographs and pictures of peers interacting or doing an activity together.
    - watch videos of social interactions with the sound turned off. Discuss feelings associated with the nonverbal cues. (30)
    - observe various school and playground activities and discuss feelings being exhibited.
    - role-play different social interactions and express one's self with appropriate facial expressions and body positions.
    - play "Charades." Act out a message using a variety of nonverbal cues to portray a feeling and ask the other students to interpret it.

  - practice the proper use of <u>social boundaries</u> (proximity to others) when communicating (arm's length).
    - try to carry on a conversation standing too close or too far from the other student.
    - discuss how violating a classmate's personal space makes the peer feel uncomfortable.

  - discuss, role-play, and rehearse appropriate <u>touching rules</u> (e.g., touch only close friends and family members except for an appropriate, firm handshake; never initiate tickling or touching of others).

    > 🐾 *Do not penalize students with **TS** and/or **OCD** for touching tics and obsessions. Ask permission to talk to health care professional for accommodations.*

    - practice the proper use of social boundaries when communicating (arm's length).

  - Encourage the parents to use the social interactions of others that are occurring in such places as malls, amusement parks, restaurants, sporting events, and airports as a means of discussing both positive and negative interactions.

- Use the "feeling thermometer" to enhance interpretation of feelings, reactive behaviors and consequences. (50, 51)

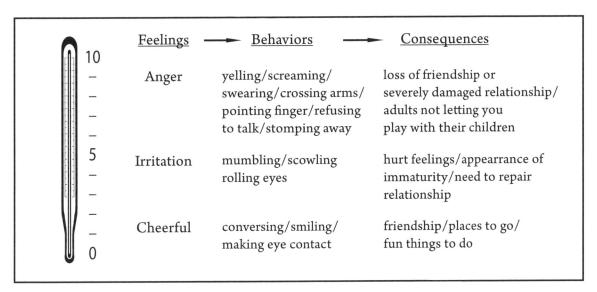

Figure 27.4. Feeling Thermometer

  - Provide a template of the "Feeling Thermometer" to be completed after a negative incident and assist completion. (Appendix p. 403)
- Help the student consider the <u>needs of the listener</u>. Students with **ADHD** frequently do not self-monitor their communications. (44, 45)

Suggest that the student:

  - cue the listener to the topic of discussion.
  - state the new topic when changing subjects.
  - provide background information to a listener who is unfamiliar with the topic.
  - focus on the main idea rather than stressing details.
  - use complete sentences as opposed to meaningless, disconnected fragments of a story. Address the who, what, when, where, how, and why of the event.
  - attend to the rhythm and modulation of speech (too fast/too slow, too loud/too soft) and the effect they have on the listener's interest and understanding.
  - think about everyday situations and practice what might be said to be polite/impolite, assertive/aggressive, sensitive/insensitive, friendly/aloof, formal/informal, direct/vague, etc.
  - take turns speaking.
  - watch for cues indicating when it is time for the listener to speak.

Section VII

- stop and clarify communications when misunderstood.

  🐾 *Assure the student that being misunderstood is very common.*

- rephrase or revise an unclear word or sentence.

- make clarifying statements: "I might not have made myself clear. Let me try again."

- ask questions to make sure the other person understood.

- role-play situations in which misunderstandings occur (e.g., use of imprecise language, unclear comments, improper referents, omission of pertinent information) then re-enact the situation with comments that are clear and understandable.

• Develop accurate perceptions of how others might view the student so that feedback can be used to self-correct. (25)

  🐾 *Students with **ADHD** may have difficulty interpreting and understanding how others characterize them except when peers react intensely with either excitement or anger.*

Suggest that the student:

- discuss a range of traits that are appropriate for same-age peers.

- think about how others might feel and what they might say about the student, recognizing that one's own feelings are often clues to the feelings of others.

- determine whether the feelings are consistent with the affect being projected.

- assess whether those characteristics would be appealing to peers.

- state whether that image accurately describes the student.

- evaluate and tell which personal behaviors feel appropriate and which ones feel inappropriate.

- ask a trusted adult for feedback concerning behaviors which make the adult feel uncomfortable.

- consider whether the student's image needs improvement.

• Teach the student how to monitor social interactions and not try to develop a friendship too rapidly or intensely. (25)

Suggest that the student:

- discuss the difference between various types of relationships (close friend/acquaintance, parent/teacher, male/female).

- count the number of times contact is made with a new friend (several times a day, once a day, once a week).

- determine if the number of contacts made by the student is similar to the number of reciprocal contacts made by the friend.

- define appropriate same sex topics.

Chapter 27

MEMORY PROBLEMS

Review interventions for Memory Problems in Chapter 14.

SHORT-TERM MEMORY PROBLEMS

Difficulty with Working Memory

The following behaviors serve as general indicators. The student will not exhibit every characteristic listed. These behaviors may also be indicative of other problems.

> Missing or forgetting words/phrases/sentences/meaning of peer's communication
> Having difficulty following topic shifts during conversations
> Having trouble retrieving/processing possible responses before speaking
> Forgetting what was going to be said while speaking
> Interrupting speaker so as to not forget what one wants to say
> Having difficulty processing complex social situations
> Being unable to integrate verbal/nonverbal cues in quick paced/changing social interactions
> Having difficulty processing both the obvious and abstract meanings of social interactions
> Being unable to generate/analyze alternatives to problem situations
> Having trouble remembering behavior in past in order to adapt current behavior

The student with working memory problems often has difficulty handling unfamiliar, complex social situations. To process an interaction and engage in a conversation, the student must quickly and simultaneously attend to and interpret verbal and nonverbal cues, process the ongoing social situation, consider possible responses and their consequences, make a decision, and respond appropriately.

Interventions

- Increase attention (pp. 97-102) and improve executive skills (pp. 107-130) so that they can be <u>automatically</u> applied in complex social situations.

- Use, as needed, the recommendations offered throughout this chapter to enhance working memory (e.g., organization/sequencing, inflexibility, self-monitoring, use of feedback, self-correction).

- Provide frequent opportunities for spontaneous social interactions.

- Organize small groups of students to discuss topics.

    ○ Provide advance notice of the topic.

    ○ Brainstorm with the student what is known about the subject prior to the group discussion

    ○ Facilitate interactions if the student is having difficulty processing and keeping up with pace of the discussion.

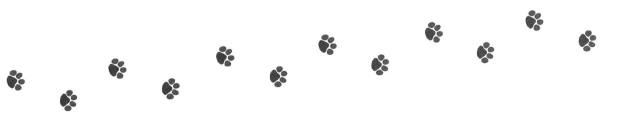

Section VII

LONG-TERM MEMORY PROBLEMS

Difficulty Retrieving (Recalling)

The following behaviors serve as general indicators. The student will not exhibit every characteristic listed. These behaviors may also be indicative of other problems.

- Exhibiting fluent and articulate speech in spontaneous situations, but having difficulty responding when expected to speak
- Possessing age adequate vocabulary, but having trouble finding words to use in social conversations
- Being unable to substitute alternative vocabulary word when cannot retrieve specific word to use
- Making inappropriate word substitutions/repeating words
- Responding to what is said with inappropriate silences and delays
- Having trouble using precise language
- Using ambiguous referents ("thing"/"stuff," "he"/"she" rather than specific names of objects/persons)
- Using filler words ("um"/"er"/"well"/"you know"/"I know it, but I can't think of it"/"I forget")
- Struggling to recall specifics of emotionally charged social situations
- Struggling to remember social routines and procedures (e.g., greeting and departing skills/how to ask for a date/perform certain dance steps)
- Being unable to retrieve previously taught strategies for specific social settings

Interventions

- Recognize that retrieval problems may make the student unwilling to participate in social conversations.

- Provide extra time to respond.

- Suggest breathing when searching for words, rather than filling the time with rapid, irrelevant verbalizations.

- Recommend delaying a response when needed ("Let me think about that for a minute.").

- Expand the student's vocabulary so that alternative words are available when needed.

References

REFERENCES

Section I: Awareness

Chapter 1: Attention Deficit Hyperactivity Disorder

1. American Psychiatric Association. (2000). Diagnostic and Statistical Manual of Mental Disorders, Fourth Edition, Text Revision. Washington, DC: American Psychiatric Association.
2. Barkley, R. A. (2006). Attention-Deficit Hyperactivity Disorder (3rd ed.): A Handbook for Diagnosis and Treatment. New York, NY: Guilford Press.
3. Carlson, C. L. and Mann, M. (2002). Sluggish cognitive tempo predicts a different pattern of impairment in attention deficit hyperactivity disorder, predominantly inattentive type. Journal of Clinical Child and Adolescent Psychology, 31, 123-129.
4. Communicable Disease Center. (2005). Mental health in the United States: Prevalence of diagnosis and medication treatment for attention-deficit/hyperactivity disorder – United States. Morbidity and Mortality Weekly Report, 54, 842-847. www.cdc.gov
5. Costello, E. J., Mustillo, S., Erkanli, A., et al. (2003). Prevalence and development of psychiatric disorders in childhood and adolescence. Archives of General Psychiatry, 60, 837-847.
6. Froehlich, T. E., Lanphear, B. P., Epstein, J. N., et al. (2007). Prevalence, recognition, and treatment of attention-deficit/hyperactivity disorder in a national sample of US children. Archives of Pediatric and Adolescent Medicine, 161, 857-864.
7. Costello, E. J., Angold, A., Burns, B. J., et al. (1996). The Great Smokey Mountains study of youth: Goals, designs, methods, and prevalence of DSM-III-R disorders. Archives of General Psychiatry, 53, 1129-1136.
8. Baumgaertel, A., Wolraich, M. L., and Dietrich, M. (1995). Comparison of diagnostic criteria for attention deficit disorders in a German elementary school sample. Journal of the American Academy of Child and Adolescent Psychiatry, 34, 629-638.
9. Carlson, C. L. and Mann, M. (2000). Attention-deficit/hyperactivity disorder, predominately inattentive subtype. Child and Adolescent Psychiatric Clinics of North America, 9, 499-510.
10. Carlson, C. L., Tamm, L., and Miranda, G. (1997). Gender differences in children with ADHD, ODD, and co-occurring ADHD/ODD identified in a school population. Journal of the American Academy of Child and Adolescent Psychiatry, 36, 1706-1714.
11. Gaub, M. and Carlson, C. L. (1997). Behavioral characteristics of DSM-IV ADHD subtypes in a school-based population. Journal of Abnormal Child Psychology, 25, 103-111.
12. Wolraich, M. L., Hannah, J. N., Baumgaertel, A., and Feurer, I. D. (1998). Examination of DSM-IV criteria for attention deficit/hyperactivity disorder in a country-wide sample. Journal of Developmental and Behavioral Pediatrics, 19, 162-168.
13. Wolraich, M. L., Hannah, J. N., Pinnock, T. Y., et al. (1996). Comparison of diagnostic criteria for attention-deficit hyperactivity disorder in a country-wide sample. Journal of the American Academy of Child and Adolescent Psychiatry, 35, 319-324.
14. Nolan, E. E., Gadow, K. D., and Sprafkin, J. (2001). Teacher reports of DSM-IV ADHD, ODD, and CD symptoms in schoolchildren. Journal of the American Academy of Child and Adolescent Psychiatry, 40, 241-249.
15. Faraone, S. V., Biederman, J., Weber, W., and Russell, R. L. (1998). Psychiatric, neuropsychological, and psychosocial features of DSM-IV subtypes of attention-deficit/hyperactivity disorder: Results from a clinically referred sample. Journal of the American Academy of Child and Adolescent Psychiatry, 37, 185-193.
16. Cuffe, S. P., McKeown, R. E., Jackson, K. L., et al. (2001). Prevalence of attention-deficit/hyperactivity disorder in a community sample of older adolescents. Journal of the American Academy of Child and Adolescent Psychiatry, 40, 1037-1044.

17. Peterson, B. S., Pine, D. S., Cohen, P., and Brook, J. S. (2001). Prospective, longitudinal study of tic, obsessive-compulsive, and attention-deficit/hyperactivity disorders in an epidemiological sample. Journal of the American Academy of Child and Adolescent Psychiatry, 40, 685-695.
18. Faraone, S. V. (2005). How prevalent is ADHD in adults? Attention, December, 29-33.
19. Weiss, M., Hechtman, L. T., and Weiss, G. (1999). ADHD in Adulthood: A Guide to Current Theory, Diagnosis, and Treatment. Baltimore, MD: John Hopkins University Press.
20. Murphy, K. R. and Barkley, R. A. (1996). Prevalence of DSM-IV symptoms of ADHD in adult licensed drivers: Implications for clinical diagnosis. Journal of Attention Disorders, 1, 147-161.
21. Kessler, R. C., Berglund, P., Demler, O., et al. (2005). Lifetime prevalence and age-of-onset distributions of DSM-IV disorders in the National Comorbidity Survey Replication. Archives of General Psychiatry, 62, 593-602.
22. Goldstein, S. and Gordon, M. (2003). Gender issues and ADHD: Sorting fact from fiction. The ADHD Report, 11 (4), 7-11, 16.
23. Gaub, M. and Carlson, C. L. (1997). Gender differences in ADHD: A meta-analysis and critical review. Journal of the American Academy of Child and Adolescent Psychiatry, 36, 1036-1045.
24. Kessler, R. C., Adler, L., Barkley, R., et al. (2006). The prevalence and correlates of adult ADHD in the United States: Results from the national comorbidity survey replication. American Journal of Psychiatry, 163, 716-723.
25. Gershon, J. (2002). A meta-analysis review of gender differences in ADHD. Journal of Attention Disorders, 5, 241-154.
26. Biederman, J., Mick, E., Faraone, S. V., et al. (2002). Influence of gender on attention deficit hyperactivity disorder in children referred to a psychiatric clinic. American Journal of Psychiatry, 159, 36-42.
27. Applegate, B., Lahey, B. B., Hart, E. L., et al. (1997). Validity of the age-of-onset criterion for ADHD: A report from the DSM-IV field trials. Journal of the American Academy of Child and Adolescent Psychiatry, 36, 1211-1221.
28. Goodyear, P. and Hynd, G. W. (1992). Attention-deficit disorder (AD/HD) and without (ADD/WO) hyperactivity: Behavioral and neuropsychological differentiation. Journal of Clinical Child Psychology, 21, 273-305.
29. Szatmari, R., Offord, D. R., and Boyle, M. H. (1989). Ontario Child Health Study: Prevalence of attention deficit disorder with hyperactivity. Journal of Child Psychology and Psychiatry, 30, 219-230.
30. Biederman, J., Faraone, S., Milberger, S., et al. (1996). A prospective 4-year follow-up study of attention-deficit hyperactivity and related disorders. Archives of General Psychiatry, 53, 437-446.
31. Cartwright-Hatton, S., McNicol, K., and Doubleday, E. (2006). Anxiety in a neglected population: Prevalence of anxiety disorders in preadolescent children. Clinical Psychology Review, 26, 817-833.
32. Mayes, S. D., Calhoun, S. L., and Crowell, E. W. (2000). Learning disabilities and ADHD: Overlapping spectrum disorders. Journal of Learning Disabilities, 33, 417-424.
33. Semrud-Clikeman, M., Biedeman, J., Sprich-Buckminster, S., et al. (1992). Comorbidity between ADDH and learning disability: A review and report in a clinically referred sample. Journal of the American Academy of Child and Adolescent Psychiatry, 31, 439-448.
34. Interagency Committee of Learning Disabilities. (1987). Learning Disabilities: A Report to Congress. Washington, DC: National Institute of Child Health and Human Development. U. S. Department of Health and Human Services.
35. Reschly, D. J., Hosp, J. L., and Schmied, C. M. (2003). And Miles to Go... : State SLD Requirements and Authoritative Recommendations. Report of the National Research Center on Learning Disabilities (NRCLD). Washington, DC: US Department of Education, Office of Special Education Programs.
36. Barkley, R. A., Fischer, M., Edelbrock, C. S., and Smallish, L. (1990). The adolescent outcome of hyperactive children diagnosed by research criteria. I. An 8-year prospective follow-up study. Journal of the American Academy of Child and Adolescent Psychiatry, 29, 546-557.
37. Gittelman, R., Mannuzza, S., Shenker, R., and Bonagura, N. (1985). Hyperactive boys almost grown up: I. Psychiatric status. Archives of General Psychiatry, 42, 937-947.

Reference

38. Biederman, J., Faraone, S., Milberger, S., et al. (1996). Predictors of persistence and remission of ADHD into adolescence: Results from a four-year prospective follow-up study. Journal of the American Academy of Child and Adolescent Psychiatry, 35, 343-351.
39. Mannuzza, S. and Klein, R. G. (2000). Long-term prognosis in attention-deficit hyperactivity disorder. Child and Adolescent Psychiatric Clinics of North America, 9, 711-726.
40. Mick, E., Faraone, S. V., and Biederman, J. (2004). Age-dependent expression of attention-deficit/hyperactivity disorder symptoms. Psychiatric Clinics of North America, 27, 215-224.
41. Mannuzza, S., Klein, R. G., Bonagura, N., et al. (1991). Hyperactive boys almost grown up: V. Replication of psychiatric status. Archives of General Psychiatry, 48, 77-83.
42. Biederman, J., Mick, E., and Faraone, S. V. (1998). Normalized functioning in youths with persistent attention-deficit/hyperactivity disorder. Journal of Pediatrics, 133, 544-551.
43. Brotman, M. A., Schmajuk, M., Rich, B. A., et al. (2006). Prevalence, clinical correlates, and longitudinal course of severe mood dysregulation in children. Biological Psychiatry, 60, 991-997.
44. Angold, A., Costello, E. J., and Erkanli, A. (1999). Comorbidity. Journal of Child Psychology and Psychiatry, 40, 57-87.
45. U.S. Department of Health and Human Services. (1999). Mental Health: A Report of the Surgeon General-Executive Summary. Rockville, MD: U.S. Department of Health and Human Services, Substance Abuse and Mental Health Services Administration, Center for Mental Health Services, National Institutes of Health, Nation Institute of Mental Health.
46. Lewinsohn, P. M., Klein, D. N., and Seeley, J. R. (1995). Bipolar disorders in a community sample of old adolescents: Prevalence, phenomenology, comorbidity, and course. Journal of the American Academy of Child and Adolescent Psychiatry, 34, 454-463.
47. Barkley, R. A., Fischer, M., Smallish, L., and Fletcher, K. (2006). Young adult outcome of hyperactive children: Adaptive functioning in major life activities. Journal of the American Academy of Child and Adolescent Psychiatry, 45, 192-202.
48. Weiss, G. and Hechtman, L. T. (1993). Hyperactive Children Grown Up (2nd ed.). New York, NY: Guilford Press.
49. Barkley, R. A., Geuvrement, D. C., Anastopoulos, A. D., et al. (1993). Driving-related risks and outcomes of attention deficit hyperactivity disorder in adolescents and young adults: A 3 to 5-year follow-up survey. Pediatrics, 92, 212-218.
50. Barkley, R. A. (2004). Driving impairments in teens and adults with attention-deficit/hyperactivity disorder. Child and Adolescent Psychiatric Clinics of North America, 27, 233-260.
51. Milberger, S., Biederman, J., Faraone, S. V., et al. (1997). ADHD is associated with early initiation of cigarette smoking in children and adolescents. Journal of the American Academy of Child and Adolescent Psychiatry, 36, 37-44.
52. Faraone, S. V. and Wilens, T. (2003). Does stimulant treatment lead to substance use disorders? Journal of Clinical Psychiatry, 64, 9-13.
53. Biederman, J. (2003). Pharmacotherapy for attention-deficit/hyperactivity disorder (ADHD) decreases the risk for substance abuse: Findings from a longitudinal follow-up of youths with and without ADHD. Journal of Clinical Psychiatry, 64, 3-8.
54. Flory, K., Molina, B. S. G., Pelham, W. E., et al. (2007). ADHD and risky sexual behavior. The ADHD Report, 15(3), 1-4.
55. Fischer, M. and Barkley, R. A. (2007). The persistence of ADHD into adulthood: (Once again) It depends on whom you ask. The ADHD Report, 15(4), 7-9, 12-16.
56. Barkley, R. A., Murphy, K. R., Fischer, M. (2007). Adults with ADHD: Clinic-referred cases vs. children grown up. The ADHD Report, 15(5), 1-7, 13.
57. Biederman, J. (2004). Impact of Comorbidity in adults with attention-deficit/hyperactivity disorder. Journal of Clinical Psychiatry, 65 (supplement 3), 3-7.
58. Mannuzza, S., Klein, R. G., Bessler, M. A., et al. (1998). Adult psychiatric status of hyperactive boys grown up. American Journal of Psychiatry, 155, 493-498.

59. Biederman, J., Faraone, S. V., Spencer, T., et al. (1993). Patterns of psychiatric comorbidity, cognition, and psychosocial functioning in adults with attention deficit hyperactivity disorder. American Journal of Psychiatry, 150, 1792-1798.
60. Mannuzza, S., Klein, R. G., Bessler, A., et al. (1993). Adult outcome of hyperactive boys: Educational achievement, occupational rank, and psychiatric status. Archives of General Psychiatry, 50, 565-576.
61. Murphy, K. and Barkley, R. A. (1996). Attention deficit hyperactivity disorder adults: Comorbidities and adaptive impairments. Comprehensive Psychiatry, 37, 393-401.
62. Mannuzza, S., Klein, R. G., and Moulton, J. L. (2003). Does stimulant treatment place children at risk for adult substance abuse? A controlled, prospective follow-up study. Journal of Child and Adolescent Psychopharmacology, 13, 273-282.
63. Faraone, S. V., Biederman, J., Wilens, T. E., and Adamson, J. (2007). A naturalistic study or the effects of pharmacotherapy on substance use disorders among ADHD adults. Psychological Medicine, 37, 1743-1752.
64. Mannuzza, S., Klein, R. G., Bessler, A., et al. (1997). Educational and occupational outcome of hyperactive boys grown up. Journal of the American Academy of Child and Adolescent Psychiatry, 36, 1222-1227.
65. Biederman, J., Faraone, S. V., Spencer, T. J., et al. (2006). Functional impairments in adults with self-reports of diagnosed ADHD: A controlled study of 1001 adults in the community. Journal of Clinical Psychiatry, 67, 524-540.

Chapter 2: Tic Disorders

1. Costello, E. J., Mustillo, S., Erkanli, A., et al. (2003). Prevalence and development of pschiatric disorders in childhood and adolescence. Archives of General Psychiatry, 60, 837-844.
2. Kurlan, R., McDermott, M. P., Deeley, C., et al. (2001). Prevalence of tics in schoolchildren and association with placement in special education. Neurology, 57, 1383-1388.
3. Peterson, B. S., Pine, D. S., Cohen, P., and Brook, J. S. (2001). Prospective, longitudinal study of tic, obsessive-compulsive, and attention-deficit/hyperactivity disorders in an epidemiological sample. Journal of the American Academy of Child and Adolescent Psychiatry, 40, 685-695.
4. Zohar, A. H., Apter, A., King, R. A., et al. (1999). Epidemiological studies. In Leckman, J. F. and Cohen, D. J. editors: Tourette's Syndrome–Tics, Obsessions, Compulsions: Developmental Psychopathology and Clinical Care. New York, NY: John Wiley & Sons.
5. American Psychiatric Association. (2000). Diagnostic and Statistical Manual of Mental Disorders, Fourth Edition, Text Revision. Washington, DC: American Psychiatric Association.
6. Costello, E. J., Angold, A., Burns, B. J., et al. (1996). The Great Smokey Mountains study of youth: Functional impairment and serious emotional disturbance. Archives of General Psychiatry, 53, 1137-1143.
7. Freeman, R. D., Fast, D. K., Burd, L., et al. (2000). An international perspective on Tourette syndrome: Selected findings from 3500 individuals in 22 countries. Developmental Medicine and Child Neurology, 42, 436-447.
8. Banaschewski, T., Woerner, W., and Rothenberger, A. (2003). Premonitory sensory phenomena and suppressibility of tics in Tourette syndrome: Developmental aspects in youth and adolescents. Developmental Medicine and Child Neurology, 45, 700-703.
9. Woods, D. W., Piacentini, J., Himle, M. B., and Chang, S. (2005). Premonitory Urge for Tics Scale (PUTS): Initial psychometric results and examination of the premonitory urge phenomenon in youth with tic disorders. Journal of Developmental and Behavioral Pediatrics, 26, 397-403.
10. Dornbush, M. P. and Pruitt, S. K. (1995). Teaching the Tiger. Duarte, CA: Hope Press.
11. Apter, A., Pauls, D. L., Bleich, A., et al. (1993). An epidemiological study of Gilles de la Tourette's syndrome in Israel. Archives of General Psychiatry, 50, 734-738.
12. Zohar, A. H., Ratzoni, G., Pauls, D. L., et al. (1992). An epidemiological study of obsessive-compulsive disorder and related disorders in Israeli adolescents. Journal of the American Academy of Child and Adolescent Psychiatry, 31, 1057-1061.

13. Spencer, T., Biederman, J., Coffey, B., et al. (1999). The 4-year course of tic disorders in boys with attention-deficit/hyperactivity disorder. Archives of General Psychiatry, 56, 842-847.
14. Walkup, J. T., Khan, S., Schuerholz, L., et al. (1999). Phenomenology and natural history of tic-related ADHD and learning disabilities. In Leckman, J. F. and Cohen, D. J. editors: Tourette's Syndrome–Tics, Obsessions, Compulsions: Developmental Psychopathology and Clinical Care. New York, NY: John Wiley & Sons.
15. Leckman, J. F., King, R. A., and Cohen, D. J. (1999). Tics and tic disorders. In Leckman, J. F. and Cohen, D. J. editors: Tourette's Syndrome–Tics, Obsessions, Compulsions: Developmental Psychopathology and Clinical Care. New York, NY: John Wiley & Sons.
16. Spencer, T., Biederman, J., Harding, M., et al. (1998). Disentangling the overlap between Tourette's disorder and ADHD. Journal of Child Psychology and Psychiatry, 39, 1037-1044.
17. Peterson, B. S. (1996). Considerations of natural history and pathophysiology in the psychopharmacology of Tourette's syndrome. Journal of Clinical Psychiatry, 54 (Supplement 1), 24-34.
18. Bruun, R. D. and Budman, C. L. (1997). The course and prognosis of Tourette syndrome. Neurologic Clinics of North America, 15, 291-298.
19. Bruun, R. D. and Budman, C. L. (2005). The natural history of Gilles de la Tourette syndrome. In Kurlan, R. editor: Handbook of Tourette's Syndrome and Related Tic and Behavioral Disorders (2nd ed.). New York, NY: Marcel Dekker.
20. King, R. A., Leckman, J. F., Scahill, L., and Cohen, D. J. (1999). Obsessive-compulsive disorder, anxiety, and depression. In Leckman, J. F. and Cohen, D. J. editors: Tourette's Syndrome–Tics, Obsessions, Compulsions: Developmental Psychopathology and Clinical Care. New York, NY: John Wiley & Sons.
21. Packer, L. E. (1997). Social and educational resources for patients with Tourette syndrome. Neurologic Clinics of North America, 15, 457-473.
22. Como, P. G. (2005). Neuropsychological function in Tourette's syndrome. In Kurlan, R. editor: Handbook of Tourette's Syndrome and Related Tic and Behavioral Disorders (2nd ed.). New York, NY: Marcel Dekker.
23. Coffey, B. J., Frisone, D., and Gianini, L. (2005). Anxiety and other comorbid emotional disorders. In Kurlan, R. editor: Handbook of Tourette's Syndrome and Related Tic and Behavioral Disorders (2nd ed.). New York, NY: Marcel Dekker.
24. Kurlan, R., Como, P. G., Miller, B., et al. (2002). The behavioral spectrum of tic disorders. A community-based study. Neurology, 59, 414-420.
25. Cartwright-Hatton, S., McNicol, K., and Doubleday, E. (2006). Anxiety in a neglected population: Prevalence of anxiety disorders in preadolscent children. Clinical Psychology Review, 26, 817-833.
26. Coffey, B. J. and Park, K. S. (1997). Behavioral and emotional aspects of Tourette syndrome. Neurologic Clinics of North America, 15, 277-289.
27. Spencer, T., Biederman, J., Coffey, B., et al. (2001). Tourette disorder and ADHD. In Cohen, D. J., Goetz, C. G., and Jankovic, J. editors: Tourette Syndrome. Philadelphia, PA: Lippincott, Williams, and Wilkens.
28. Budman, C. L., Rockmore, L., and Bruun, R. D. (2005). Aggressive symptoms and Tourette's syndrome. In Kurlan, R. editor: Handbook of Tourette's Syndrome and Related Tic and Behavioral Disorders (2nd ed.). New York, NY: Marcel Dekker.
29. Abwender, D. A., Como, P. G., Kurlan, R., et al. (1996). School problems in Tourette's syndrome. Archives of Neurology, 53, 509-511.
30. Singer, H. S., Schuerholz, L. J., and Denckla, M. B. (1995). Learning difficulties in children with Tourette syndrome. Journal of Child Neurology, 10 (1), S58-S61.
31. Bloch, M. H., Peterson, B. S., Scahill, L., et al. (2006). Adulthood outcome of tic and obsessive-compulsive symptom severity in children with Tourette syndrome. Archives of Pediatric and Adolescent Medicine, 160, 65-69.

32. Leckman, J. F., Zhang, H., Vitale, A., et al. (1998). Course of tic severity in Tourette syndrome: The first two decades. Pediatrics, 102, 14-19.
33. Pappert, E. J., Goetz, C. G., Louis, E. D., et al. (2003). Objective assessments of longitudinal outcome in Gilles de la Tourette's syndrome. Neurology, 61, 936-940.

Chapter 3: Obsessive-Compulsive Disorder

1. American Psychiatric Association. (2000). Diagnostic and Statistical Manual of Mental Disorders, Fourth Edition, Text Revision. Washington, DC: American Psychiatric Association.
2. Adapted from Dornbush, M. P. and Pruitt, S. K. (1995). Teaching the Tiger. Duarte, CA: Hope Press.
3. Riddle, M. A., Scahill, L., King, R., et al. (1990). Obsessive-compulsive disorder in children and adolescents: Phenomenology and family history. Journal of the American Academy of Child and Adolescent Psychiatry, 29, 766-772.
4. Hanna, G. L. (1995). Demographic and clinical features of obsessive-compulsive disorder in children and adolescents. Journal of the American Academy of Child and Adolescent Psychiatry, 34, 19-27.
5. Geller, D. A., Biederman, J., Griffin, S., et al. (1996). Comorbidity of juvenile obsessive-compulsive disorder with disruptive behavior disorders. Journal of the American Academy of Child and Adolescent Psychiatry, 35, 1637-1646.
6. Geller, D. A., Biederman, J., Faraone, S., et al. (2001). Developmental aspects of obsessive-compulsive disorder: Findings in children, adolescents, and adults. Journal of Nervous and Mental Disease, 189, 471-477.
7. Geller, D. A. (1998). Juvenile obsessive-compulsive disorder. In Jenike, L., Baer, L., and Minichiello, W. E. editors: Obsessive-Compulsive Disorders: Practical Management, (3rd ed.). St. Louis, MO: Mosby.
8. Costello, E. J., Angold, A., Burns, B. J., et al. (1996). The Great Smokey Mountains study of youth: Goals, designs, methods, and prevalence of DSM-III-R disorders. Archives of General Psychiatry, 53, 1129-1136.
9. Costello, E. J., Mustillo, S., Erkanli, A., et al. (2003). Prevalence and development of psychiatric disorders in childhood and adolescence. Archives of General Psychiatry, 60, 837-844.
10. Geller, D. A., Biederman, J., Jones, J., et al. (1998). Is juvenile obsessive-compulsive disorder a developmental subtype of the disorder? A review of the pediatric literature. Journal of the American Academy of Child and Adolescent Psychiatry, 37, 420-427.
11. Peterson, B. S., Pine, D. S., Cohen, P., and Brook, J. S. (2001). Prospective, longitudinal study of tic, obsessive-compulsive, and attention-deficit/hyperactivity disorders in an epidemiological sample. Journal of the American Academy of Child and Adolescent Psychiatry, 40, 685-695.
12. Zohar, A. H. (1999). The epidemiology of obsessive-compulsive disorder in children and adolescents. Child and Adolescent Psychiatric Clinics of North America, 8, 445-460.
13. Valleni-Basile, L. A., Garrison, C. Z., Waller, J. L., et al. (1996). Incidence of obsessive-compulsive disorder in a community sample of young adolescents. Journal of the American Academy of Child and Adolescent Psychiatry, 35, 898-906.
14. Apter, A., Fallon, T. J., King, R. A., et al. (1996). Obsessive-compulsive characteristics: From symptoms to syndrome. Journal of the American Academy of Child and Adolescent Psychiatry, 35, 907-912.
15. Kessler, R. C., Adler, L., Barkley, R., et al. (2006). The prevalence and correlates of adult ADHD in the United States: Results from the National Comorbidity Survey Replication. American Journal of Psychiatry, 163, 716-723.
16. Biederman, J., Faraone, S., Milberger, S., et al. (1996). A prospective 4-year follow-up study of attention-deficit hyperactivity and related disorders. Archives of General Psychiatry, 53, 437-446.
17. Kurlan, R., McDermott, M. P., Deeley, C., et al. (2001). Prevalence of tics in schoolchildren and association with placement in special education. Neurology, 57, 1383-1388.
18. Coffey, B. J. and Park, K. S. (1997). Behavioral and emotional aspects of Tourette syndrome. Neurologic Clinics of North America, 15, 277-289.

Reference

19. Rasmussen, S. A. and Eisen, J. L. (1998). The epidemiology and clinical features of obsessive-compulsive disorder. In Jenike, M. A., Baer, L., and Minichiello, W. E. editors: <u>Obsessive-Compulsive Disorders: Practical Management (3rd ed.)</u>. St. Louis, MO: Mosby.
20. King, R. A., Leonard, H., March, J., et al. (1998). Practice parameters for the assessment and treatment of children and adolescents with obsessive-compulsive disorder. <u>Journal of the American Academy of Child and Adolescent Psychiatry, 37 (Supplement 10)</u>, 27S-45S.
21. Piacentini, J., Bergman, R. L., Keller, M., and McCracken, J. (2003). Functional impairment in children and adolescents with obsessive-compulsive disorder. <u>Journal of Child and Adolescent Psychopharmacology, 13 (Supplement 1)</u>, S61-S69.
22. Swedo, S. E., Rapoport, J. L., Leonard, H., et al. (1989). Obsessive-compulsive disorder in children and adolescents. Clinical phenomenology of 70 consecutive cases. <u>Archives of General Psychiatry, 46</u>, 335-341.
23. Swedo, S. E. and Rapoport, J. L. (1989). Phenomenology and differential diagnosis of obsessive-compulsive disorder in children and adolescents. In Rapoport, J. L. editor: <u>Obsessive-Compulsive Disorder in Children and Adolescents</u>. Washington, DC: American Psychiatric Press.
24. Cartwright-Hatton, S., McNicol, K., and Doubleday, E. (2006). Anxiety in a neglected population: Prevalence of anxiety disorders in preadolescent children. <u>Clinical Psychology Review, 26</u>, 817-833.
25. Geller, D. A., Biederman, J., Faraone, S. V., et al. (2002). Attention-deficit/hyperactivity disorder in children and adolescents with obsessive-compulsive disorder: Fact or artifact? <u>Journal of the American Academy of Child and Adolescent Psychiatry, 41</u>, 52-58.
26. Sukhodolsky, D. G., Rosario-Campos, M. C., Scahill, L., et al. (2005). Adaptive, emotional, and family functioning of children with obsessive-compulsive disorder and comorbid attention deficit hyperactivity disorder. <u>American Journal of Psychiatry, 162</u>, 1125-1132.
27. Zohar, A. H., Ratzoni, G., Pauls, D. L., et al. (1992). An epidemiological study of obsessive-compulsive disorder and related disorders in Israeli adolescents. <u>Journal of the American Academy of Child and Adolescent Psychiatry, 31</u>, 1057-1061.
28. Miguel, E. C., Coffey, B. J., Baer, L., et al. (1995). Phenomenology of intentional repetitive behaviors in obsessive-compulsive disorder and Tourette's syndrome. <u>Journal of Clinical Psychiatry, 56</u>, 246-255.
29. Leckman, J. F., Walker, D. E., Goodman, W. K., et al. (1994). "Just right" perceptions associated with compulsive behavior in Tourette's syndrome. <u>American Journal of Psychiatry, 151</u>, 675-680.
30. Miguel, E. C., Rosario-Campos, M. C., Shavitt, R. G., et al. (2001). The tic-related obsessive-compulsive disorder phenotype and treatment implications. In Cohen, D. J., Goetz, C. G., and Jankovic, J. editors: <u>Tourette Syndrome</u>. Philadelphia, PA: Lippencott, Williams and Wilkens.
31. King, R. A., Findley, D., Scahill, L., et al. (2005). Obsessive-compulsive disorder in Tourette's syndrome. In Kurlan, R. editor: <u>Handbook of Tourette's Syndrome and Related Tic and Behavioral Disorders (2nd ed.)</u>. New York, NY: Marcel Dekker.
32. Douglass, H. M., Moffitt, T. E., Dar, R., et al. (1995). Obsessive-compulsive disorder in a birth cohort of 18-year-olds: Prevalence and predictors. <u>Journal of the American Academy of Child and Adolescent Psychiatry, 34</u>, 1424-1431.
33. U.S. Department of Health and Human Services. (1999). <u>Mental Health: A Report of the Surgeon General-Executive Summary</u>. Rockville, MD: U.S. Department of Health and Human Services, Substance Abuse and Mental Health Services Administration, Center for Mental Health Services, National Institutes of Health, National Institute of Mental Health.
34. Leonard, H. L., Swedo, S. E., Lenane, M. C., et al. (1993). A 2- to 7-year follow-up study of 54 obsessive-compulsive children and adolescents. <u>Archives of General Psychiatry, 50</u>, 429-439.
35. Kessler, R. C., Berglund, P., Demler, O., et al. (2005). Lifetime prevalence age-of-onset distributions of DSM-IV disorders in the National Comorbidity Survey Replication. <u>Archives of General Psychiatry, 62</u>, 593-602.
36. Stewart, S. E., Geller, D. A., Jenike, M., et al. (2004). Long-term outcome of pediatric obsessive-compulsive disorder: A meta-analysis and qualitative review of the literature. <u>Acta Psychiatrica Scandinavica, 110</u>, 4-13.

Section VIII

Chapter 4: Arousal/Processing Speed/Attention/Inhibition

1. Anderson, V. A., Anderson, P., Northam, E., et al. (2001). Development of executive functions through late childhood and early adolescence in an Australian sample. Developmental Neuropsychology, 20, 385-406.
2. Korkman, M., Kemp, S. L., and Kirk, U. (2001). Effects of age on neurocognitive measures of children 5 to 12: A cross-sectional study on 800 children from the United States. Developmental Neuropsychology, 20, 331-354.
3. McKay, K. E., Halperin, J. M., Schwartz, S. T., and Sharma, V. (1994). Developmental analysis of three aspects of information processing: Sustained attention, selective attention, and response organization. Developmental Neuropsychology, 10, 121-132.
4. Klenberg, L., Korkman, M., and Lahti-Nuuttila, P. (2001). Differential development of attention and executive functions in 3- to 12-year-old Finnish children. Developmental Neuropsychology, 20, 407-428.
5. Welsh, M. C. (2002). Developmental and clinical variations in executive functions. In Molfese, D. L. and Molfese, V. J. editors: Developmental Variations in Learning: Applications to Social, Executive Function, Language, and Reading Skills. Mahwah, NJ: Lawrence Erlbaum Associates.

Chapter 5: Executive Functions

1. Denckla, M. B. (1996). A theory and model of executive function: A neuro-psychological perspective. In Lyon, G. R. and Krasnegor, N. A. editors: Attention, Memory, and Executive Function. Baltimore, MD: Paul. H. Brooks Publishing.
2. Denckla, M. B. (2000). Learning disabilities and attention-deficit/hyperactivity disorder in adults: Overlap with executive dysfunction. In Brown, T. E. editor: Attention-Deficit Disorders and Comorbidities in Children, Adolescents, and Adults. Washington, DC: American Psychiatric Press.
3. Lezak, M. D. (1995). Neuropsychological Assessment (3rd ed.). New York, NY: Oxford University Press.
4. Welch, M. C. and Pennington, B. F. (1988). Assessing frontal lobe functioning in children: Views from developmental psychology. Developmental Neuropsychology, 4, 199-230.
5. Brown, T. E. (2008). Executive functions: Describing six aspects of a complex syndrome. Attention, 15, 12-17.
6. Gioia, G. A., Isquith, P. K., and Guy, S. C. (2000). Behavior Rating Inventory of Executive Function. Odessa, FL: Psychological Assessment Resources.
7. Welsh, M. C. (2002). Developmental and clinical variations in executive functions. In Molfese, D. L. and Molfese, V. J. editors: Developmental Variations in Learning: Applications to Social, Executive Function, Language, and Reading Skills. Mahwah, NJ: Lawrence Erlbaum Associates.
8. Klenberg, L., Korkman, M., and Lahti-Nuuttila, P. (2001). Differential development of attention and executive functions in 3- to 12-year-old Finnish children. Developmental Neuropsychology, 20, 407-428.
9. Anderson, V. A., Anderson, P., Northam, E., et al. (2001). Development of executive functions through late childhood and early adolescence in an Australian sample. Developmental Neuropsychology, 20, 385-406.
10. Korkman, M., Kemp, S. L., and Kirk, U. (2001). Effects of age on neurocognitive measures of children 5 to 12: A cross-sectional study on 800 children from the United States. Developmental Neuropsychology, 20, 331-354.

Chapter 6: Memory

1. Baddeley, A. D. (1986). Working Memory. New York, NY: Oxford University Press.
2. Baddeley, A. D. (1996). Exploring the central executive. The Quarterly Journal of Experimental Psychology, 49A, 5-28.

3. Baddeley, A. D. (2000). The episodic buffer: A new component of working memory. Trends in Cognitive Sciences, 4, 417-423.
4. Hutton, U. M. Z. and Towse, J. N. (2001). Short-term memory and working memory as indices of children's cognitive skills. Memory, 9, 383-394.
5. Luciana, M., Conklin, H. M., Hooper, C. J., and Yarger, R. S. (2005). The development of nonverbal working memory and executive control processes in adolescents. Child Development, 76, 697-712.
6. Conklin, H. M., Luciana, M., Hooper, C. J., and Yarger, R. S. (2007). Working memory performance in typically developing children and adolescents: Behavioral evidence of protracted frontal lobe development. Developmental Neuropsychology, 31, 103-128.
7. Welsh, M. C. (2000). Developmental and clinical variations in executive functions. In Molfese, D. L. and Molfese, V. J. editors: Developmental Variations in Learning: Applications to Social, Executive Function, Language, and Reading Skills. Mahwah, NJ: Lawrence Erlbaum Associates.
8. Gathercole, S. E. (1998). The development of memory. Journal of Child Psychology and Psychiatry and Allied Disciplines, 39, 3-27.
9. Bruer, J. T. (1993). Schools for Thought: A Science of Learning in the Classroom. Cambridge, MA: MIT Press.
10. Stickgold, R. and Walker, M. P. (2005). Memory consolidation and reconsolidation: What is the role of sleep? Trends in Neurosciences, 28, 408-415.
11. Ward, H., Shum, D., McKinlay, L., et al. (2005). Development of prospective memory: Tasks based on the prefrontal-lobe model. Child Neuropsychology, 11, 527-549.
12. Case R. (1995). Capacity-based explanations of working memory growth: A brief history and reevaluation. In Weinert, F. S. and Schneider, W. editors: Memory Performance and Competencies: Issues in Growth and Development. Mahwah, NJ: Lawrence Erlbaum Associates.
13. Pressley, M. and Van Meter, P. (1994). What is memory development the development of? A 1990's theory of memory and cognitive development 'twixt 2 and 20. In Morris, P. and Gruneberg, M. editors: Theoretical Aspects of Memory (2nd ed.). New York, NY: Routledge.

SECTION II: RESOURCES

Chapter 7: Medication/Therapeutic Interventions/Educational and Community Resources

1. Dornbush, M. P. and Pruitt, S. K. (1995). Teaching the Tiger. Duarte, CA: Hope Press.
2. MTA Cooperative Group. (1999). A 14-month randomized clinical trial of treatment strategies for attention-deficit/hyperactivity disorder. Archives of General Psychiatry, 56, 1073-1086.
3. Arnold, L. E., Swanson, J. M., Hechtman, L., et al. (2008). Understanding the 36-month MTA follow-up findings in context. Attention, 15, 15-18.
4. March, J. S. (1995). Cognitive-behavioral psychotherapy for children and adolescents with OCD: A review and recommendations for treatment. Journal of the American Academy of Child and Adolescent Psychiatry, 34, 7-18.
5. Watson, H. J. and Rees, C. S. (2008). Meta-analysis of randomized, controlled treatment trials for pediatric obsessive-compulsive disorder. Journal of Child Psychology and Psychiatry, 49, 489-498.
6. Piacentini, J. (1999). Cognitive behavioral therapy of childhood OCD. Child and Adolescent Psychiatric Clinics of North America, 8, 599-616.
7. Storch, E. A., Merlo, L. J., Larson, M. J., et al. (2008). Impact of comorbidity on cognitive-behavioral therapy response in pediatric obsessive-compulsive disorder. Journal of the American Academy of Child and Adolescent Psychiatry, 47, 583-592.
8. March, J., Foa, E., Gammon, P. (2004). Cognitive-behavior therapy, sertraline, and their combination for children and adolescents with obsessive-compulsive disorder: The Pediatric OCD Treatment Study (POTS) randomized controlled trial. Journal of the American Medical Association, 292, 1969-1976.
9. Johnston, H. F. and March, J. S. (1993). Obsessive-compulsive disorder in children and adolescents. In Reynolds, W. editor: Internalizing Disorders in Children and Adolescents. New York, NY: John Wiley & Sons.

Section VIII

10. Azrin, N. H. and Nunn, R. G. (1973). Habit-reversal: A method of eliminating nervous habits and tics. <u>Behaviour Research and Therapy</u>, <u>11</u>, 619-628.
11. Piacentini, J. and Chang, S. (2005). Habit reversal training for tic disorders in children and adolescents. <u>Behavior Modification</u>, <u>29</u>, 803-822.
12. Peterson, A. L. (2007). Psychosocial management of tics and intentional repetitive behaviors associated with Tourette syndrome. In Woods, D. W., Piacentini, J. C., and Walkup, J. T. editors: <u>Treating Tourette Syndrome and Tic Disorders</u>. New York, NY: Guilford Press.
13. Woods, D. W., Miltenberger, R. G., and Lumley, V. A. (1996). Sequential application of major habit-reversal components to treat motor tics in children. <u>Journal of Applied Behavior Analysis</u>, <u>29</u>, 483-493.
14. Carr, J. E. and Chong, I. M. (2005). Habit reversal treatment of tic disorders: A methodological critique of the literature. <u>Behavior Modification</u>, <u>29</u>, 858-875.
15. Hoag, M. J. and Burlingame, G. M. (1997). Evaluating the effectiveness of child and adolescent group treatment: A meta-analytic review. <u>Journal of Clinical Child Psychology</u>, <u>26</u>, 234-246.

SECTION III: INTERVENTIONS

Chapter 8: Classroom Modifications/Accommodations

1. Dornbush, M. P. and Pruitt, S. K. (1995). <u>Teaching the Tiger</u>. Duarte, CA: Hope Press.
2. Packer, L. E. (2005). Tic-related school problems: Impact on functioning, accommodations, and interventions. <u>Behavior Modification</u>, <u>29</u>, 876-899.
3. U.S. Department of Health and Human Services: Health Resources and Services Administration (HRSA). www.stopbullyingnow.hrsa.gov
4. Nasel, T. R., Overpeck, M., Pilla, R. S., et al. (2001). Bullying behaviors among U.S. youth: Prevalence and association with psychosocial adjustment. <u>Journal of the American Medical Association</u>, <u>285</u>, 2094-2100.
5. Bradshaw, C. P., Sawyer, A. L., and O'Brennan, L. M. (2007). Bullying and peer victimization at school: Perceptual differences between students and school staff. <u>School Psychology Review</u>, <u>36(3)</u>, 361-382.
6. Unnever, J. D. and Cornell, D. G. (2003). Bullying, self-control, and ADHD. <u>Journal of Interpersonal Violence</u>, <u>18</u>, 129-147.
7. Leff, S. S., Kupersmidt, J. B., Patterson, C. J., and Power, T. J. (1999). Factors influencing teacher identification of peer bullies and victims. <u>School Psychology Review</u>, <u>28</u>, 505-517.
8. Davidson, L. M. and Demaray, M. K. (2007). Social support as a moderator between victimization and internalizing-externalizing distress from bulling. <u>School Psychology Review</u>, <u>36(3)</u>, 383-405.
9. Olweus, D. and Limber, S. (1999). Bullying prevention program. In Elliott, D. S. (series editor): <u>Blueprints for Violence Prevention: Book Nine, Bullying Prevention Program</u>. Boulder, CO: Institute of Behavioral Science, Regents of the University of Colorado.
10. Vreeman, R. C. and Carroll, A. E. (2007). A systematic review of school-based interventions to prevent bullying. <u>Archives of Pediatric and Adolescent Medicine</u>, <u>161</u>, 78-88.
11. Soderlund, G., Sikstrom, S., and Smart, A. (2007). Listen to the noise. Noise is beneficial for cognitive performance in ADHD. <u>Journal of Child Psychology and Psychiatry</u>, <u>48</u>, 840-847.
12. Abikoff, H., Courtney, M. E., Szeibel, P. J., and Koplewicz, H. S. (1996). The effects of auditory stimulation on the arithmetic performance of children with ADHD and nondisabled children. <u>Journal of Learning Disabilities</u>, <u>29</u>, 238-246.

Chapter 9: Student Interventions

1. Dornbush, M. P. and Pruitt, S. K. (1995). <u>Teaching the Tiger</u>. Duarte, CA: Hope Press.
2. Seligman, M. E. (1974). Depression and learned helplessness. In Friedman, R. and Katz, M. M. editors: <u>The Psychology of Depression: Contemporary Theory and Research</u>. Washington, DC: Winston-Wiley.

3. Herman, K. C. and Ostrander, R. (2007). The effects of attention problems on depression: Developmental, academic, and cognitive pathways. School Psychology Quarterly, 22(4), 483-510.
4. Gickling, E. and Armstrong, D. L. (1978). Levels of instructional difficulty as related to on-task behavior, task completion, and comprehension. Journal of Learning Disabilities, 11, 559-566.
5. Pruitt, S. K. (1995). Trick Book. Teaching the Tiger. Duarte, CA: Hope Press.
6. Dunn, R. and Dunn, K. (1992). Teaching Elementary Students Through Their Individual Learning Styles: Practical Approaches for Grades 3-6. Boston, MA: Allyn and Bacon.
7. Dunn, R. and Dunn, K. (1993). Teaching Secondary Students Through Their Individual Learning Styles: Practical Approaches for Grades 7-12. Boston, MA: Allyn and Bacon.
8. Lovelace, M. K. (2005). Meta-analysis of experimental research based on the Dunn and Dunn model. Journal of Educational Research, 98, 176-182.
9. Gardner, H. (1983). Frames of Mind: The Theory of Multiple Intelligences. New York, NY: Basic Books, HarperCollins Publishers.
10. Gardner, H. (1991). The Unschooled Mind: How Children Think and How Schools Should Teach. New York, NY: Basic Books, HarperCollins Publishers.
11. Armstrong, T. (2000). In Their Own Way: Discovering and Encouraging Your Child's Personal Learning Style - Revised. Los Angeles, CA: Putnam Publishing Group.
12. Armstrong, T. (1999). 7 Kinds of Smart: Identifying and Developing Your Multiple Intelligences - Revised. New York, NY: Penguin Group.
13. Inspiration Software (1988-to present). Inspiration and Kidspiration Portland, OR: Author. Available from Inspiration Software, Inc., 7412 SW Beaverton Hillsdale Hwy., Suite 102, Portland, OR 97225-2167. Available at www.inspiration.com.
14. Marcotte A. C. and Stern, C. (1997). Qualitative analysis of graphomotor output in children with attentional disorders. Child Neuropsychology, 3, 147-153.
15. Mayes, S. D. and Calhoun, S. L. (2007). Learning, attention, writing, and processing speed in typical children and children with ADHD, autism, anxiety, depression, and oppositional defiant disorder. Child Neuropsychology, 13, 469-493.
16. Schultz, R. T., Carter, A. S., Scahill, L., and Leckman, J. F. (1999). Neuropsychological findings. In Leckman, J. F. and Cohen, D. J. editors: Tourette's Syndrome - Tics, Obsession, Compulsions: Developmental Pathology and Clinical Care. New York, NY: John Wiley & Sons.
17. Schultz, R. T., Evans, D. W., and Wolff, M. (1999). Neuropsychological models of childhood obsessive-compulsive disorder. Child and Adolescent Psychiatric Clinics of North America, 8, 513-531.
18. Jimerson, S. R. (2001). Meta-analysis of grade retention research: Implications for practice in the 21st century. School Psychology Review, 30, 420-437.
19. Jimerson, S. R. (2004). Is grade retention educational malpractice? Empirical evidence from meta-analyses examining the efficacy of grade retention. In Walberg, H. J., Reynolds, A. J., and Wang, M. C. editors: Can Unlike Students Learn Together? Grade Retention, Tracking, and Grouping. Greenwich, CT: Information Age Publishing.
20. Jimerson, S. R. and Ferguson, P. (2007). A longitudinal study of grade retention: Academic and behavioral outcomes of retained students through adolescence. School Psychology Quarterly, 22(30), 314-339.

Chapter 10: Underarousal/Slow Cognitive Processing Speed

1. Healy, D. and Rucklidge, J. J. (2006). An investigation into the relationship among ADHD symptomatology, creativity, and neuropsychological functioning in children. Child Neuropsychology, 12, 421-438.
2. Rucklidge, J. J. and Tannock, R. (2002). Neuropsychological profiles of adolescents with ADHD. Effects of reading difficulties and gender. Journal of Child Psychology and Psychiatry, 43, 1-16.

3. Mayes, S. D. and Calhoun, S. L. (2007). Learning, attention, writing, and processing speed in typical children and children with ADHD, autism, anxiety, depression, and oppositional defiant disorder. Child Neuropsychology, 13, 469-493.
4. Carlson, C. L. and Mann, M. (2002). Sluggish cognitive tempo predicts a different pattern of impairment in attention deficit hyperactivity disorder, predominately inattentive type. Journal of Clinical Child and Adolescent Psychology, 31, 123-129.
5. Goodyear, P. and Hynd, G. W. (1992). Attention-deficit disorder with (ADD/H) and without (ADD/WO) hyperactivity: Behavioral and neuropsychological differentiation. Journal of Clinical Child Psychology, 21, 273-305.
6. Nigg, J. T., Blaskey, L. G., Huang-Pollock, C. L., and Rappley, M. D. (2002). Neuropsychological executive functions and DSM-IV ADHD subtypes. Journal of the American Academy of Child and Adolescent Psychiatry, 41, 59-66.
7. Weiler, M. D., Bernstein, J. H., Bellinger, D. C., and Waber, D. P. (2000). Processing speed in children with attention deficit/hyperactivity disorder, inattentive type. Child Neuropsychology, 6, 218-234.
8. Barkley, R. A. (2006). Attention-Deficit Hyperactivity Disorder (3rd ed.): A Handbook for Diagnosis and Treatment. New York, NY: Guilford Press.
9. Singer, H. S., Schuerholz, L. J., and Denckla, M. B. (1995). Learning difficulties in children with Tourette syndrome. Journal of Child Neurology, 10, S58-S61.
10. Schultz, R. T., Carter, A. S., Scahill, L., and Leckman, J. F. (1999). Neuropsychological findings. In Leckman, J. F. and Cohen, D. J. editors: Tourette's Syndrome–Tics, Obsession, Compulsions: Developmental Psychopathology and Clinical Care. New York, NY: John Wiley & Sons.
11. Schultz, R. T., Evans, D. W., and Wolff, M. (1999). Neuropsychological models of childhood obsessive-compulsive disorder. Child and Adolescent Psychiatric Clinics of North American, 8, 513-531.
12. Hoben, T. F. (2004). Sleep and its disorders in children. Seminars in Neurology, 24, 327-340.
13. Dornbush, M. P. and Pruitt, S. K. (1995). Teaching the Tiger. Duarte, CA: Hope Press.
14. Wilbarger, P. and Wilbarger J. (1991). Sensory Defensiveness in Children aged 2-12: An Intervention Guide for Parents and Other Caregivers. Denver, CO: Avanti Educational Programs.
15. Wilbarger, P. (1995). The sensory diet: Activity programs based on sensory processing theory. American Occupational Association Sensory Integration Special Interest Section Newsletter, 18, 1-3.
16. Williams, M. S. and Shellenberger, S. (1994). How Does Your Engine Run? Albuquerque, NM: Therapy Works.
17. Stickgold, R. and Walker, M. P. (2005). Memory consolidation and reconsolidation: What is the role of sleep? Trends in Neurosciences, 28, 408-415.
18. Walker, M. P. and Stickgold, R. (2004). Sleep-dependent learning and memory consolidation. Neuron, 44, 121-133.
19. Rauchs, G., Desgranges, B., Foret, J., and Eustache, F. (2005). The relationship between memory systems and sleep stages. Journal of Sleep Research, 14, 123-140.
20. Gruber, R., Sadeh, A., and Raviv, A. (2000). Instability of sleep patterns in children with attention-deficit/hyperactivity disorder. Journal of the American Academy of Child and Adolescent Psychiatry, 39, 495-501.
21. Owens, J. A., Maxim, R., Nobile, C., et al. (2000). Parental and self-report of sleep in children with attention-deficit/hyperactivity disorder. Archives of Pediatric and Adolescent Medicine, 154, 549-555.
22. Lecendreux, M., Konofal, E., Bouvard, M., et al. (2000). Sleep and alertness in children with ADHD. Journal of Child Psychology and Psychiatry, 41, 803-812.
23. Rothenberger, A., Kostanecka, T., Kinkelbur, J., et al. (2001). Sleep and Tourette syndrome. In Cohen, D. J., Goetz, C. G., and Kankovic, J. editors: Tourette Syndrome. Philadelphia, PA: Lippincott, Williams, & Wilkins.
24. Kostanecka-Endress, T., Banaschewski, T., Kinkelbur, J., et al. (2003). Disturbed sleep in children with Tourette syndrome. A polysomnographic study. Journal of Psychosomatic Research, 55, 23-29.

25. Allen, R. P., Singer, H. S., Brown, J. E., and Salam, M. M. (1992). Sleep disorders in Tourette syndrome: A primary or unrelated problem? Pediatric Neurology, 8, 275-280.
26. Cortese, S., Konofal, E., Yateman, N., et al. (2006). Sleep disturbances in children with ADHD. The ADHD Report, 14(3), 6-11.
27. Golan, N., Shahar, E., Ravid, S., and Pillar, G. (2004). Sleep disorders and daytime sleepiness in children with attention-deficit/hyperactivity disorder. Sleep, 27, 261-266.
28. Stein, D., Pat-Horenczyk, R., Blank, S., et al. (2002). Sleep disturbances in adolescents with symptoms of attention-deficit/hyperactivity disorder. Journal of Learning Disabilities, 35, 268-275.
29. Ring, A. Stein, D., Barak, Y., et al. (1998). Sleep disturbances in children with attention-deficit/hyperactivity disorder: A comparative study with healthy siblings. Journal of Learning Disabilities, 31, 572-578.
30. Marcotte, A., Thacher, P. V., Butters, M., et al. (1998). Parental report of sleep problems in children with attentional and learning disorders. Journal of Behavioral Pediatrics, 19, 178-186.
31. Owens, J., Sangal, R. B., Allen, A. J., et al. (2004). Sleep of children with ADHD compared to healthy controls. Sleep, 27, Abstract Supplement, A91.
32. Packer, L. E. and Pruitt, S. K. (2002-2008). Sleep Survey. Challenging Kids, Inc.
33. Steenari, M. R., Vuontela, V., Paavonen, E. J., et al. (2003). Working memory and sleep in 6- to 13-year-old schoolchildren. Journal of the American Academy of Child and Adolescent Psychiatry, 42, 85-92.
34. Wolfson, A. R. and Carskadon, M. A. (1998). Sleep schedules and daytime functioning in adolescents. Child Development, 69, 875-887.
35. Aronen, E. T., Paavonen, E. J., Fjallberg, M., et al. (2000). Sleep and psychiatric symptoms in school-age children. Journal of the American Academy of Child and Adolescent Psychiatry, 39, 502-508.
36. Buick, J. V. (2004). Television viewing, computer game playing, and Internet use and self-reported time to bed and time out of bed in secondary school children. Sleep, 27, 101-104.
37. Buick, J. V. (2007). Adolescent use of mobile phones for calling and for sending text messages after lights out: Results from a prospective cohort study with a one-year follow up. Sleep, 30, 1220-1223.
38. Kratochvil, C. J., Lake, M., Pliszka, S. R., and Walkup, J. T. (2005) Pharmacological management of treatment-induced insomnia in ADHD. Journal of the American Academy of Child and Adolescent Psychiatry, 44, 499-501.
39. Cohrs, S., Rasch, T., Altmeyer, S., et al. (2001). Decreased sleep quality and increased sleep related movements in patients with Tourette's syndrome. Journal of Neurological and Neurosurgical Psychiatry, 70, 192-197.

Chapter 11: Anxiety/"Storms"/Overarousal

1. Roblek, T. and Piacentini, J. (2005). Cognitive-behavior therapy for childhood anxiety disorders. Child and Adolescent Psychiatric Clinics of North America, 14, 863-876.
2. Ginsburg, G. S., Riddle, M. A., and Davies, M. (2006). Somatic symptoms in children and adolescents with anxiety disorders. Journal of the American Academy of Child and Adolescent Psychiatry, 45, 1179-1187.
3. Jensen, P. S. and Cantwell, D. (1997). Comorbidity in ADHD. Implications for research, practice, and DSM 5. Journal of the American Academy of Child and Adolescent Psychiatry, 35, 1065-1079.
4. Tannock, R. and Schachar, R. (1995). Differential-effects of methylphenidate on working-memory in children with and without comorbid anxiety. Journal of the American Academy of Child and Adolescent Psychiatry, 43, 886-896.
5. Carlson, C. L. and Mann, M. (2002). Sluggish cognitive tempo predicts a different pattern of impairment in the attention deficit/hyperactivity disorder, predominately inattentive type. Journal of Clinical Child and Adolescent Psychology, 31, 123-129.
6. Hartman, C. A., Willcutt, W. G., Rhee, S. H., and Pennington, B. F. (2004). The relation between sluggish cognitive tempo and DSM IV ADHD. Journal of Abnormal Child Psychology, 35, 491-503.

Section VIII

7. Brown, T. E. (2000). Attention-Deficit Disorders and Comorbidities in Children, Adolescents, and Adults. Washington, DC: American Psychiatric Press.
8. Jensen, P. S., Hinshaw, S. P., Kraemer, H. C., et al. (2001). ADHD comorbidity findings from the MTA study: Comparing comorbid subgroups. Journal of the American Academy of Child and Adolescent Psychiatry, 40, 147-158.
9. Dornbush, M. P. and Pruitt, S. K. (1995). Teaching the Tiger. Duarte, CA: Hope Press.
10. Pruitt, S. K. (1983). "Storms." Staff grand rounds. Parkaire Consultants, Atlanta, GA.
11. Mick, E., Spencer, T., Woznick, J., and Biederman, J. (2005). Heterogeneity of irritability in attention-deficit/hyperactivity disorder subjects with and without mood disorders. Biological Psychiatry, 58, 576-582.
12. Biederman, J., Faraone, S., Milberger, S., et al. (1996). A prospective 4-year follow-up study of attention-deficit hyperactivity and related disorders. Archives of General Psychiatry, 53, 437-446.
13. Budman, C. L., Bruun, R., Park, K., et al. (2000). Explosive outbursts in children with Tourettte's disorder. Journal of the American Academy of Child and Adolescent Psychiatry, 39, 1270-1276.
14. Stephens, R. J. and Sandor, P. (1999). Aggressive behavior in children with Tourette syndrome and comorbid attention-deficit hyperactivity disorder and obsessive-compulsive disorder. Canadian Journal of Psychiatry, 44, 1036-1042.
15. Budman, C. L., Rockmore, L., and Sossin, M. (2003). Clinical phenomenology of episodic rage in children with Tourette syndrome. Journal of Psychosomatic Research, 55, 59-65.
16. Platzman, K. A. and Pruitt, S. K. (2003). Is It Naughty of Neurological. Handout at Grand Rounds. Parkaire Consultants. Atlanta, GA.
17. Sukhodolsky, D. G., Scahill, L., Zhang, H., et al. (2003). Disruptive behavior in children with Tourette's syndrome: Association with ADHD comorbidity, tic severity, and functional impairment. Journal of the American Academy of Child and Adolescent Psychiatry, 42, 98-105.
18. Geller, D. A., Biederman, J., Faraone, S., et al. (2001). Developmental aspects of obsessive-compulsive disorder: Findings in children, adolescents, and adults. Journal of Nervous and Mental Disease, 189, 471-477.
19. Meichenbaum, D. H. and Goodman, J. (1971). Training impulsive children to talk to themselves: A means of developing self-control. Journal of Abnormal Psychology, 77, 115-126.
20. Mary Jane Trotti. (2006). Parkaire Consultants. Atlanta, GA.
21. Pruitt, S. K. (1990). "Graceful Exit." Staff Development Course-Impact of Neurological Disorders on Education, Behavior, and Socialization. Atlanta, GA: State of Georgia.
22. Giler, J. Z. (2000). Socially ADDept. Santa Barbara, CA: CES Publications.
23. Wagner, A. P. (2002). What to Do When Your Child Has Obsessive-Compulsive Disorder. Strategies and Solutions. Rochester, NY: Lighthouse Press.
24. Chansky, T. E. (2000). Freeing Your Child from Obsessive-Compulsive Disorder. New York, NY: Three Rivers Press.
25. Pruitt, S. K. (1992). "Public Hangings." Staff Development Course-Impact of Neurological Disorders on Education, Behavior, and Socialization. Atlanta, GA: State of Georgia.

Chapter 12: Inattention/Impulsivity/Hyperactivity

1. Sherman, E. M. S., Shepard, L., Joschko, M., and Freeman, R. D. (1998). Sustained attention and impulsivity in children with Tourette syndrome: Comorbidity and confounds. Journal of Clinical and Experimental Neuropsychology, 20, 644-657.
2. Dornbush, M. P. and Pruitt, S. K. (1995). Teaching the Tiger. Duarte, CA: Hope Press.
3. Geffner, D., Lucker, J. R., and Koch, W. (1996). Evaluation of auditory discrimination in children with ADD and without ADD. Child Psychiatry and Human Development, 26, 169-179.
4. Soderlund, G., Sikstrom, S., and Smart, A. (2007). Listen to the noise: Noise is beneficial for cognitive performance in ADHD. Journal of Child Psychology and Psychiatry, 48, 840-847.

5. Ozonoff, S., Strayer, D. L., McMahon, W. M., and Filloux, F. (1998). Inhibitory deficits in Tourette syndrome: A function of comorbidity and symptom severity. Journal of Child Psychiatry, 39, 1109-1118.
6. Wilbarger, P. and Wilbarger J. (1991). Sensory Defensiveness in Children aged 2-12: An Intervention Guide for Parents and Other Caregivers. Denver, CO: Avanti Educational Programs.
7. Wilbarger, P. (1995). The sensory diet: Activity programs based on sensory processing theory. American Occupational Association Sensory Integration Special Interest Section Newsletter, 18, 1-3.
8. Williams, M. S. and Shellenberger, S. (1994). How Does Your Engine Run? Albuquerque, NM: Therapy Works.

Chapter 13: Executive Dysfunction

1. Mahone, E. M., Cirion, P. T., Cutting, L. E., et al. (2002). Validity of the behavior rating inventory of executive function in children with ADHD and/or Tourette syndrome. Archives of Clinical Neuropsychology, 17, 643-662.
2. Pennington, B. F. and Ozonoff S. (1996). Executive functions and developmental psychopathology. Journal of Child Psychology and Psychiatry, 37, 51-87.
3. Shallice, T., Marzocchi, G. M., Coser, S., et al. (2002). Executive function profile of children with attention deficit hyperactivity disorder. Developmental Neuropsychology, 21, 43-71.
4. Martel, M., Nikolas, M., and Nigg, J. T. (2007). Executive function in adolescents with ADHD. Journal of the American Academy of Child and Adolescent Psychiatry, 46, 1437-1444.
5. Fischer, M., Barkley, R. A., Edelbrock, C. S., and Smallish, L. (1990). The adolescent outcome of hyperactive children diagnosed by research criteria: II. Academic, attentional, and neuropsychological status. Journal of Consulting and Clinical Psychology, 58, 580-588.
6. Seidman, L. J., Biedermen, J., Faraone, S. V., et al. (1997). Toward defining a neuropsychology of attention-deficit hyperactivity disorder: Performance of children and adolescents from a large clinically referred sample. Journal of Consulting and Clinical Psychology, 65, 150-160.
7. Biederman, J., Petty, C. R., Doyle, A. E., et al. (2008). Stability of executive function deficits in girls with ADHD: A prospective longitudinal followup study into adolescence. Developmental Neuropsychology, 33, 44-61.
8. Fischer, M., Barkley, R. A., Smallish, L., and Fletcher, K. (2005). Executive functioning in hyperactive children as young adults: Attention, inhibition, response perseveration, and the impact of comorbidity. Developmental Neuropsychology, 27, 107-133.
9. Seidman, L. J., Biederman, J., Weber, W., et al. (1998). Neuropsychological function in adults with attention-deficit hyperactivity disorder. Biological Psychiatry, 44, 260-268.
10. Sherman, E. M. S., Shepard, L., Joschko, M., and Freeman, R. D. (1998). Sustained attention and impulsivity in children with Tourette syndrome: Comorbidity and confounds. Journal of Clinical and Experimental Neuropsychology, 20, 644-657.
11. Ozonoff, S., Strayer, D. L., McMahon, W. M., and Filloux, F. (1998). Inhibitory deficits in Tourette syndrome: A function of comorbidity and symptom severity. Journal of Child Psychiatry, 39, 1109-1118.
12. Channon, S., Pratt, P., and Robertson, M. M. (2003). Executive function, memory, and learning in Tourette's syndrome. Neuropsychology, 17, 247-254.
13. de Groot, C. M., Yeates, K. O., Baker, G. B., and Bornstein, R. A. (1997). Impaired neuropsychological functioning in Tourette's syndrome subjects with co-occurring obsessive-compulsive and attention deficit symptoms. Journal of Neuropsychiatry and Clinical Neurosciences, 9, 267-272.
14. Schultz, R. T., Evans, D. W., and Wolff, M. (1999). Neuropsychological models of childhood obsessive-compulsive disorder. Child and Adolescent Psychiatric Clinics of North America, 8, 513-531.
15. Savage, C. R., Baer, L., Keuthen, N. J., et al. (1999). Organizational strategies mediate nonverbal memory impairment in obsessive-compulsive disorder. Biological Psychiatry, 45, 905-916.

16. Pruitt, S. K. (1995). "Get a Clue." Staff Development Course "Clueless." Atlanta, GA: State of Georgia.
17. Pruitt, D. G. and Pruitt, S. K. (2001). "P. L. A. N." Adapted from Staff Development Course. Atlanta, GA: State of Georgia.
18. Inspiration Software (1988-to present). Inspiration and Kidspiration Portland, OR: Author. Available from Inspiration Software, Inc., 7412 SW Beaverton Hillsdale Hwy., Suite 102, Portland, OR 97225-2167. Available at www.inspiration.com
19. Pruitt, D. G. (2006). Parkaire Consultants. Atlanta, GA.
20. Siklos, S. and Kerns, K. A. (2004). Assessing multitasking in children with ADHD using a modified Six Elements Test. *Archives of Clinical Neuropsychology*, 19, 347-361.
21. Savage, C. R. (1998). Neuropsychology of obsessive-compulsive disorder: Research findings and treatment implications. In Jenike, M. A., Baer, L., and Minichiello, W. E. editors: *Obsessive-Compulsive Disorders: Practical Management*. St. Louis, MO: Mosby, Inc.
22. Dornbush, M. P. and Pruitt, S. K. (1995). *Teaching the Tiger*. Duarte, CA: Hope Press.
23. Packer, L. E. and Pruitt, S. K. (2002-2008). Organizational Skills Survey. Challenging Kids, Challenged Teachers!, Inc.
24. Levine, M. D. (1994). *Educational Care: A System for Understanding and Helping Children with Learning Problems at Home and in School*. Cambridge, MA: Educators Publishing Service, Inc.
25. Cappella, B., Gentile, J. R., and Juliano, D. B. (1977). Time estimation by hyperactive and normal children. *Perceptual and Motor Skills*, 44, 787-790.
26. Meaux, J. B. and Chelonis, J. J. (2003). Time perception differences in children with and without ADHD. *Journal of Pediatric Health Care*, 17, 64-71.
27. Toplak, M. E., Rucklidge, J. J., Hetherington, R., et al. (2003). Time perception deficits in attention-deficit/hyperactivity disorder and comorbid reading difficulties in child and adolescent samples. *Journal of Child Psychology and Psychiatry*, 44, 888-903.
28. Rommelse, N. N. J., Oosterlaan, J., Buitelaar, J., et al. (2007). Time reproduction with ADHD and their nonaffected siblings. *Journal of the American Academy of Child and Adolescent Psychiatry*, 46, 582-590.
29. Barkley, R. A. (1997). Behavioral inhibition, sustained attention, and executive functions: Constructing a unifying theory of ADHD. *Psychological Bulletin*, 121, 65-94.
30. Mullins, C., Bellgrove, M. A., Gill, M., and Robertson, I. H. (2005). Variability in time reproduction: Difference in ADHD combined and inattentive subtypes. *Journal of the American Academy of Child and Adolescent Psychiatry*, 44, 169-176.
31. Smith, A., Taylor, E., Rogers, J. W., et al. (2002). Evidence for a pure time perception deficit in children with ADHD. *Journal of Child Psychology and Psychiatry*, 43, 529-542.
32. Head, D., Bolton, D., and Hymas, N. (1989). Deficit in cognitive shifting ability in patients with obsessive-compulsive disorder. *Biological Psychiatry*, 25, 928-937.
33. Barkley, R. A. (2006). *Attention-Deficit/Hyperactivity Disorder (3rd ed.)* New York, NY: Guilford Press.
34. Carter, E. W., Clark, N. M., Cushing, L. S., and Kennedy, C. H. (2005). Moving from elementary to middle school: Supporting a smooth transition for students with severe disabilities. *Teaching Exceptional Children*, 37, 8-14.
35. Hoza, B., Gerdes, A. C., Hinshaw, S. P., et al. (2004). Self-perceptions of competence in children with ADHD and comparison children. *Journal of Consulting and Clinical Psychology*, 72, 382-391.
36. Owens, J. S. and Hoza, B. (2003). The role of inattention and hyperactivity/impulsivity in the positive illusory bias. *Journal of Consulting and Clinical Psychology*, 71, 680-691.
37. Meichenbaum, D. H. and Goodman, J. (1971). Training impulsive children to talk to themselves: A means of developing self-control. *Journal of Abnormal Psychology*, 77, 115-126.

Reference

Chapter 14: Memory Problems

1. Alloway, T. P., Gathercole, S. E., and Adams, A. (2005). Working memory and phonological awareness as predictors of progress towards early learning goals at school entry. British Journal of Developmental Psychology, 23, 417-426.
2. Gathercole, S. E., Pickering, S. J., Knight, C., and Stegmann, Z. (2004). Working memory skills and educational attainment: Evidence from national curriculum assessment at 7 and 14 years of age. Applied Cognitive Psychology, 18, 1-16.
3. Hutton, U. M. Z. and Towse, J. N. (2001). Short-term memory and working memory as indices of children's cognitive skills. Memory, 9, 383-394.
4. Kofler, M. J., Rapport, M. D., Bolden, J., and Altro, T. A. (2008). Working memory as a core deficit in ADHD: Preliminary findings and implications. ADHD Report, 16(6), 8-9, 12-14.
5. Martinussen, R., Hayden, J., Hoog-Johnson, S., and Tannock, R. (2005). A meta-analysis of working memory impairments in children with attention-deficit/hyperactivity disorder. Journal of the American Academy of Child and Adolescent Psychiatry, 44, 377-384.
6. Karatekin, C. (2004). A test of the integrity of the components of Baddeley's model of working memory in attention-deficit/hyperactivity disorder (ADHD). Journal of Child Psychology and Psychiatry, 45, 912-926.
7. Cornoldi, C., Marzocchi, G. M., Belotti, M., et al. (2001). Working memory interference control deficit in children referred by teachers for ADHD symptoms. Child Neuropsychology, 7, 230-240.
8. Bull, R. and Scerif, G. (2001). Executive functioning as a predictor of children's mathematics ability: Inhibition, switching, and working memory. Developmental Neuropsychology, 19, 273-293.
9. Stevens, J., Quittner, A. L., Zuckerman, J. B., and Moore, S. (2002). Behavioral inhibition, self-regulation of motivation, and working memory in children with attention-deficit hyperactivity disorder. Developmental Neuropsychology, 21, 117-139.
10. Cain, K., Oakhill, J., and Bryant, P. (2004). Children's reading comprehension ability: Concurrent prediction by working memory, verbal ability, and component skills. Journal of Educational Psychology, 96, 31-42.
11. McInnes, A., Humphries, T., Hoog-Johnson, S., and Tannock, R. (2003). Listening comprehension and working memory are impaired in attention-deficit hyperactivity disorder irrespective of language impairment. Journal of Abnormal Child Psychology, 31, 427-443.
12. Mahone, E. M., Cirino, P. T., Cutting, L. E., et al. (2002). Validity of the behavior rating inventory of executive function in children with ADHD and/or Tourette syndrome. Archives of Clinical Neuropsychology, 17, 643-662.
13. Schultz, R. T., Evans, D. W., and Wolff, M. (1999). Neuropsychological models of childhood obsessive-compulsive disorder. Child and Adolescent Psychiatric Clinics of North America, 8, 513-531.
14. Dornbush, M. P. and Pruitt, S. K. (1995). Teaching the Tiger. Duarte, CA: Hope Press.
15. Levine, M. D. (1994). Educational Care. A System for Understanding and Helping Children with Learning Problems at Home and at School. Cambridge, MA: Educators Publishing Service.
16. Bruer, J. T. (1993). Schools for Thought: A Science of Learning in the Classroom. Cambridge, MA: MIT Press.
17. Ogle, D. S. (1986). K-W-L: A teaching model that develops active reading of expository text. The Reading Teacher, 39, 564-570.
18. Pruitt, S. K. and Rhinehart, V. (1979). Mother Vowel's House. Parkaire Consultants. Atlanta, GA.
19. Gathercole, S. E. (1998). The development of memory. Journal of Child Psychology and Psychiatry and Allied Disciplines, 39, 3-27.
20. O'Neill, M. E. and Douglas, V. I. (1991). Study strategies and story recall in attention deficit disorders and reading disability. Journal of Abnormal Child Psychology, 19, 671-692.
21. Savage, C. R., Baer, L., Keuthen, N. J., et al. (1999). Organizational strategies mediate nonverbal memory impairment in obsessive-compulsive disorder. Biological Psychiatry, 45, 905-916.

Section VIII

22. Stickgold, R. and Walker, M. P. (2005). Memory consolidation and reconsolidation: What is the role of sleep? Trends in Neurosciences, 28, 408-415.
23. Evans, J. J., Wilson, B. A., Schuri, U., et al. (2000). A comparison of "errorless" and "trial-and-error" learning methods for teaching individuals with acquired memory deficits. Neuropsychological Rehabilitation, 10, 67-101.
24. Kessels, R. P. C. and de Haan, E. H. F. (2003). Implicit learning in memory rehabilitation: A meta-analysis on errorless learning and vanishing cues methods. Journal of Clinical and Experimental Neuropsychology, 25, 805-814.
25. National Training Laboratories. (1960+). Learning Pyramid. Bethel, ME.
26. Atkinson, R. C. and Shriffin, R. M. (1968). Human memory: A proposed system and its control processes. The Psychology of Learning and Motivation: Advances in Research and Theory (Volume 2). New York, NY: Academic Press.
27. Russell, P. (1979). The Brain Book. New York, NY: E. P. Dutton.
28. Von Restorff, H. (1933). Uber die Wirkung von Bereichsbildungen im Spurenfeld (The effects of field information on the trace field). In Spence, K. and Spence, J. editors: Psychologie Forschung, 18, 299-334.
29. Yohe, T. G. (1972). Schoolhouse Rock Songs. ABC television from 1983-1985. Distributed on DVD in 2002 by Buena Vista Home Video.
30. French, B. F., Zentall, S. S., and Bennett, D. (2003). Short-term memory of children with and without characteristics of attention deficit hyperactivity disorder. Learning and Individual Differences, 13, 205-225.
31. Ebbinghaus, H. (1885/1913). Memory: A Contribution to Experimental Psychology. Translated 1913: Ruyer, D. H. and Bussenius, C. E. New York, NY: Teachers College Press.
32. Counseling Services. University of Waterloo. Retrieved from the World Wide Web 7/7/04. www.adm.uwaterloo.ca/infocs/Study/Curve
33. Cutting, L. E., Koth, C. W., Mahone, E. M., and Denckla, M. B. (2003). Evidence for unexpected weakness in learning in children with attention-deficit/hyperactivity disorder without reading disabilities. Journal of Learning Disabilities, 36, 259-269.
34. Kourakis, I. E., Katachanakis, C. N., Vlahonikolis, I. G., and Paritsis, N. K. (2004). Examination of verbal memory and recall time in children with attention deficit hyperactivity disorder. Developmental Neuropsychology, 26, 565-570.
35. Clark, C., Prior, M., and Kinsella, G. J. (2000). Do executive deficits differentiate between adolescents with ADHD and oppositional defiant/conduct disorder? A neuropsychological study using the Six Elements Test and Hayling Sentence Completion Test. Journal of Abnormal Child Psychology, 28, 403-414.
36. Kerns, K. A. and Price, K. J. (2001). An investigation of prospective memory in children with ADHD. Child Neuropsychology, 7, 162-171.
37. Siklos, S. and Kerns, K. A. (2004). Assessing multitasking in children with ADHD using a modified Six Elements Test. Archives of Clinical Neuropsychology, 19, 347-361.
38. Kliegel, M., Ropeter, A., and Mackinlay, R. (2006). Complex prospective memory in children with ADHD. Child Neuropsychology, 12, 407-419.
39. Cornoldi, C., Barbieri, A., Gaiani, C., and Zocchi, S. (1999). Strategic memory deficits in attention deficit disorder with hyperactivity participants: The role of executive processes. Developmental Neuropsychology, 15, 53-71.

Section IV: Academic Interventions

Chapter 15: Oral Expression

1. Tannock, R., Purvis, K. L., and Schachar, R. J. (1993). Narrative abilities in children with attention deficit hyperactivity disorder and normal peers. Journal of Abnormal Child Psychology, 21, 103-117.

2. Purvis, K. L. and Tannock, R. (1997). Language abilities in children with attention deficit hyperactivity disorder, reading disabilities, and normal controls. Journal of Abnormal Child Psychology, 25, 133-144.
3. Zentall, S. S. (1988). Production deficiencies in elicited language but not in spontaneous verbalizations of hyperactive children. Journal of Abnormal Child Psychology, 16, 657-673.
4. Geffner, D. (2006). Language and auditory processing problems in ADHD. The ADHD Report, 14 (3), 1-6.
5. Mathers, M. E. (2006). Aspects of language in children with ADHD. Applying functional analysis to explore language use. Journal of Attention Disorders, 9, 523-533.

Chapter 16: Listening Comprehension

1. Ogle, D. S. (1986). K-W-L: A teaching model that develops active reading of expository text. The Reading Teacher, 39, 564-570.
2. Social Anxiety Disorder. Retrieved from the World Wide Web on 2/22/07. www.massgeneral.org/schoolpsychiatry
3. McInnes, A., Humphries, T., Hoog-Johnson, S., and Tannock, R. (2003). Listening comprehension and working memory are impaired in attention-deficit hyperactivity disorder irrespective of language impairment. Journal of Abnormal Child Psychology, 31, 427-443.

Chapter 17: Basic Reading Skills

1. Fletcher, J. M. (2002). Neuropsychology of Reading and Learning Disabilities: What We Know From Research. Presented at the International Dyslexia Association Conference. Atlanta, GA.
2. Report of the National Reading Panel. (2000). Teaching Children to Read: An evidence-Based Assessment of the Scientific Research Literature and Its Implications for Reading Instruction. Washington, DC: U.S. Department of Health and Human Services, Public Health Service, National Institutes of Health, National Institute of Child Health and Human Development. www.nationalreadingpanel.org
3. Shaywitz, S. (2004). Overcoming Dyslexia: A New and Complete Science-Based Program for Reading Problems at Any Level. New York, NY: Alfred A. Knopf.
4. Semrud-Clikeman, M., Biederman, J., Sprich-Buckminster, S., et al. (1992). Comorbidity between ADDH and learning disability: A review and report in clinically referred sample. Journal of American Academy of Child and Adolescent Psychiatry, 31, 439-448.
5. Singer, H. S., Schuerholz, L. J., and Denckla, M. B. (1995). Learning difficulties in children with Tourette syndrome. Journal of Child Neurology, 10, 558-561.
6. Morris, R. D., Stuebing, K. K., Fletcher, J. M., Shaywitz, S. E., et al. (1998). Subtypes of reading disability: Variability around a phonological core. Journal of Educational Psychology, 90, 1-27.
7. Recording for the Blind & Dyslexic (RFB&D). National Headquarters. 20 Roszel Road. Princeton, NJ 08540. www.rfbd.org
8. Gardner, H. (1985). Frames of Mind: The Theory of Multiple Intelligences. New York, NY: Basic Books, HarperCollins Publishers.
9. Gardner, H. (1991). The Unschooled Mind: How Children Think and How Schools Should Teach. New York, NY: Basic Books, HarperCollins Publishers.
10. Armstrong, T. (2000). In Their Own Way: Discovering and Encouraging Your Child's Personal Learning Style-Revised. Los Angeles, CA: Putnam Publishing Group.
11. Armstrong, T. (1999). 7 Kinds of Smart: Identifying and Developing Your Multiple Intelligences - Revised. New York, NY: Penguin Group.
12. Catts, H. W., Gillispie, M., Leonard, L. B., et al. (2002). The role of speed of processing, rapid naming, and phonological awareness in reading achievement. Journal of Learning Disabilities, 35, 509-524.
13. Swanson, H. L., Howard, C. B., and Saez, L. (2006). Do different components of working memory underlie different subgroups of reading disabilities? Journal of Learning Disabilities, 39, 252-269.

Section VIII

14. Dowhower, S. (1994). Repeated reading revisited: Research into practice. <u>Reading and Writing Quarterly: Overcoming Learning Disabilities</u>, 10, 343-358.
15. Gickling, E. E. and Armstrong, D. L. (1978). Levels of instructional difficulty as related to on-task behavior, task completion, and comprehension. <u>Journal of Learning Disabilities</u>, 11, 559-566.
16. Willcutt, E. G. and Pennington, B. F. (2000). Comorbidity of reading disability and attention-deficit/hyperactivity disorder: Differences by gender and subtype. <u>Journal of Learning Disabilities</u>, 33, 179-191.
17. Dornbush, M. P. and Pruitt, S. K. (1995). <u>Teaching the Tiger</u>. Duarte, CA: Hope Press.
18. Swanson, H. L. and Sachse-Lee, C. (2001). A subgroup analysis of working memory in children with reading disabilities: Domain-general or domain-specific deficiency? <u>Journal of Learning Disabilities</u>, 34, 249-263.
19. Ackerman, P. T., Anhalt, J. M., and Dykman, R. A. (1986). Arithmetic automatization failure in children with attention and reading disorders: Associations and sequela. <u>Journal of Learning Disabilities</u>, 19, 222-232.
20. Beck, I. L., Perfetti, C. A., and Mskoewn, M. G. (1982). Effects of long-term vocabulary instruction on lexical access and reading comprehension. <u>Journal of Educational Psychology</u>, 74, 506-521.
21. Wilson, B. A., Baddeley, A., Evans, J. J., and Shiel, A. J. (1994). Errorless learning in the rehabilitation of memory impaired people. <u>Neuropsychological Rehabilitation</u>, 4, 307-326.
22. Evans, J. J., Wilson, B. A., Schuri, U., et al. (2000). A comparison of "errorless" and "trial-and-error" learning methods for teaching individuals with acquired memory deficits. <u>Neuropsychological Rehabilitation</u>, 10, 67-101.
23. Adams, M. J. (1990). <u>Beginning to Read: Thinking and Learning About Print</u>. Cambridge, MA: MIT Press.
24. Wolf, M. and Bowers, P. G. (1999). The "double deficit hypothesis" for developmental dyslexias. <u>Journal of Educational Psychology</u>, 91, 1-24.

Chapter 18: Reading Comprehension

1. Mayes, S. D., Calhoun, S. L., and Crowell, E. W. (2000). Learning disabilities and ADHD: Overlapping spectrum disorders. <u>Journal of Learning Disabilities</u>, 33, 417-424.
2. Report of the National Reading Panel. (2000). <u>Teaching Children to Read: An evidence-Based Assessment of the Scientific Research Literature and Its Implications for Reading Instruction</u>. Washington, DC: U.S. Department of Health and Human Services, Public Health Service, National Institutes of Health, National Institute of Child Health and Human Development. www.nationalreadingpanel.org
3. Gardner, H. (1985). <u>Frames of Mind: The Theory of Multiple Intelligences</u>. New York, NY: Basic Books, HarperCollins Publishers.
4. Gardner, H. (1991). <u>The Unschooled Mind: How Children Think and How Schools Should Teach</u>. New York, NY: Basic Books, HarperCollin Publishers.
5. Armstrong, T. (2000). <u>In Their Own Way: Discovering and Encouraging Your Child's Personal Learning Style-Revised</u>. Los Angeles, CA: Putnam Publishing Group.
6. Armstrong, T. (1999). <u>7 Kinds of Smart: Identifying and Developing Your Multiple Intelligences - Revised</u>. New York, NY: Penguin Group.
7. Gickling, E. and Armstrong, D. L. (1978). Levels of instructional difficulty as related to on-task behavior, task completion, and comprehension. <u>Journal of Learning Disabilities</u>, 11, 559-566.
8. Boyle, E. A., Rosenberg, M. S., Connelly, V. J., et al. (2003). Effects of audio texts on the acquisition of secondary-level content by students with mild disabilities. <u>Learning Disability Quarterly</u>, 26, 203-214.
9. Rowe, K. J. and Rowe, K. S. (1992). The relationship between inattentiveness in the classroom and reading achievement: An explanatory study. <u>Journal of the American Academy of Child and Adolescent Psychiatry</u>, 31, 357-367.
10. Dornbush, M. P. and Pruitt, S. K. (1995). <u>Teaching the Tiger</u>. Duarte, CA: Hope Press.

11. Jennings, M. K. and Pruitt, S. K. (1994). How to read a chapter. Teaching the Tiger. Duarte, CA: Hope Press.
12. Kim, A. H., Vaughn, S., Wanzek, J., and Wei, S. (2004). Graphic organizers and their effects on the reading comprehension of students with LD: A synthesis of research. Journal of Learning Disabilities, 37, 105-118.
13. Inspiration Software (1988-to present). Inspiration and Kidspiration. Portland, OR: Author. Available from Inspiration Software, Inc., 7412 SW Beaverton Hillsdale Hwy., Suite 102, Portland, OR 97225-2167. Available at www.inspiration.com.
14. Cain, K., Oakhill, J., and Bryant, P. (2004). Children's reading comprehension ability: Concurrent prediction by working memory, verbal ability, and component skills. Journal of Educational Psychology, 96, 31-42.
15. Swanson, H. L., Howard, C. B., and Saez, L. (2006). Do different components of working memory underlie different subgroups of reading disabilities? Journal of Learning Disabilities, 39, 252-269.
16. O'Neill, M. E. and Douglas, V. I. (1991). Study strategies and story recall in attention deficit and reading disability. Journal of Abnormal Psychology, 19, 671-692.
17. Lorch, E. P., O'Neil, K., Berthiaume, K. S., et al. (2004). Story comprehension and the impact of studying on recall in children with attention deficit hyperactivity disorder. Journal of Clinical Child and Adolescent Psychology, 33, 506-515.

Chapter 19: Written Expression/Long Term Reports

1. Mayes, S. D., Calhoun, S. L., and Crowell, E. W. (2000). Learning disabilities and ADHD: Overlapping spectrum disorders. Journal of Learning Disabilities, 33, 417-424.
2. Singer, H. S., Schuerholz, L. J., and Denckla, M. B. (1995). Learning difficulties in children with Tourette syndrome. Journal of Child Neurology, 10, 558-561.
3. Piacentini, J., Bergman, R. L., Keller, M., and McCracken, J. (2003). Functional impairment in children and adolescents with obsessive-compulsive disorder. Journal of Child and Adolescent Psychopharmacology, 13 (Supplement 1), S61-S69.
4. Stanford, P. and Siders, J. A. (2001). E-pal writing! Teaching Exceptional Children, 34, 21-24.
5. Dornbush, M. P. and Pruitt, S. K. (1995). Teaching the Tiger. Duarte, CA: Hope Press.
6. Marcotte, A. C. and Stern, C. (1997). Qualitative analysis of graphomotor output in children with attentional disorders. Child Neuropsychology, 3(2), 147-153.
7. Tseng, M. H., Henderson, A., Chow, S. M. K., and Yao, G. (2004). Relationship between motor proficiency, attention, impulse, and activity in children with ADHD. Developmental Medicine and Child Neurology, 46, 381-388.
8. Schultz, R. T., Carter, A. S., Scahill, L., and Leckman, J. F. (1999). Neuropsychological findings. In Leckman, J. F. and Cohen, D. J. editors: Tourette's Syndrome–Tics, Obsession, Compulsions: Developmental Psychopathology and Clinical Care. New York, NY: John Wiley & Sons.
9. Schultz, R. T., Evans, D. W., and Wolff, M. (1999). Neuropsychological models of obsessive-compulsive disorder. Child and Adolescent Psychiatric Clinics of North America, 8, 513-531.
10. Quilin, T. (2004). Speech recognition technology and students with writing difficulties: Improving fluency. Journal of Educational Psychology, 96, 337-346.
11. Manus, R. (2002). Teaching Students to Spell High-Use Words for Everyday Writing. Presented at the International Dyslexia Association Conference. Atlanta, GA.
12. Franklin Electronic Publishers, Inc. One Franklin Plaza. Burlington, NJ 08016-4907. Available at www.franklin.com
13. Chalk, J. C., Hagan-Burke, S., and Burke, M. D. (2005). The effects of self-regulated strategy development on the writing process for high school students with learning disabilities. Learning Disability Quarterly, 28, 75-87.

Section VIII

14. Inspiration Software (1988-to present). Inspiration and Kidspiration Portland, OR: Author. Available from Inspiration Software, Inc., 7412 SW Beaverton Hillsdale Hwy., Suite 102, Portland, OR 97225-2167. Available at www.inspiration.com.
15. Pruitt, S. K. (1992). Written expression editing strip. Staff Development Course. Atlanta, GA: State of Georgia.
16. Schumaker, J. B., Deshler, D. D., Nolan, S., et al. (1981). Error monitoring: A learning strategy for improving academic performance of LD adolescents. Research Report, 32, Lawrence, KS: University of Kansas Institute for Research in Learning Disabilities.
17. Kirk, L. (2006). Parkaire Consultants. Atlanta, GA.
18. Swanson, H. L. and Berninger, V. W. (1996). Individual differences in children's working memory and writing skill. Journal of Experimental Child Psychology, 63, 358-385.

Chapter 20: Math Caluculation

1. Semrud-Clikeman, M., Biederman, J., Sprich-Buckminster, S., et al. (1992). Comorbidity between ADHD and learning disability: A review and report in a clinically referred sample. Journal of the American Academy of Child and Adolescent Psychiatry, 31, 439-448.
2. Mayes, S. D., Calhoun, S. L., and Crowell, E. W. (2000). Learning disabilities and ADHD: Overlapping spectrum disorders. Journal of Learning Disabilities, 33, 417-424.
3. Geary, D. C. (2004). Mathematics and learning disabilities. Journal of Learning Disabilities, 37, 4-15.
4. Barbaresi, W. J., Katusic, S. K., Colligan, R. C., et al. (2005). Math learning disorder: Incidence in a population-based birth cohort, 1976-1982, Rochester, Minn. Ambulatory Pediatrics, 5, 281-289.
5. Singer, H. S., Schuerholz, L. J., and Denckla, M. B. (1995). Learning difficulties in children with Tourette syndrome. Journal of Child Neurology, 10, 558-561.
6. Schultz, R. T., Carter, A. S., Gladstone, M., et al. (1998). Visual-motor, visuoperceptual, and fine motor functioning in children with Tourette syndrome. Neuropsychology, 12, 134-145.
7. Dornbush, M. P. and Pruitt, S. K. (1995). Teaching the Tiger. Duarte, CA: Hope Press.
8. Marcotte, A. C. and Stern, C. (1997). Qualitative analysis of graphomotor output in children with attentional disorders. Child Neuropsychology, 3(2), 147-153.
9. Schultz, R. T., Carter, A. S., Scahill, L., and Leckman, J. F. (1999). Neuropsychological findings. In Leckman, J. F. and Cohen, D. J. editors: Tourette's Syndrome–Tics, Obsession, Compulsions: Developmental Psychopathology and Clinical Care. New York, NY: John Wiley & Sons.
10. Schultz, R. T., Evans, D. W., and Wolff, M. (1999). Neuropsychological models of obsessive-compulsive disorder. Child and Adolescent Psychiatric Clinics of North America, 8, 513-531.
11. Fuchs, L. S., Fuchs, D., Compton, D. L., et al. (2006). The cognitive correlates of third grade skill in arithmetic, algorithmic computation, and arithmetic words problems. Journal of Educational Psychology, 98, 29-43.
12. Bull, R. and Johnston, R. S. (1997). Children's arithmetical difficulties: Contributions from processing speed, item identification, and short-term memory. Journal of Experimental Child Psychology, 65, 1-24.
13. Carlson, C. L. and Mann, M. (2002). Sluggish cognitive tempo predicts a different pattern of impairment in attention deficit hyperactivity disorder, predominately inattentive type. Journal of Clinical Child and Adolescent Psychology, 31, 123-129.
14. Marshall, R. M., Schafer, V. A., O'Donnell, L., et al. (1999). Arithmetic disabilities and ADD subtypes: Implications for DSM-IV. Journal of Learning Disabilities, 32, 239-247.
15. Fuchs, L. S., Compton, D. L., Fuchs, D., et al. (2005). The prevention, identification, and cognitive determinants of math difficulty. Journal of Educational Psychology, 97, 493-513.
16. Isaacs, A. C. and Carroll, W. M. (1999). Strategies for basic-fact instruction. Teaching Children Mathematics, 5, 508-515.
17. Tournaki, N. (2003). The differential effects of teaching addition through strategy instruction versus drill and practice to students with and without learning disabilities. Journal of Learning Disabilities, 36, 449-458.

18. Bull, R. and Scerif, G. (2001). Executive functioning as a predictor of children's mathematics ability: Inhibition, switching, and working memory. Developmental Neuropsychology, 19, 273-293.
19. Pruitt, S. K. (1993). Math Editing Cue.
20. Cherry, D. (1993). Error Patterns. Parkaire Consultants. Atlanta, GA.
21. www.education-world.com/a_curr/mnemonic. Adapted from Frank, A. R. and Brown, D. (1992). Self-monitoring strategies in arithmetic. Teaching Exceptional Children, 24(z), 52-53.
22. Dirty Marvin Smells Bad. (1982). Parkaire Consultants. Atlanta, GA.
23. Hitch, G. J. and McAuley, E. (1991). Working memory and children with specific arithmetical learning difficulties. British Journal of Psychology, 82, 375-386.
24. Wilson, K. M. and Swanson, H. L. (2001). Are mathematics disabilities due to a domain-general or a domain-specific working memory deficit? Journal of Learning Disabilities, 34, 237-248.
25. Ackerman, P. T., Anhalt, J. M., and Dykman, R. A. (1986). Arithmetic automatization failure in children with attention and reading disorders: Associations and sequela. Journal of Learning Disabilities, 19, 222-232.
26. Wilson, B. A., Baddeley, A., Evans, J. J., and Shiel, A. J. (1994). Errorless learning in the rehabilitation of memory impaired people. Neuropsychological Rehabilitation, 4, 307-326.
27. Evans, J. J., Wilson, B. A., Schuri, U., et al. (2000). A comparison of "errorless" and "trial-and-error" learning methods for teaching individuals with acquired memory deficits. Neuropsychological Rehabilitation, 10, 67-101.

Chapter 21: Math Reasoning

1. Fuchs, L. S., Fuchs, D., Compton, D. L., et al. (2006). The cognitive correlates of third grade skill in arithmetic, algorithmic computation, and arithmetic words problems. Journal of Educational Psychology, 98, 29-43.
2. Zentall, S. S., Smith, Y. N., Lee, Y. B., and Wieczorek, C. (1994). Mathematical outcomes of attention-deficit hyperactivity disorder. Journal of Learning Disabilities, 27, 510-519.
3. Zentall, S. S. and Ferkis, M. A. (1993). Mathematical problem solving for youth with ADHD, with and without learning disabilities. Learning Disability Quarterly, 16, 6-17.
4. Marshall, R. M., Schafer, V. A., O'Donnell, L., et al. (1999). Arithmetic disabilities and ADD subtypes: Implications for DSM-IV. Journal of Learning Disabilities, 32, 239-247.
5. Dornbush, M. P. and Pruitt, S. K. (1995). Teaching the Tiger. Duarte, CA: Hope Press.
6. Marzocchi, G. M., Lucangeli, D., De Meo, T., et al. (2002). The disturbing effect of irrelevant information on arithmetic problem solving in inattentive children. Developmental Neuropsychology, 21, 73-92.
7. Bull, R. and Scerif, G. (2001). Executive functioning as a predictor of children's mathematics ability: Inhibition, switching, and working memory. Developmental Neuropsychology, 19, 273-293.
8. Swanson, H. L., Cooney, J. B., and Brock, S. (1993). The influence of working memory and classification ability on children's word problem solution. Journal of Experimental Child Psychology, 55, 374-395.
9. Swanson, H. L. and Sachse-Lee, C. (2001). Mathematical problem solving and working memory in children with learning disabilities: Both executive and phonological processes are important. Journal of Experimental Child Psychology, 79, 294-321.
10. Black, B. (1994). The Hand Trick. St. Jude's Catholic School. Altanta, GA
11. Bush, D. M. (2006). Parkaire Consultants. Atlanta, GA.

Section V: Study Skills

Chapter 22: Notetaking

1. Marcotte, A. C. and Stern, C. (1997). Qualitative analysis of graphomotor output in children with attentional disorders. Child Neuropsychology, 3(2), 147-153.

Section VIII

2. Mayes, S. D. and Calhoun, S. L. (2007). Learning, attention, writing, and processing speed in typical children and children with ADHD, autism, anxiety, depression, and oppositional defiant disorder. Child Neuropsychology, 13, 469-493.
3. Tseng, M. H., Henderson, A., Chow, S. M. K., and Yao, G. (2004). Relationship between motor proficiency, attention, impulse, and activity in children with ADHD. Developmental Medicine and Child Neurology, 46, 381-388.
4. Schultz, R. T., Carter, A. S., Scahill, L., and Leckman, J. F. (1999). Neuropsychological findings. In Leckman, J. F. and Cohen, D. J. editors: Tourette's Syndrome – Tics, Obsession, Compulsions: Developmental Psychopathology and Clinical Care. New York, NY: John Wiley & Sons.
5. Schultz, R. T., Evans, D. W., and Wolff, M. (1999). Neuropsychological models of obsessive-compulsive disorder. Child and Adolescent Psychiatric Clinics of North America, 8, 513-531.
6. Healy, D. and Rucklidge, J. J. (2006). An investigation into the relationship among ADHD symptomatology, creativity, and neuropsychological functioning in children. Child Neuropsychology, 12, 421-438.
7. Rucklidge, J. J. and Tannock, R. (2002). Neuropsychological profiles of adolescents with ADHD. Effects of reading difficulties and gender. Journal of Child Psychology and Psychiatry, 43, 1-16.
8. Carlson, C. L. and Mann, M. (2002). Sluggish cognitive tempo predicts a different pattern of impairment in attention deficit hyperactivity disorder, predominately inattentive type. Journal of Clinical Child and Adolescent Psychology, 31, 123-129.
9. Goodyear, P. and Hynd, G. W. (1992). Attention-deficit disorder with (ADD/H) and without (ADD/WO) hyperactivity: Behavioral and neuropsychological differentiation. Journal of Clinical Child Psychology, 21, 273-305.
10. Nigg, J. T., Blaskey, L. G., Huang-Pollock, C. L., and Rappley, M. D. (2002). Neuropsychological executive functions and DSM-IV ADHD subtypes. Journal of the American Academy of Child and Adolescent Psychiatry, 41, 59-66.
11. Weiler, M. D., Bernstein, J. H., Bellinger, D. C., and Waber, D. P. (2000). Processing speed in children with attention deficit/hyperactivity disorder, inattentive type. Child Neuropsychology, 6, 218-234.
12. Barkley, R. A. (2006). Attention-Deficit Hyperactivity Disorder (3rd ed.): A Handbook for Diagnosis and Treatment. New York, NY: Guilford Press.
13. Singer, H. S., Schuerholz, L. J., and Denckla, M. B. (1995). Learning difficulties in children with Tourette syndrome. Journal of Child Neurology, 10, S58-S61.
14. Schultz, R. T., Carter, A. S., Scahill, L., and Leckman, J. F. (1999). Neuropsychological findings. In Leckman, J. F. and Cohen, D. J. editors: Tourette's Syndrome–Tics, Obsession, Compulsions: Developmental Psychopathology and Clinical Care. New York, NY: John Wiley & Sons.
15. Schultz, R. T., Evans, D. W., and Wolff, M. (1999). Neuropsychological models of childhood obsessive-compulsive disorder. Child and Adolescent Psychiatric Clinics of North America, 8, 513-531.
16. Pauk, W. (1989). The Cornell Notetaking Technique. Cornell University. Ithaca, NY.
17. McInnes, A., Humphries, T., Hoog-Johnson, S., and Tannock, R. (2003). Listening comprehension and working memory are impaired in attention-deficit hyperactivity disorder irrespective of language impairment. Journal of Abnormal Child Psychology, 31, 427-443.
18. Russell, P. (1979). The Brain Book. New York, NY: E. P. Dutton.
19. Ebbinghaus, H. (1885/1913). Memory: A Contribution to Experimental Psychology. Trans. Ruyer, D. H. and Bussenius, C. E. New York, NY: Teachers College Press.

Chapter 23: Homework

1. Packer, L. E. and Pruitt, S. K. (2002-2008). Homework Survey. Challenging Kids, Challenged Teachers!, Inc.
2. Dornbush, M. P. and Pruitt, S. K. (1995). Teaching the Tiger. Duarte, CA: Hope Press.
3. National Education Association (NEA). Retrieved from the World Wide Web on 2/24/06. www.nea.org

Reference

Chapter 24: Test Preparation

1. Russell, P. (1979). The Brain Book. New York, NY: E. P. Dutton.
2. Dornbush, M. P. and Pruitt, S. K. (1995). Teaching the Tiger. Duarte, CA: Hope Press.

SECTION VI: TESTS

Chapter 25: Tests

1. Lang, S. C., Elliott, S. N., Bolt, D. M., and Kratochwill, T. R. (2008). The effects of testing accommodations of students' performances and reactions to testing. School Psychology Quarterly, 23, 107-124.
2. Schulte, A. G., Elliott, S. N., and Kratochwill, T. R. (2001). Experimental analysis of the effects of testing accommodations on students' standardized achievement test scores. School Psychology Review, 30, 527-547.
3. Tindal G. and Fuchs, L. (1999). A Summary of Research on Testing Accommodations: What We Know So Far. Lexington, KY: University of Kentucky Mid-South Regional Resource Center.

Chapter 26. Test-Taking Strategies

1. Scruggs, T. E. and Mastropieri, M. A. (1992). Teaching Test-Taking Skills. Helping Students Show What They Know. Brookline, MA: Brookline Books.
2. Test Taking Tips. Retrieved from the World Wide Web on 3/4/05. www.testtakingtips.com/test
3. Test Taking Strategies. Counseling and Psychological Services. University of North Carolina. Retrieved from the World Wide Web on 3/4/05. www.caps.unc.edu/TestTake
4. Study Guides and Strategies. University of St. Thomas. Retrieved from the World Wide Web on 2/12/04. www.studygs.net/tsttak4
5. Dornbush, M. P. and Pruitt, S. K. (1995). Teaching the Tiger. Duarte, CA: Hope Press.

SECTION VII: SOCIAL COMPETENCE

Chapter 27: Social Skills Interventions

1. Greene, R. W., Biederman, J., Faraone, S. V., et al. (1996). Toward a new psychometric definition of social disability in children with attention-deficit hyperactivity disorder. Journal of the American Academy of Child and Adolescent Psychiatry, 35, 571-578.
2. Biederman, J., Mick, E., and Faraone, S. V. (1998). Normalized functioning in youths with persistent attention-deficit/hyperactivity disorder. Journal of Pediatrics, 133, 544-551.
3. Greene, R. W., Biederman, J., Faraone, S. V., et al. (1997). Adolescent outcome of boys with attention-deficit/hyperactivity disorder and social disability: Results from a 4-year longitudinal follow-up study. Journal of Consulting and Clinical Psychology, 65, 758-767.
4. Greene, R. W., Biederman, J., Faraone, S. V., et al. (2001). Social impairment in girls with ADHD: Patterns, gender comparisons, and correlates. Journal of the American Academy of Child and Adolescent Psychiatry, 40, 704-710.
5. Gaub, M. and Carlson, C. L. (1997). Behavioral characteristics of DSM-IV ADHD subtypes in a school-based population. Journal of Abnormal Child Psychology, 25, 103-111.
6. Pfiffner, L. J., Calzada, E., and McBurnett, K. (2000). Interventions to enhance social competence. Child and Adolescent Psychiatric Clinics of North America, 9, 689-709.
7. Barkley, R. A. (1997). Behavioral inhibition, sustained attention, and executive functions: Constructing a unifying heory of ADHD. Psychological Bulletin, 121, 65-94.
8. Landau, S., Milich, R., and Diener, M. B. (1998). Peer relations of children with attention-deficit hyperactivity disorder. Reading and Writing Quarterly: Overcoming Learning Difficulties, 14, 83-105.
9. Zumple, H. J. and Landau, S. (2002). Peer problems, Attention, April, 32-35.

10. Ollendick, T. H., Greene, R. W., Francis, G., et al. (1991). Sociometric status: Its stability and validity among neglected, rejected, and popular children. Journal of Child Psychology and Psychiatry, 32, 525-534.
11. Ollendick, T. H., Weist, M. D., Borden, M. C., and Greene, R. W. (1992). Sociometric status and academic, behavioral, and psychological adjustment: A five year longitudinal study. Journal of Consulting and Clinical Psychology, 60, 80-87.
12. Bagwell, C. L., Molina, B., Pelham, W. E., and Hosa, B. (2001). Attention- deficit hyperactivity disorder and problems in peer relations: Predictions from childhood to adolescence. Journal of the American Academy of Child and Adolescent Psychiatry, 40, 1285-1292.
13. Maedgen, J. W. and Carlson, C. L. (2000). Social functioning and emotional regulation in attention deficit hyperactivity disorder subtypes. Journal of Clinical Child Psychology, 29, 30-42.
14. Kurlan, R., Como, P. G., Miller, B., et al. (2002). The behavioral spectrum of tic disorders. A community-based study. Neurology, 59, 414-420.
15. Bawden, H. N., Stokes, A., Camfield, P. R., et al. (1998). Peer relationship problems in children with Tourette's disorder or diabetes mellitus. Journal of Child Psychology and Psychiatry, 39, 663-668.
16. Stokes, A., Bawden, H. N., Camfield, P. R., et al. (1991). Peer Problems in Tourette's disorder. Pediatrics, 87, 936-942.
17. Carter, A. S., O'Donnell, D. A., Scahill, L., et al. (2000). Social and emotional adjustment in children affected with Gilles de la Tourette's syndrome: Associations with ADHD and family functioning. Journal of Child Psychology and Psychiatry, 41, 215-223.
18. Sukhodolsky, D. G., Scahill, L., Zhang, H., et al. (2003). Disruptive behavior in children with Tourette's syndrome: Association with ADHD comorbidity, tic severity, and functional impairment. Journal of the American Academy of Child and Adolescent Psychiatry, 42, 98-105.
19. Hanna, G. L. (1995). Demographic and clinical features of obsessive-compulsive disorder in children and adolescents. Journal of the American Academy of Child and Adolescent Psychiatry, 34, 19-27.
20. Piacentini, J., Bergman, R. L., Keller, M., and McCraken, J. (2003). Functional impairment in children and adolescents with obsessive-compulsive disorder. Journal of Child and Adolescent Psychopharmacology, 12 (1), S61-S69.
21. Sukhodolsky, D. G., do Rosario-Campos, M. C., Scahill, L., et al. (2005). Adaptive, emotional, and family functioning of children with obsessive- compulsive disorder. American Journal of Psychiatry, 162, 1125-1132.
22. Obsessive-Compulsive Foundation. www.ocfoundation.org
23. Storch, E. A., Ledley, D. R., Lewin, A. B., et al. (2006). Peer victimization in children with obsessive-compulsive disorder: Relations with symptoms of psychopathology. Journal of Clinical Child and Adolescent Psychology, 35, 446-455.
24. Geller, D. A., Biederman, J., Faraone, S. V., et al. (2002). Attention-deficit/hyperactivity disorder in children and adolescents with obsessive-compulsive disorder: Fact or artifact? Journal of the American Academy of Child and Adolescent Psychiatry, 41, 52-58.
25. Dornbush, M. P. and Pruitt, S. K. (1995). Teaching the Tiger. Duarte, CA: Hope Press.
26. Greene, R. W. and Ablon, J. S. (2001). What does the MTA study tell us about effective pyschosocial treatment for ADHD? Journal of Clinical Child Psychology, 30, 114-121.
27. Lavoie, R. D. (2005). It's So Much Work to Be Your Friend. Helping the Child with Learning Disabilities Find Social Success. New York, NY: Touchstone.
28. Pfiffner, L. J. (2003). Psychosocial treatment for ADHD–Inattentive type. ADHD Report, 11 (5), 1-8.
29. Mehrabian, A. (1971). Silent Messages. Belmont, CA: Wadsworth.
30. Nowicki, S. and Duke, M. P. (1992). Helping the Child Who Doesn't Fit In. Atlanta, GA: Peachtree Publishers.
31. Born, G. (2006). Parkaire Consultants. Atlanta, GA.
32. Social Anxiety Disorder. Retrieved from the World Wide Web on 2/22/07. www.massgeneral.org/schoolpsychiatry

Reference

33. Carlson, C. L. and Mann, M. (2002). Sluggish cognitive tempo predicts a different pattern of impairment in the attention deficit hyperactivity disorder, predominately inattentive type. Journal of Clinical Child and Adolescent Psychology, 31, 123-129.
34. Weiler, M. D., Bernstein, J. H., Bellinger, D. C., and Waber, D. P. (2000). Processing speed in children with attention deficit/hyperactivity disorder, inattentive type. Child Neuropsychology, 6, 218-234.
35. Singer, H. S., Schuerholz, L. J., and Denckla, M. B. (1995). Learning difficulties in children with Tourette syndrome. Journal of Child Neurology, 10, S58-S61.
36. Schultz, R. T., Carter, A. S., Scahill, L., and Leckman, J. F. (1999). Neuropsychological findings. In Leckman, J. F. and Cohen, D. J. editors: Tourette's Syndrome – Tics, Obsession, Compulsions: Developmental Psychopathology and Clinical Care. New York, NY: John Wiley & Sons.
37. Schultz, R. T., Evans, D. W., and Wolff, M. (1999). Neuropsychological models of childhood obsessive-compulsive disorder. Child and Adolescent Psychiatric Clinics of North American, 8, 513-531.
38. Biederman, J., Monuteaux, M. C., Doyle, A. E., et al. (2004). Impact of executive function deficits and attention-deficit/hyperactivity disorder (ADHD) on academic outcomes in children. Journal of Consulting and Clinical Psychology, 72, 757-766.
39. Diamantopoulou, S., Rydell, A. M., Thorell, L. B., and Bohlin, G. (2008). Impact of executive functioning and symptoms of attention deficit hyperactivity disorder on children's peer relations and school performance. Developmental Neuropsychology, 32, 521-542.
40. Oram, J., Fine, J., Okamoto, C., and Tannock, R. (1999). Assessing the language of children with attention deficit hyperactivity disorder. American Journal of Speech-Language Pathology, 8, 72-80.
41. Mary Jane Trotti. (2006). Parkaire Consultants. Atlanta, GA.
42. Gray, C. A. (1998). Social skills and comic strip conversations with students with Asperger syndrome and high functioning autism. In Schopler, E., Mesibov, G. B., and Kunce, L. J. editors: Asperger Syndrome or High-Functioning Autism?. New York: Plenum Press.
43. Zentall, S. S. (1988). Production deficiencies in elicited language but not in the spontaneous verbalizations of hyperactive children. Journal of Abnormal Child Psychology, 16, 657-673.
44. Tannock, R., Purvis, K. L., and Schachar, R. J. (1993). Narrative abilities in children with attention deficit hyperactivity disorder and normal peers. Journal of Abnormal Child Psychology, 21, 103-117.
45. Purvis, K. L. and Tannock, R. (1997). Language abilities in children with attention deficit hyperactivity disorder, reading disabilities, and normal controls. Journal of Abnormal Child Psychology, 25, 133-144.
46. Dimitrovsky, L., Spector, H., Levy-Shiff, R., and Vakill, E. (1998). Interpretation of facial expressions of affect in children with learning disabilities with verbal and nonverbal deficits. Journal of Learning Disabilities, 31, 286-292.
47. Corbett, B. and Glidden, H. (2000). Processing affective stimuli in children with attention-deficit hyperactivity disorder. Child Neuropsychology, 6, 144-155.
48. Cadesky, E. B., Mota, V. L., and Schachar, gR. J. (2000). Beyond words: How do children with ADHD and/or conduct problems process nonverbal information about affect? Journal of the American Academy of Child and Adolescent Psychiatry, 39, 1160-1167.
49. Boakes, J., Chapman, E., Houghton, S., and West, J. (2008). Facial affect interpretation in boys with attention deficit/hyperactivity disorder. Child Neuropsychology, 14, 82-96.
50. Wagner, A. P. (2005). Worried No More. Help and Hope for Anxious Children. Lighthouse Point, FL: Lighthouse Press.
51. Chansky, T. E. (2000). Freeing Your Child from Obsessive-Compulsive Disorder. New York NY: Three Rivers Press.

APPENDIX

Comorbid Disorders

 The presence of the following disorders should be determined by a health care professional specifically trained to diagnose and treat psychological conditions. If the student appears to meet the criteria for one or more of the disorders, it is recommended that the student be referred for an evaluation.

Oppositional Defiant Disorder (ODD)

Students with ODD exhibit defiant, argumentative, and resistant behaviors in opposition to the demands made by others, particularly parents and teachers. Poor frustration tolerance and negative, hostile, angry moods are common. Behaviors associated with ODD include: temper outbursts, verbal or physical aggression, stubbornness, continual testing of limits, and an unwillingness to negotiate or compromise. The students have low self-esteem and blame others for their own mistakes.

 Clinical experience suggests that many students need further evaluation to determine whether the ODD symptoms are due to undiagnosed neurological disorders and require treatment.

Conduct Disorder (CD)

The essential feature of this disorder is "a persistent pattern of conduct in which the basic rights of others and major age-appropriate societal norms are violated." The problems associated with this disorder are more serious than those associated with ODD. CD behaviors include: overly aggressive behavior towards animals and peers (bullying, physical aggression, cruelty); destruction of property; fire-setting; antisocial behaviors (breaking and entering, theft, vandalism); lying and cheating; and/or serious violation of rules (staying out late past a given curfew, truancy, running away from home). There is often a lack of concern for others and a lack of remorse. School suspension and expulsion are common. Cigarette smoking, drugs, alcohol, and sexual problems may be associated with the disorder.

Antisocial Personality Disorder

Antisocial personality disorder develops during the late teenage years. Behaviors consistent with a conduct disorder have been present before the age of 15. The condition is characterized by a lack of concern for the moral or legal standards of the society. Adults with this disorder manipulate, exploit, or violate the rights of others. Their behavior is often criminal and they are sometimes called psychopaths or sociopaths. Symptoms include: acting impulsively; stealing, fighting, and breaking the law; disregarding the safety for self and others; conning for pleasure or profit; repeatedly lying or using aliases; having poor work habits; failing to honor financial obligations; and lacking guilt or rationalizing the pain inflicted on others.

Major Depression

Students who are severely depressed must exhibit five of the following symptoms: depressed or irritable mood most of the day, diminished interest or pleasure in activities, changes in weight or appetite, sleep disturbance, psychomotor agitation or retardation, fatigue or lethargy, feelings of worthlessness or guilt, diminished concentration, and recurrent thoughts of death or suicide.

Section IX

Bipolar Disorder (Manic-Depression)

Students with mood disorders experience alternating periods of depression and mania that last from a few hours to a few days. Whereas depression is accompanied by episodes of severe irritability, sadness, and low energy, mania is associated with a persistent state of elation or agitation and heightened energy. Manic symptoms may include: inflated self-esteem (grandiose belief in one's own abilities); decreased need for sleep (feels rested after only a few hours of sleep); flight of ideas or racing thoughts; distractibility, hyperactivity, and agitation; overtalkative or pressured talking; excessive involvement in multiple projects and activities; explosive, lengthy, and often destructive rages ("storms"); and/or inappropriate or precocious sexual behavior.

Anxiety Disorders

Anxiety or unrealistic worry is the defining feature of an anxiety disorder. Students who are excessively fearful and overestimate the level of danger often experience impairment in day-to-day functioning. There are several types of anxiety disorders. Students may have one or more of the following:.

Agoraphobia

Agoraphobia is the fear of being in a place or situation where escape is difficult (or embarrassing) or help is not available. Situations that are avoided may include: attending school, being alone or in crowds, riding the bus, and going on field trips or to performances. In these circumstances, students may experience diarrhea, vomiting, and feeling sick. Students with severe cases sometimes become depressed and are unable to leave home.

Generalized Anxiety Disorder

An overanxious disorder of childhood is a condition of excessive anxiety and chronic, unrealistic, and uncontrolled worry. Students are anxious almost every day about both important and unimportant problems, situations, events, and activities. These worries interfere with normal routines, school, and social interactions. The students are distracted by their worries and find it difficult to stop thinking about them. They feel restless, tense, and irritable; complain of headaches, stomachaches, and other physical symptoms; and often have sleep disturbances.

Panic Disorder

Students with panic disorder experience a sudden feeling or attack of overwhelming dread or intense fear that something terrible is happening. Panic attacks are accompanied by physical sensations of shortness of breath, chills or hot flashes, sweating, heart palpitations, chest pains, difficulty swallowing, trembling or shaking, dizziness, and/or nausea. The attacks often are associated with a fear of going crazy or dying. Repeated panic attacks lead to a fear of reoccurring episodes and loss of control. Students often begin to avoid situations where they fear a panic attack may occur and assistance will not be available.

Separation Anxiety

Separation anxiety or fear of being away from home or one's parents can be secondary to a panic disorder, agoraphobia, social anxiety disorder, or the occurrence of a stressful event (e.g., divorce, death in the family). Students with the disorder may be afraid to go places without parents (sleep at friend's house, attend a birthday party, go to camp). They may follow their parents around the house and try to sleep with them or their siblings. When anticipating a separation, they often develop physical symptoms such as headaches, diarrhea, nausea, vomiting, or breathlessness. During a separation, they may worry that something terrible will happen to the parent (e.g., accident, illness, fire, crime).

Appendix

Social Phobia (Social Anxiety Disorder)

Students with social anxiety disorders are painfully shy, timid, uneasy, and self-conscious when exposed to unfamiliar people or to possible judgment by others. They cling to parents and fear other children as well as adults at an age when it is no longer normal. Symptoms may include: crying, freezing, becoming panicky, shrinking back, withdrawing, or having a tantrum. Social anxiety is sometimes called performance anxiety or the fear of being humiliated or embarrassed by saying or doing something foolish or inappropriate. The students may worry about being required to interact socially with classmates, respond orally in class, read aloud, or write on the blackboard. Some may refuse to attend school for these reasons.

Specific Phobia

A specific phobia is the fear of specific objects or situations that is excessive and out of proportion to the actual danger. Common fears include: thunderstorms, the dark, enclosed spaces, driving, flying, choking, sight of blood, animals, reptiles, and insects. The phobic situations are avoided or accompanied with intense anxiety or distress.

- *For a more indepth discussion of the comorbid disorders consult* <u>Challenging Kids, Challenged Teachers</u>*! by Leslie E. Packer, Ph. D. and Sheryl K. Pruitt, M. Ed., ET/P (working title, manuscript in press. Bethesda, MD: Woodbine House)*

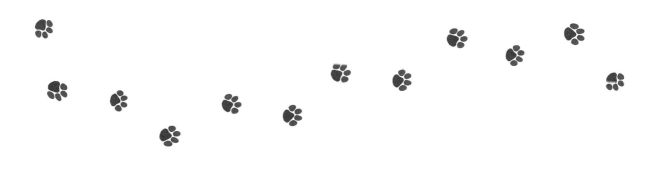

Get A Clue

G | **GOAL(S)**
E | Examine Task/Activity/Problem _____
_____
T | Think of Goal _____
_____

A | ACT

C | Create PLANS

    P | Propose Solutions _____
_____
_____

    L | List Priorities _____
_____
_____

    A | Analyze Strategies _____
_____
_____

    N | Note Organization/ _____
          Sequence
_____
_____

    S | Set Timelines _____
_____
_____

L | Launch Plans
U | Use Best Strategy _____
E | Evaluate/Edit _____

Plan

P | Propose Goal _____
_____
_____
_____
_____
_____

L | List and Analyze Strategies _____
_____
_____
_____
_____
_____
_____

A | Analyze Best Strategy _____
_____
_____
_____
_____
_____

N | Notice Errors and Edit _____
_____
_____
_____
_____
_____

Section IX

THE STORY OF MOTHER VOWEL

After the consonant sounds have been mastered, "The Story of Mother Vowel" helps the student learn and retrieve the abstract sounds associated with the short (baby) vowel sounds in a meaningful context. The student quickly learns the story and enjoys retelling it.

🐾 *As you read the story below, use the hand signals indicated for each vowel.*

Mother Vowel and her babies live on a farm. The names of the babies are "a," "e," "i," "o," and "u." The babies are too young to talk and only make sounds. Poor Mother Vowel never knows what they want!

One day Baby "a" was hungry and saw an apple tree. Pointing to the tree with her arm raised up in the air, Baby "a" began to shout "aaaaaaaaaaaaaaa" as in the beginning sound in the word "apple." Mother Vowel was thrilled to know that Baby "a" would raise her arm and say, "aaaaaaaaaaaaaa" every time she wanted an apple.

Hand signal: Raise hand and wave as trying to reach an apple.
Sit next to the student in front of a mirror to demonstrate how the mouth forms the vowels (e.g., pulls back when making the short (baby) vowel sound "aaaaaaaaaaaaaaa").

Baby "e" loved scrambled eggs. Mother Vowel scrambled a dozen eggs and placed them on the table. All of a sudden the phone rang in the kitchen. While Mother Vowel was talking on the telephone, Baby "e" climbed on the table and ate all of the eggs. When Mother Vowel returned from the kitchen, Baby "e" was holding his stomach and saying, "eeeeeeeeeeeeeeh" as in beginning sound in the word "egg." His stomach hurt so much that every time his mother tried to serve him eggs, he would hold his stomach and moan, "eeeeeeeeeeeeeeh!"

Hand signal: Hold stomach with both hands and lean over as if in pain.

Baby "i" was standing on the rail of the fence and looking down at the pigs in the pig sty. All of a sudden he slipped and fell head first into the sty. He was covered with mud from his head to his toes! He ran straight to Mother Vowel and cried, "iiiiiiiiiiiicky, iiiiiiiiiiicky, iiiiiiiiiiicky" while shaking the mud off his hands. As he said "icky," the skin on his nose wrinkled up. *(Make a wrinkled nose. Ask the student to do the same thing and feel the wrinkles on both noses.)* Whenever Baby "i" saw the pigs, he would shake his hands, wrinkle his nose, and say, "icky, icky, icky."

Hand signal: Wrinkle nose and shake hands as if shaking off mud.

Mother Vowel took Baby "o" to the fish store. When Baby "o" saw a little octopus, she said, "aaahhhhhhhhhhhh." From that day on, every time she saw an octopus, she would say, "aaahhhhhhhhhhhh."

Hand signal: Place right fist on top of left hand. Wiggle fingers of left hand.

There was one very mischievous baby. Baby "u" crawled into Mother Vowel's closet. He saw her sewing kit and pulled out the scissors. Baby "u" then spotted her umbrella and began cutting it up. Mother Vowel came in the room and went to the closet to get her umbrella. She saw what Baby "u" was doing and shook her finger at him and said, "UH, UH, UH." From then on, every time it rained and Mother Vowel got her umbrella, Baby "u" would shake his finger and say, "UH, UH, UH."

Hand signal: Shake finger as if scolding the baby.

 As the student decodes words, use hand signals to cue the appropriate sound and/or provide additional time for retrieval of known sounds.

Abstract decoding rules may also be difficult for the student to learn. Therefore, it is important to teach fewer rules and place them in a meaningful context.

For example:

- When baby (short) vowels are not old enough to walk by themselves, they need to hold their parents' (consonants) hands. One baby walking with a parent on each side makes the baby (short) sound as in "hat," "met," "sit," "hot," and "nut."

- After the baby vowel has become "more grown up" and learned his own name (long vowel), he is able to go walking with his vowel friends. For example, if two vowels are walking together, only the first vowel speaks and says his name while the other vowel is polite and remains silent as in "paint," "heat," and "coat."

- Two consonants are close cousins of the Vowel family – "y" and "w." Cousin "y" has trouble deciding if he is a consonant or a vowel so he has two hats, one black (consonant) and one red (vowel). He wears his black hat at the beginning of a word and makes the consonant sound. He wears his red hat and acts like a "grown up" (long) vowel in a word like in "by" or "guy" or is silent following an "a" such as in "day."

- Cousin "w" is a scamp! He likes to make all the rules go crazy. He pretends to be a vowel when he follows "o" and makes the baby say her "grown-up" (long) name, such as in "snow." At other times, he is mean and pinches her until she says "ow!" like in "how." Cousin "w" then feels sorry for what he did and asks his friend "a" to help make her feel better by saying "awwwwwwwwwwwwww" like in the word "paw."

- Neighbor "r" from the consonant family likes to play tiger games. He chases "e," "i," and "u" all over the farm while growling his baby sound "rrrrrrrrrrrrrrrrr!" like in the words "her," "dirt," or "hurt."

    Hand signal: Bend pointer finger to make a tiger's claw.

- As the vowels get older, romance blooms! Neighbor "r" falls in love with "a" and says his grown-up name, as in "car." Thus, "r" can say either his baby name "rrrrrrrrrrrrrrrr" or his grown-up name.

Sheryl K. Pruitt, M.Ed., ET/P and Vickie Rhinehart at Parkaire Consultants, Inc. 1988

Dolch Basic Sight Vocabulary Words

(High-Frequency Words/Sight Words)

Listed in order of descending frequency

I	II	III	IV	V	VI	VII
the	be	if	every	play	always	kind
to	have	now	pretty	who	drink	both
and	go	long	jump	been	once	sit
he	we	no	green	may	soon	which
a	am	came	four	stop	made	fall
I	then	ask	away	off	run	carry
you	little	very	old	never	gave	small
it	down	an	by	seven	open	under
of	do	over	their	eight	has	read
in	can	yours	here	cold	find	why
was	could	its	saw	today	only	own
said	when	ride	call	fly	us	found
his	did	into	after	myself	three	wash
that	what	just	well	round	our	slow
she	so	blue	think	tell	better	hot
for	see	red	ran	much	hold	because
on	not	from	let	keep	buy	far
they	were	good	help	give	funny	live
but	get	any	make	work	warm	draw
had	them	about	going	first	ate	clean
at	like	around	sleep	try	full	grow
him	one	want	brown	new	those	best
with	this	don't	yellow	must	done	upon
up	my	how	five	start	use	these
all	would	know	six	black	fast	sing
look	me	right	walk	white	say	together
is	will	put	two	ten	light	please
her	yes	too	or	does	pick	thank
there	big	got	before	bring	hurt	wish
some	went	take	eat	goes	pull	many
out	are	where	again	write	out	shall
as	come					

Name: _____ Date: _____

Story Organizer

Title:
[   ]

Who? (people/subjects)	

| **Where?** (places) | |

| **When?** (time) | |

| **What?** (actions/events) | |

| **How?** (cause/effect) | |

| **Why?** (reasons) | |

| **Solutions** | |

| **Outcome** | |

Name: _____ Date: _____

Problem/Solution

Title:
☐

Problem	Who had the problem? What was the problem?
Causes	Why was there a problem?
Effects	What was the effect?
Solutions	Attempted Solutions: Results 1. 1. 2. 2.
Outcome	

Summary: _____
_____
_____

Name: _____ Date: _____

Sequence

Title:
[   ]

Stage/Step/Event

1 [   ]

2 [   ]

3 [   ]

What was the beginning stage/step/event?	
How did they lead to each other?	
Outcome	

Summary: _____
_____
_____

Name: _____ Date: _____

Information/Description

Title:
[ ]

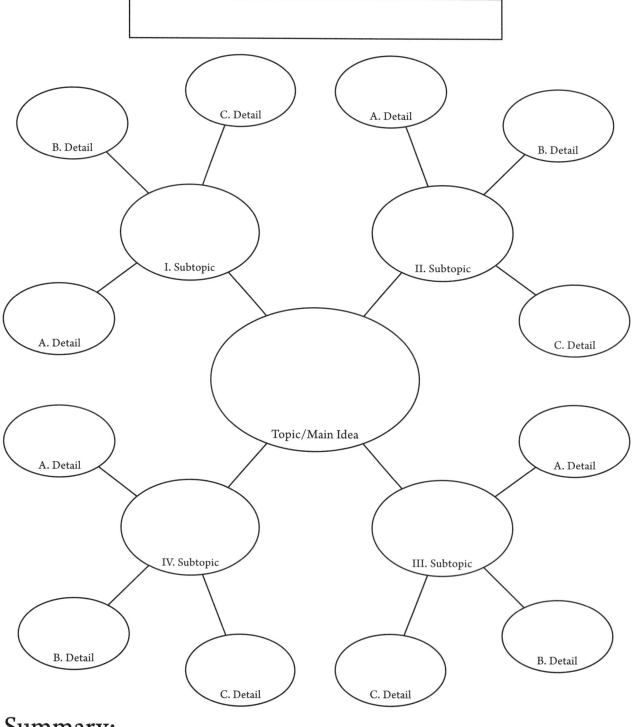

Summary: _____
_____
_____

Name: _____ Date: _____

Main Ideas/Facts Chart

Title: ☐

Introductory Paragraph	Paragraph 2	Paragraph 3	Paragraph 4	Concluding Paragraph
Topic	Main Idea of Paragraph	Main Idea of Paragraph	Main Idea of Paragraph	Topic Restatement
Ideas to be Developed	Supporting Facts	Supporting Facts	Supporting Facts	Most Important Facts

This page may be reprinted for classroom and personal, noncommercial use only. *Tigers, Too* © 2009 by Marilyn P. Dornbush, Ph.D, and Sheryl K. Pruitt, M.Ed., ET/P.

Name: _____ Date: _____

Compare/Contrast (Similarities/Differences)

Subject 1: _____   Subject 2: _____

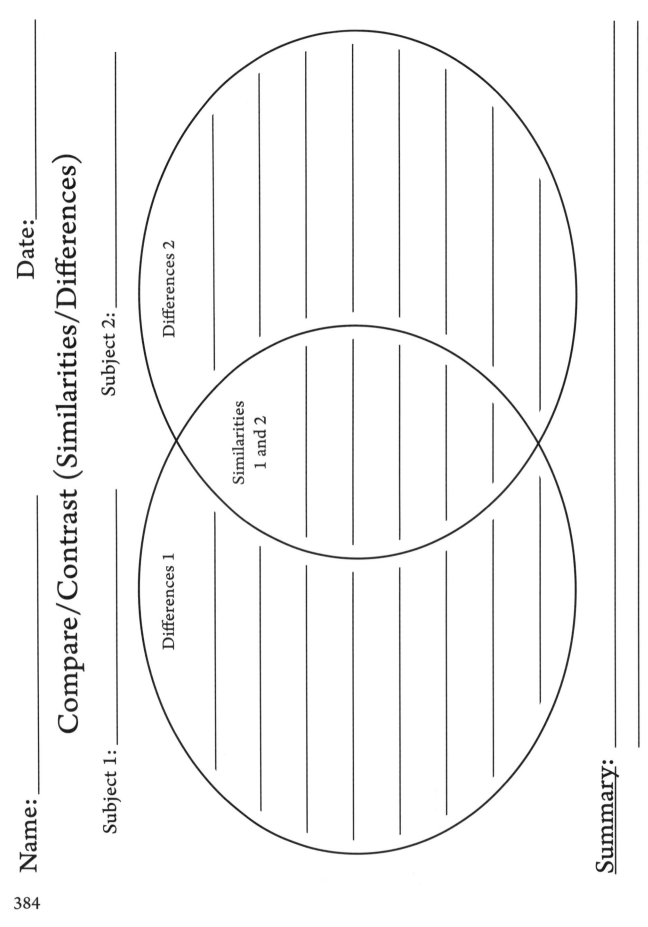

Summary: _____

Name: _____ Date: _____

Compare/Contrast (Similarities/Differences)

Subject 1: _____   Subject 2: _____

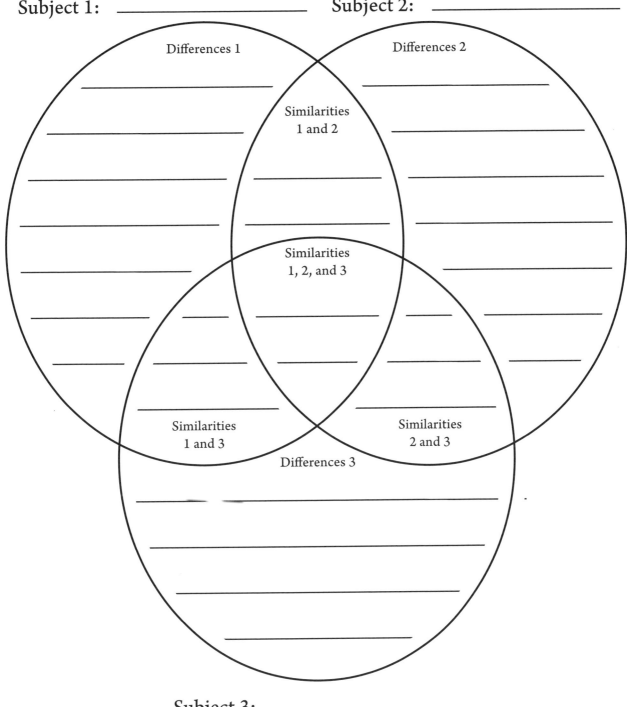

Subject 3: _____

Summary: _____
_____
_____

Name: _____ Date: _____

Opinions/Facts

Title:
☐

Opinions   Facts

Summary: _____
_____
_____

Name: _____ Date: _____

Cycle of Stages/Steps/Events

Title:

Stage/Step/Event 1

Stage/Step/Event 2

Stage/Step/Event 4

Stage/Step/Event 3

What were the important stages/steps/events?	1. 2. 3. 4.
How were they related?	
How/Why did they keep the cycle going?	

Summary: _____
_____
_____

Name: _____ Date: _____

Cause and Effect

Title:

[ ]

Cause ⟶ Effect

Cause	Effect
What happened? Why did it happen?	What was the result? What was the consequence?

Outcome | [ ]

Summary: _____
_____
_____

Revision Checklist for Narrative Writing

<u>First Paragraph</u>	Did you capture the reader's attention and make the reader want to read further?	Yes	No
<u>Character(s)</u>	Who was the main character?		
	_____		
	Who were other important characters?		
	_____		
	_____		
	_____		
	Did you adequately describe of the characters?	Yes	No
	Did the dialogue develop the characters' personalities and advance the plot?	Yes	No
<u>Setting</u>	Did you tell <u>where</u> the story took place?	Yes	No
	Did you tell <u>when</u> the story took place?	Yes	No
	Did your <u>setting</u> enhance the story?	Yes	No
	Did you frequently refer to the setting?	Yes	No
	Did you use <u>descriptive words</u> to depict what was seen, heard, and felt?	Yes	No
<u>Plot</u>	Did you explain <u>what</u> the conflict/problem was?	Yes	No
	Did you explain <u>why</u> there was a conflict/problem?	Yes	No
<u>Outcome</u>	Did you explain <u>how</u> the conflict/problem was resolved?	Yes	No
	Did you include an appropriate ending/solution (not abrupt/leave the reader with many questions)?	Yes	No

** If you circled "No" to any of the above questions, revise that part before turning in your paper.

Revision Checklist for Expository Writing

<u>First Paragraph</u>	Did you clearly <u>state the topic</u>?	Yes	No
	Did you include three or four <u>ideas/examples</u>?	Yes	No
	Did you capture the reader's attention and make the reader want to read further?	Yes	No
	Did you end with a <u>transition sentence</u> that connected the following paragraph?	Yes	No
<u>Following Paragraphs</u>	Did you write a <u>beginning sentence</u> that stated the main idea of each paragraph?	Yes	No
	Did you include <u>facts and examples</u> to support the main idea?	Yes	No
	Did you include a few <u>quotes</u> from authorities?	Yes	No
	Did you reference the quotes?	Yes	No
	Did you include some <u>illustrations</u> to explain the main idea and details?	Yes	No
	Did you <u>sequence the ideas</u> so they made sense and related to each other?	Yes	No
	Were there any words or sentences that did not need to be included?	Yes	No
	Did you use a <u>variety of words</u> rather than the same words over and over again?	Yes	No
	Did you use <u>adjectives</u> and <u>adverbs</u>?	Yes	No
	Did you <u>summarize</u> at the end of the paragraph?	Yes	No
	Did you <u>rephrase the main idea</u> in words that are different from those used in the first paragraph?	Yes	No
<u>Concluding Paragraph</u>	Did you <u>summarize</u> important ideas presented?	Yes	No
	Did you end with a <u>concluding statement</u>?	Yes	No

** If you circled "No" to any of the above questions, revise that part before turning in your paper.

PROOFREADING CHECKLIST

Did you capitalize the:	Yes	No
Title?	Yes	No
First word in each sentence?	Yes	No
Word "I"?	Yes	No
Proper names of people and places?	Yes	No
Did you put a period at the end of each sentence?	Yes	No
Did you put question marks at the end of each question?	Yes	No
Did you put quotation marks around people's words?	Yes	No
Did you put commas in a sequence of people, places?	Yes	No
Did you use apostrophes for contractions and possessives?	Yes	No
Did you check your spelling?	Yes	No
Did you use complete sentences?	Yes	No
Did you make the subjects and verbs agree with each other (singular/plural)?	Yes	No
Were the verb tenses consistent throughout the paper?	Yes	No
Could you read the essay aloud without stumbling over words?	Yes	No
Was your handwriting legible?	Yes	No
Did you provide enough space between the words?	Yes	No
Did you make the overall appearance of the paper neat?	Yes	No

** If you circled "No" to any of the above questions, correct that part before turning in your paper.

ADDITION FACTS STRATEGIES

Present these strategies to the students in the order listed below.

To Add:	Strategy
0	The answer is the other number.
1	Go up one. If not automatic: Practice with manipulatives. Practice rote counting. Play games to drill "What number comes after _____?"
2	Go up two. Start counting audibly – for 5 + 2, think "5" and say, "6…7." Or, use 2 dots to count up: 5 + 2. Gradually fade auditory and visual cues.
10	Put a "1" in front of the other number. Do examples and have students discover the pattern. Use visual cues and then fade.
9	Add 10 and go down one. Demonstrate with manipulatives so students see why it works. Start by writing the number you get when 10 is added; gradually fade visual cue.
the doubles: 9+9=18 8+8=16 7+7=14 6+6=12 5+5=10	First, be sure students can count by 2's efficiently. Use manipulatives to demonstrate the relationship between these facts. Write this set of facts as shown, with 9 + 9 at the top. Help students to visualize the facts in order. When students have learned one fact, use it to help them remember the next one. Ex: "If 5 + 5 = 10, what is 6 + 6?" Use similar principles for 3 + 3 and 4 + 4.
the doubles plus one: 3+4=7 4+5=9 5+6=11 6+7=13 7+8=15 8+9=17	Be sure "the doubles" are automatic before going on to this strategy. Use manipulatives to demonstrate. Ex: "You know 5 + 5 = 10. Let's add one more. 5 + 6 must be 11." Use the cue, "Which one of the doubles is it next to?" Teach the student to verbalize, "That's easy! I know 6 + 6 = 12, so 6 + 7 must be 13." Even after students begin to get the answer automatically, have them tell you their thinking process. It reduces impulsivity and teaches self-checking.
ways to make 10: 10+0=10 9+1=10 8+2=10 7+3=10 6+4=10 5+5=10	These combinations are very important! Knowing them automatically will help with subtraction, adding columns, making change and more. Drill using fingers, abacus, and games with number pairs which add up to 10, etc. Be sure to include practice with one missing addend: 9 + ___ = 10.
5+7 5+8	To solve 5 + 7, think, "5 + 5 = 10 and 2 more is 12." To solve 5 + 8, think, "5 + 5 = 10 and 3 more is 13."
3+5 3+6 3+8 4+7	When students have mastered the above strategies, only a few facts remain. Help students come up with strategies that work best for them. Ex: for 6 + 8, think of 6 + 6 and go up 2; for 4 + 7, think of 3 + 7 and go up 1

Compiled by Donna Cherry, 1993

MULTIPLICATION FACTS STRATEGIES

Present these strategies to the students in the order listed below.
*Master one strategy before going on to another.
*Remind students to cue themselves, "What's my strategy?" before giving an answer.

To Add:	Strategy:
0	The answer is always 0.
1	The answer is the other number.
2	Double the other number. See addition strategies for doubles. This method is more efficient than counting by 2's and prepares students for the 4's strategy below.
5	Look at the clock. For example, when the big hand is on the 6, it is 30 minutes after, so 5 x 6 = 30. Pointing to numerals on the classroom clock, ask students, "If the big hand is on the ___, it is how many minutes after?" Drill the 3, 6, 9 and 12 first. Then work on the numbers in between. Later, practice using a quickly drawn clock. Finally, encourage students to visualize the clock and solve multiplication problems.
9	Finger trick. Palms down, assign a number to each finger from 1-10 (left to right). For 9 x 4, bend down finger number 4. There will be 3 fingers to the left of the bent finger, and 6 fingers to the right, so the answer is 36. Try other examples. Practice until students can solve automatically – without counting fingers. (source unknown)
10	Write the other number and put a zero after it. Later, fade the visual cue.
11	Write the number twice. If students have been exposed to 2 digit multiplication, show them why this works.

Drill the above strategies until the student uses them efficiently before going on to the more difficult strategies below. There are only 15 more facts to master!

3	Count by 3's. Begin with manipulatives – count objects in groups of threes. Then, count on fingers by 3's. Palms down, assign a number to each finger from 1-10 (left to right). As students count, have them wiggle the appropriate finger. Help them associate each finger with the corresponding multiplication problem Ex: For 3 x 8, the student will wiggle the 8th finger and say, "24".
4 4x4=16 4x6=24 4x7=28 4x8=32	Double the other number. Then double again. Ex: 4 x 7 is the same as saying: 7 + 7 = 14, and then 14 + 14 = 28. Since student have already mastered the doubles, the first step is easy. Most students will need to write down the second step until more automatic. Gradually fade the visual cues.
6x4=24 6x6=36 6x8=48	Say in rhythm. Notice that students now have 2 strategies for 6 x 4 (see 4's trick).
7x8=56	Think of the two numbers before 7 and 8. Say, "5...6...7...8." The 5 and 6 give you the answer (56).
8x8=64	Starting with 8, count backwards by 2's: 6, 4 – the answer is 64 or "8 x 8 fell on the floor, when it got up it was 64". (Leslie Seeley)
That leaves: 7x6=42 7x7=49	Help students invent a strategy for these. Or, practice with backward chaining: Write problem and answer on dry erase board in color of student's choice. Student says the whole problem (i.e.: 7 x 7 = 49). Teacher erases the last numeral. Student replaces the numeral and says the whole problem again. Repeat the procedure, with the teacher erasing the last two, then three, then four characters, etc. Continue until the student can say and write the problem without prompts. If a student makes an error at any point, begin again. Note: Try backward chaining with erasable markers on windows. Or, try using shaving cream on a table. (source unknown).

Compiled by Donna Cherry, 1993

This page may be reprinted for classroom and personal, noncommercial use only.
Tigers, Too © 2009 by Marilyn P. Dornbush, Ph.D., and Sheryl K. Pruitt, M.Ed., ET/P.

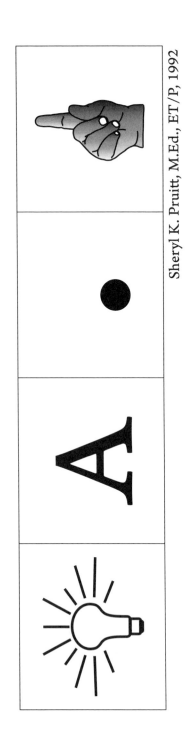

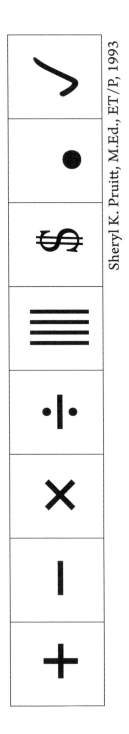

Dirty ÷
Marvin ×
Smells −
Bad →

Does ÷
McDonalds ×
Sell −
Cheese
Burgers →

(source unknown)

Parkaire Consultants, Inc. 1982

MATH EDITING CHECKLIST FOR COMPUTATIONS

Did you <u>copy</u> the problem correctly?　　　　　　　　　　　　　　Yes　　No

Did you <u>line up and space</u> the numbers properly?　　　　　　　Yes　　No

Did you <u>estimate</u> the answer?　　　　　　　　　　　　　　　　　Yes　　No

Did you use the correct <u>operation</u>?　　　　　　　　　　　　　　Yes　　No

Did you remember the <u>math facts</u> correctly?　　　　　　　　　Yes　　No

Did you miss the answer by one number?　　　　　　　　　　　　Yes　　No

Did you guess at the answer?　　　　　　　　　　　　　　　　　　Yes　　No

Did you regroup (<u>carry</u>) in addition/multiplication problems?　　Yes　　No

Was the answer more than 9?　　　　　　　　　　　　　　　　　　Yes　　No

Did you regroup (<u>borrow</u>) in subtraction problems?　　　　　　Yes　　No

Was the top number smaller than the bottom number?　　　　　Yes　　No

Did you remember the <u>sequence of division</u> problems correctly?　Yes　　No

Did you keep the division problems lined up correctly?　　　　　Yes　　No

Is your <u>handwriting legible</u>?　　　　　　　　　　　　　　　　　Yes　　No

** If you circled "No" to any of the above questions, correct that part before turning in your paper.

Math Words And Corresponding Symbols

positive, plus, add	+	equals, is equal to	=
minus, subtract, negative	−	not equal, is not equal to	≠
times, multiply	×	less than	<
divide	÷	more than	>
percent	%	is less than or equal to	≤
approximately, about, more/less	≈	is more than or equal to	≥
degree	°	is similar to	∼
parentheses	( )	is parallel to	∥
brackets	[ ]	is congruent to	≅
braces	{ }	infinity	∞
absolute Value Bars	∥	angle	∠
dollars	$	right angle	∟
inches	″	triangle	△
feet	′	perpendicular	⊥
pi, 3.141592653589	π	the sum of	Σ
square root	√	factorial	!
is an element of	∈	is to (ratio)	:
is not an element of	∉	numeric constant 2.71828	e
is a subset of	⊂ ⊆	line AB	$\overline{AB}$
is not a subset	⊄ ⊈	segment AB	$\overleftrightarrow{AB}$
the set of	∪	ray AB	$\overrightarrow{AB}$
the intersection of	∩	therefore	∴

Name: _____   Date: _____

Ready The Plane For The Math's 4 C's

Mark Each Box As Completed

Ready

☐ Read Problem   ☐ Examine Cue Words   ☐ Ask Question   ☐ Draw Picture   ☐ You Are Ready For Take-off

Plane

☐ Propose Solutions   ☐ Locate Important Imformation   ☐ Analyze + And - Of Solutions   ☐ Name Operation(s)   ☐ Estimate

Math's Four C's

☐ Calculate   ☐ Compare To Estimate   ☐ Check   ☐ Correct

If you have not checked a box, redo that part and follow sequence again before turning in paper.

This page may be reprinted for classroom and personal, noncommercial use only. *Tigers, Too* © 2009 by Marilyn P. Dornbush, Ph.D, and Sheryl K. Pruitt, M.Ed., ET/P.

MATH EDITING CHECKLIST FOR WORD PROBLEMS

Did you <u>read</u> the problem aloud?	Yes	No
Did you locate the <u>cue words</u>?	Yes	No
Did you ask for <u>unknown words</u> to be explained?	Yes	No
Did you <u>paraphrase</u> the problem/question?	Yes	No
Did you locate the <u>relevant</u> information?	Yes	No
Did you cross out the <u>irrelevant</u> information?	Yes	No
Did you make a <u>drawing</u>, diagram, or chart?	Yes	No
Did you decide on the <u>correct operation(s)</u>?	Yes	No
Did you <u>estimate</u> the answer?	Yes	No
Did you <u>calculate</u> the answer?	Yes	No
Did you <u>compare</u> the answer with the estimate?	Yes	No
Did you <u>reread</u> the problem?	Yes	No
Did you <u>check</u> the answer?	Yes	No
Did you <u>correct</u> the answer when needed?	Yes	No
Is your <u>handwriting legible</u>?	Yes	No

** If you circled "No" to any of the above questions, correct that part before turning in your paper.

Class Notes

Name: _____ Date: _____

Subject: _____

Recall Column	Notetaking Column

SHORTHAND SYMBOLS FOR NOTETAKING

Add/Plus/Positive	+	Information	info
And/Or	&	Individual	ind
Around/About/Approximately/Circa	ca	More important than/Most important	>imp/*imp
At	@		
Background	bkgd	Increases/Decreases	↑/↓
Be	b	More than/Less than	>/<
Because	b/c	Maximum/Minimum	max/min
Before	b/4	Minus/Negative	−
Causes/Results in/Leads to/Produces	→	Number	#
Comes from/Is result of/Is consequence of	←	Page/Pages	p/pp
		Question/Answer	Q/A
Change	chg	Read	rd
Compare/In comparison/In relation to	cmp	Right/Left	rt/lft
Definition	def	That is	i.e.
Difference	diff	Versus/Against/Opposed to	vs
Equal to/Same as	=	What	?
Not equal to/Is not	≠	Which	wh/
Especially	esp	With	w/
Et cetera	etc.	Without	w/o
Example	ex	Within	w/i
Following	ff	Word/Words	wd/wds
For example	e.g.	Write	wrt
Important	imp	Years	yrs

Feeling Words

MAD	SAD	GLAD	SCARED
Angry	Blue	Cheerful	Afraid
Annoyed	Bummed out	Contented	Anxious
Cross	Depressed	Delighted	Bothered
Enraged	Despairing	Ecstatic	Cautious
Furious	Disappointed	Enthusiastic	Fearful
Frustrated	Discouraged	Excited	Frightened
Hateful	Dismal	Fantastic	Horrified
Impatient	Down	Great	Intimidated
Incensed	Forlorn	Happy	Jumpy
Irate	Gloomy	Hopeful	Nervous
Irritated	Glum	Joyful	Panicked
Put out	Grieving	Lively	Petrified
Raging	Hopeless	Merry	Rattled
Resentful	Hurt	Optimistic	Shaky
Seething	Low	Pleased	Startled
Sore	Melancholic	Positive	Stressed
Stormy	Miserable	Proud	Terrified
Teed Off	Sorrowful	Satisfied	Threatened
Terrible	Sorry	Thankful	Uneasy
Upset	Unhappy	Thrilled	Uptight
Worked up	Wretched	Wonderful	Worried

Name: _____   Date: _____

Feeling ⟶   Behaviors   ⟶   Consequences

SLEEP SURVEY - PARENT REPORTING FORM

Name: _____ **Date:** _____

Subject: _____

Question	Response
What is your child's bedtime routine?	
What time on school nights does your child usually go to bed?	
Does your child need to stay up late to finish homework?	
How long does it take for your child to fall asleep?	
Once your child falls asleep, does he/she sleep through the night? If not, what are the problems?	
How many hours sleep does your child get each night of the school week?	
What time does your child usually wake up for school?	
Does your child wake up easily or do you struggle to wake him/her up?	
Does your child have difficulty getting ready for school?	
Does your child sleep in the afternoon after school? If so, for how long?	

ORGANIZATIONAL SKILLS SURVEY - PARENT REPORTING FORM

Name: _____ **Date:** _____

Subject: _____

My Child:	Never	Rarely	Some	Often	Always
is unable to keep bedroom/playroom well-organized and neat.					
misplaces/loses personal possessions, including favorite belongings.					
is unable to meet responsibilities in the home without reminders.					
is unaware of/does not know what is supposed to happen each day.					
has a poor sense of what is important and what is not.					
has trouble getting started on tasks without assistance (exclude homework).					
starts but does not finish non-school activities/projects/chores.					
is late for everything, even with frequent reminders.					
has difficulty following three-step directions without forgetting a step.					
forgets to give me notices/permission slips from school.					
has trouble planning in advance and initiating social plans with peers.					
is more a follower than a leader.					

Homework Survey - Parent Reporting Form

Name: _____ Date: _____

Subject: _____

My Child:	Never	Rarely	Some	Often	Always
fails to record homework assignment(s) independently in school.					
forgets to bring home homework planner or recorded assignment(s).					
forgets to bring home books or materials needed to complete homework assignment(s).					
does not understand/know how to do assignment(s)					
does not know when assignment(s) are due.					
underestimates/cannot allocate time required to complete each assignment.					
avoids starting homework without reminders or nagging.					
has difficulty shifting from one assignment to another.					
finds level of homework too difficult to complete independently.					
is unable to complete homework without presence of adult.					
fights about having to do/complete homework.					
cannot pack schoolbag independently and correctly.					
misplaces or loses schoolwork/homework.					
How much time is spent each day by your child completing homework?					
How much time do you spend each day helping and supervising your child to make sure that homework is completed?					
Do other factors (disabilities, after-school sports/activities, medication(s), sleep problems, etc.) interfere with the ability to complete homework? If so, list factors.					

Appendix

ORGANIZATIONS/WEB SITES

American Occupational Therapy Association (OTA)
4720 Montgomery Lane
P.O. Box 31220
Bethesda, MD 20824-1220
1-800-377-8885
(301)652-2682
(301)652-7711 FAX
website: www.aota.org

American Speech-Language-Hearing Association (ASHA)
10801 Rockville Pike
Rockville, MD 20852
1-800-638-8255
(240)333-4705 FAX
website: www.asha.org

Anxiety Disorder Association of America (ADAA)
8730 Georgia Avenue, Suite 600
Silver Spring, MD 20910
(240)485-1001
(240)485-1035 FAX
website: www.adaa.org

Children and Adults with Attention Deficit/Hyperactivity Disorder (CHADD)
8181 Professional Place, Suite 150
Landover, MD 20785
(301)306-7070
(301)306-7090 FAX
website: www.chadd.org

Council for Exceptional Children (CEC)
1110 North Glebe Road, Suite 300
Arlington, VA 22201
1-888-CEC-SPED
(703)620-3660
(703)264-9494
website: www.cec.sped.org

International Dyslexia Association (IDA)
40 York Road
Baltimore, MD 21204-5202
1-800-ABCD123
(410)321-5069
website: www.interdys.org

Learning Disabilities Association of America (LDA)
4156 Library Road
Pittsburgh, PA 15234-1349
(412)341-1515
(412)344-0224 FAX
website: www.ldaamerica.org

Section IX

Obsessive-Compulsive Foundation (OCF)
676 State Street
New Haven, CT 06511
(203)401-2070
website: www.ocfoundation.org

Obsessive-Compulsive Information Center (OCIC)
Madison Institute of Medicine
7617 Mineral Point Road, Suite 300
Madison, WI 53717
(608)827-2470
(608)827-2479 FAX
website: www.mim@miminc.org

Parents Educating Parents and Professionals
3680 Kings Highway
Douglasville, GA 30135
(770)577-7771
(770)577-7774 FAX
website: www.peppinc.org

Tourette Syndrome Association (TSA)
42-40 Bell Boulevard
Bayside, NY 11361
(718)224-2999
(718)279-9596 FAX
website: www.tsa-usa.org

Tourette Syndrome Foundation of Canada (TSFC)
5945 Airport Road, Suite 195
Mississauga, ON L4V 1R9
(416)861-8398; 1-800-361-3120
website: www.tourette.ca

National Institute of Mental Health (NIMH)
6001 Executive Boulevard
Room 8184, MSC 9663
Bethesda, MD 20892
(866)615-6464 (toll free)
(866)415-8051 (TTY toll free)
(301)443-4279 Fax
website: www.behavioralhealthlink.com

ADDITIONAL WEB SITES

All Kinds of Minds
www.allkindsofminds.org

American with Disabilities Act: Civil Rights for You
www.ldonline.org/ldindepth/adult/dale brown ada.html

Association of Educational Therapists
www.aetonline.org

Child Find (component of IDEA)
www.childfindidea.org

National Center for Learning Disabilities (NCLD)
www.NCLD.org

NICHCY (National Dissemination Center for Children with Disabilities
www.NICHCY.org

Office for Civil Rights
www.OCR@ed.gov

Parent Advocacy Coalition for Educational Rights (PACER)
www.pacer.org

Parkaire Consultants
www.parkaireconsultants.com

School Behavior: Awareness, Empathy, and Skills
www.schoolbehavior.com

Technical Assistance Alliance for Parent Centers
www.taalliance.org

Tourette Syndrome "Plus"
www.tourettesyndrome.net

U.S. Department of Education, Office of Special Education Programs
www.ed/gov/policy/speced/idea/idea2004.html

Wright's Law
For legal questions
www.wrightslaw.com

READING/MEDIA RESOURCES

General Education

A Mind at a Time
Mel D. Levine, M.D.
Simon & Schuster, 2002

All Kinds of Minds: A Young Student's Book about Learning Abilities and Learning Disorders
Mel D. Levine, M.D.
Educators Publishing Service, 1993

Attention, Memory, and Executive Function
G. Reid Lyon, Ph.D., Norman A. Krasnegor, Ph.D.
Paul H. Brooks Publishing Company, 1996

Developmental Variation and Learning Disorders
Mel D. Levine, M.D.
Educator Publishing Service, 1987

Educational Care: A System for Understanding and Helping Children with Learning Problems at Home and in School
Mel D. Levine, M.D.
Educators Publishing Service, 1994

Section IX

Executive Function in Education
Lynn Meltzer, Ph.D.
Guilford Press, 2007

Executive Skills in Children and Adolescents: A Practical Guide to Assessment and Intervention
Peg Dawson, Ed.D., Richard Guare, Ph.D.
Guilford Press, 2004

Find A Way or Make A Way: Checklists of Helpful Accommodations For Students
Leslie E. Packer, Ph.D.
Parkaire Press, 2009

Frames of Mind: The Theory of Multiple Intelligences
Howard Gardner, Ph.D.
Perseus Publishing, 1993

How Difficult Can This Be? Understanding Learning Disabilities: F.A.T. City – A Learning Disabilities Workshop (DVD)
Richard D. Lavoie, M.A., M.Ed.
Touchstone/Simon & Schuster, 1989

How to Reach and Teach All Students in the Inclusive Classroom: Practical Strategies, Lessons, and Activities (2nd Edition)
Sandra. F. Rief, M.A., Julie A. Heimburge, M.A.
Jossey-Bass, 2006

Inclusion: 750 Strategies for Success: A Practical Guide for All Educators Who Teach Students with Disabilities
Peggy A. Hammeken
Peytral Publications, 2007

Individual Classroom Plan
Becky Ottinger, Ed.
Joshua Center, 2005

In Their Own Way: Discovering and Encouraging Your Child's Learning Style – Revised
Thomas Armstrong, Ph.D.
Putnam Publishing Group, 2000

Keeping A Head in School: A Student's Guide about Learning Abilities and Learning Disorders
Mel D. Levine, M.D.
Educators Publishing Service, 1990

Learning Disabilities and Discipline (DVD)
Richard D. Lavoie, M.A., M.Ed.
Touchstone/Simon & Schuster, 1997

The Motivation Breakthrough: 6 Secrets to Turning On the Tuned-Out Child
Richard D. Lavoie, M.A., M.Ed.
Touchstone/Simon & Schuster, 2007

The Motivation Breakthrough: 6 Secrets to Turning On the Tuned-Out Child (DVD)
Richard D. Lavoie, M.A., M.Ed.
Touchstone/Simon & Schuster, 2007

The Myth of Laziness
Mel D. Levine, M.D.
Simon & Schuster, 2002

The Out-of-Sync Child: Recognizing and Coping with Sensory Processing Disorder, Revised Edition
Carol S. Kranowitz, M.A., Lucy J. Miller, Ph.D.
Berkley Publishing Group, 2006

The Out-of-Sync Child Has Fun, Revised Edition: Activities for Kids with Sensory Processing Disorder.
Carol S. Kranowitz, M.A.
Penguin Group, 2006

The Power of Resilience: Achieving Balance, Confidence, and Personal Strength in Your Life
Robert Brooks, Ph.D., Sam Goldstein, Ph.D.
McGraw-Hill, 2004

Raising Resilient Children: Fostering Strength, Hope, and Optimism in Your Child
Robert Brooks, Ph.D., Sam Goldstein, Ph.D.
McGraw-Hill, 2001

Ready or Not, Here Life Comes
Mel D. Levine, M.D.
Simon & Schuster, 2002

7 Kinds of Smart: Identifying and Developing Your Multiple Intelligences – Revised
Thomas Armstrong, Ph.D.
Penguin Group, 1999

Seven Steps to Homework Success: A Family Guide to Solving Common Homework Problems
Sydney S. Zentall, Ph.D., Sam Goldstein, Ph.D.
Specialty Press, 1998

Strategies for Teaching Students with Learning and Behavior Problems (6th Edition)
Candace S. Bos, Ph.D., Sharon Vaughn, Ph.D.
Pearson, 2006

Teacher and Child: A Book for Parents and Teachers
Haim G. Ginott, Ph.D.
Collier Books, 1993

Teaching Adolescents with Disabilities: Accessing the General Education Curriculum
Donald D. Deshler, Ph.D., Jean B. Schumaker, Ph.D..
Corwin Press, 2005

Teaching Elementary Students Through Their Individual Learning Styles: Practical Approaches for Grades 3-6
Rita Dunn, Ph.D., Kenneth Dunn, Ph.D.
Allyn and Bacon, 1992

Teaching Elementary Students Through Their Individual Learning Styles: Practical Approaches for Grades 7-12
Rita Dunn, Ph.D., Kenneth Dunn, Ph.D.
Allyn and Bacon, 1993

Thinking Smarter: Skills for Academic Success
Carla Crutsinger, M.S.
Brainworks, 1997

Section IX

The Unschooled Mind: How Children Think and How Schools Should Teach
Howard Gardner, Ph.D.
Basic Books: HarperCollins, 1991

Wrightslaw: Special Education Law, 2nd Edition
Peter W. D. Wright, ESQ., Pamela D. Wright, M.A., M.S.W.
Harbor House Law Press, 2007

SOCIAL SKILLS

50 Activities for Teaching Emotional Intelligence: Elementary School (Level I) Grades 1-5
Dianne Schilling, M.A., Susanna Palomares, M.Ed.
Innerchoice Publishing, 1996

50 Activities for Teaching Emotional Intelligence: Middle School (Level II) Grade 6-8
Dianne Schilling, M.A., Susanna Palomares, M.Ed.
Innerchoice Publishing, 1996

50 Activities for Teaching Emotional Intelligence: High School (Level III) Grades 9-12
Dianne Schilling, Susanna Palomares
Innerchoice Publishing, 1999

Helping the Child Who Doesn't Fit In Decipher the Hidden Dimensions of Social Rejection
Stephen Nowicki, Ph.D., Marshall P. Duke, Ph.D.
Peachtree Publishers, 1992

It's So Much Work to Be Your Friend: Helping the Child with Learning Disabilities Find Social Success
Richard Lavoie, M.A., M.Ed.
Touchstone: Simon & Schuster, 2005

Learning Disabilities and Social Skills: Last One Picked, First One Picked On (DVD)
Richard D. Lavoie, M.A., M.Ed.
Touchstone/Simon & Schuster, 1994

No One to Play With: Social Problems of LD and ADD Children
Betty B. Osman, Ph.D.
Academic Therapy Publications, 1989

Teaching Your Child the Language of Social Success
Marshall P. Duke, Ph.D., Stephen Nowicki, Ph.D., Elisabeth A. Martin, M.A.
Peachtree Publishers, 1996

Understanding Learning Disabilities: How Difficult Can This Be?
Richard Lavoie, M.A., M.Ed.
City Workshop (VHS tape), 1989

Appendix

TEACHERS/PARENTS/HEALTHCARE PROFESSIONALS

ATTENTION DEFICIT HYPERACTIVITY DISORDER

ADD-Friendly Ways to Organize Your Life
Judith Kolberg, B.A., Kathleen G. Nadeau, Ph.D.
Brunner-Routledge, 2002

The ADHD Book of Lists: A Practical Guide for Helping Children and Teens with Attention Deficit Disorders
Sandra. F. Rief, M.A.
Jossey-Bass, 2003

ADHD Comorbidities: Handbook for ADHD Complications in Children and Adults
Thomas E. Brown, Ph.D.
American Psychiatric Publishing, 2009

ADHD in Adolescents: Diagnosis and Treatment
Arthur L. Robin, Ph.D.
Guilford Press, 1999

AD/HD & Driving: A Guide for Parents of Teens with ADHD
J. Marlene Synder, Ph.D.
Whitefish Consultants, 2001

The ADHD Report
Russell A. Barkley, Ph.D.
Guilford Press (6 newsletters yearly)

Advice to Parents on Attention-Deficit Hyperactivity Disorder
Larry Silver, M.D
American Psychiatric Press, 1992

All About ADHD: The Complete Practical Guide for Classroom Teachers
Linda Pfiffner, Ph.D.
Scholastic Trade, 1999

Answers to Distraction
Edward M. Hallowell, M.D., John J. Ratey, M.D.
Bantam Books, 1994

Attention Deficit Disorder and the Law: A Guide for Advocates
Peter S. Lathem, J.D., Patricia H. Lathem, J.D.
JLD Communications, 1997

Attention Deficit Disorder: The Unfocused Mind in Children and Adults
Thomas E. Brown, Ph.D.
Yale University Press Health and Wellness, 2005

Attention-Deficit Disorders and Comorbidit6ies in Children, Adolescents, and Adults
Thomas E. Brown, Ph.D.
American Psychiatric Press, 2000

Attention-Deficit Hyperactivity Disorder: A Handbook for Diagnosis and Treatment (3rd edition)
Russell A. Barkley, Ph.D.
Guilford Press, 2005

Section IX

Challenging Kids, Challenged Teachers (Working Title)
Leslie E. Packer, Ph.D., Sheryl K. Pruitt, M.Ed., ET/P
Woodbine House, (In Press)

Delivered from Distraction: Getting the Most Out of Life with Attention Deficit Disorder
Edward M. Hallowell, M.D., John J. Ratey, M.D.
Random House, 2005

Dr. Larry Silver's Advice to Parents on Attention Deficit Hyperactivity Disorder
Larry B. Silver, M.D.
Times Books, 1999

Driven to Distraction: Recognizing and Coping with Attention Deficit Disorder from Childhood through Adulthood
Edward M. Hallowell, M.D., John J. Ratey, M.D.
Simon & Schuster, 1994

The Explosive Child: A New Approach for Understanding and Parenting Easily Frustrated, Chronically Inflexible Children
Ross W. Greene, Ph.D.
HarperCollins Publishers, 1998

Fathering the ADHD Child: A Book for Fathers, Mothers, and Professionals
Edward H. Jacobs, Ph.D.
Jason Aronson, Inc., 1998

Find A Way or Make A Way: Checklists of Helpful Accommodations For Students with Attention Deficit Hyperactivity Disorder, Executive Dysfunction, Mood Disorders, Tourette's Syndrome, Obsessive-Compulsive Disorder, and Other Neurological Challenges
Leslie E. Packer, Ph.D.
Parkaire Press, 2009

Managing Attention Deficit Hyperactivity Disorder in Children: A Guide for Practitioners
Sam Goldstein, Ph.D., Michael Goldstein, M.D.
John Wiley and Sons, 1998

Maybe You Know My Kid: A Parent's Guide to Identifying, Understanding, and Helping Your Child with Attention-Deficit Hyperactivity Disorder – Third Edition
Mary Cahill Fowler
Kensington Publishing, 1999

Maybe You Know My Teen: A Parent's Guide to Helping Your Adolescent with Attention Deficit Hyperactivity Disorder
Mary Cahill Fowler
Random House, 2001

The New CHADD Information and Resource Guide to AD/HD
Children and Adults with Attention-Deficit/Hyperactivity Disorder
www.chadd.org, 2006

1-2-3 Magic: Effective Discipline for Children 2-12
Thomas W. Phelan, Ph.D.
Child Management, 2004

Overcoming Underachieving: An Action Guide to Helping Your Child Succeed in School
Nancy Mather, Ph.D., Sam Goldstein, Ph.D.
John Wiley & Sons, 1998

Problem Solver Guide for Students with Adhd: Ready to Use Interventions for Elementary & Secondary Students
Harvey C. Parker, Ph.D.
Specialty Printing, Inc., 2001

Teaching Teens with ADD and ADHD: A Quick Reference Guide for Teachers and Parents
Chris A. Zeigler Dendy, M.S.
Woodbine House, 2003

Teaching the Tiger: A Handbook for Individuals Involved in the Education of Students with Attention Deficit Disorders, Tourette Syndrome, or Obsessive-Compulsive Disorder
Marilyn P. Dornbush, Ph.D., Sheryl K. Pruitt, M.Ed.
Hope Press, 1995

Teenagers with ADD: A Parents' Guide
Chris A. Zeigler Dendy, M.S.
Woodbine House, 1995

Teenagers with ADD and ADHD, Second Edition: A Guide for Parents and Professionals
Chris A. Zeigler Dendy, M.S.
Woodbine House, 2006

Treating Explosive Children: The Collaborative Problem-Solving Approach
Ross W. Greene, Ph.D., J. Stuart Ablon, Ph.D.
Guilford Press, 2006

20 Questions to Ask if Your Child Has ADHD
Mary Cahill Fowler
Career Press, 2006

Understanding Girls with AD/HD
Kathleen G. Nadeau, Ph.D., Ellen B. Littman, Ph.D., Patricia O. Quinn, M.D.
Advantage Books, 2000

Voices from Fatherhood: Fathers, Sons, and ADHD
Patrick J. Kilcarr, Ph.D., Patricia O. Quinn, M.D.
Brunner/Mazel, 1997

Tourette Syndrome

An Anthropologist on Mars, Seven Paradoxical Tales
Oliver Sacks, M.D.
Vintage, 1996

Challenging Kids, Challenged Teachers (Working Title)
Leslie E. Packer, Ph.D., Sheryl K. Pruitt, M.Ed., ET/P
Woodbine House, (In Press)

A Cursing Brain? The Histories of Tourette Syndrome
Howard I. Kushner, Ph.D.
Harvard University Press, 1999

Don't Think About Monkeys. Extraordinary Stories by People with Tourette Syndrome
Adam Ward Seligman
Hope Press, 1992

Section IX

Echolalia. An Adult's Story of Tourette Syndrome
Adam Ward Seligman
Hope Press, 1991

Find A Way or Make A Way: Checklists of Helpful Accommodations For Students with Attention Deficit Hyperactivity Disorder, Executive Dysfunction, Mood Disorders, Tourette's Syndrome, Obsessive-Compulsive Disorder, and Other Neurological Challenges
Leslie E. Packer, Ph.D.
Parkaire Press, 2009

Front of the Class: How Tourette Syndrome Made Me the Teacher I Never Had
Brad Cohen, M.Ed.
Vanderwyk & Burnham, 2005

Kevin and Me: Tourette Syndrome and the Magic Power of Music Therapy
Patricia Heenen
Hope Press, 2000

Nix Your Tics!: Eliminate Unwanted Tic Symptoms: A How-To-Guide for Young People
B. Duncan McKinlay, Ph.D., C. Psych.
Life's A Twitch! Publishing, 2008

Teaching the Tiger: A Handbook for Individuals Involved in the Education of Students with Attention Deficit Disorders, Tourette Syndrome, or Obsessive-Compulsive Disorder
Marilyn P. Dornbush, Ph.D., Sheryl K. Pruitt, M.Ed.
Hope Press, 1995

Tictionary: A Reference Guide to the World of Tourette Syndrome, Asperger Syndrome, Attention Deficit Hyperactivity Disorder, and Obsessive-Compulsive Disorder for Parents and Professionals
Becky Ottinger, Ed.
Autism Asperger Publishing Company, 2003

Tiger Trails: An Unconventional Introduction to Tourette's Syndrome
Darin M. Bush
Parkaire Press, 2009

Tourette Syndrome: The Facts
Mary Robertson, M.D., Simon Baron-Cohen, Ph.D.
Oxford University Press, 1998

Tourette Syndrome: A Practical Guide for Teachers, Parents, and Carers
Amber Carroll, Ph.D., Mary Robertson, M.D.
David Fulton Publishers, 2000

Tourette's Syndrome. Tics, Obsessions, Compulsions: Developmental Psychopathology and Clinical Care
James F. Leckman, M.D., Donald J. Cohen, M.D. (Editors)
John Wiley and Sons, 1999

Treating Tourette Syndrome and Tic Disorders: A Guide for Practitioners
Douglas W. Woods, Ph.D., John C. Piacentini, Ph.D., John T. Walkup, M.D. (Editors)
Guilford Press, 2007

Understanding Tourette Syndrome: A Handbook for Educators
Tourette Syndrome Foundation of Canada
website: www.tourette.ca, 2001

Understanding Tourette Syndrome: A Handbook for Families
Tourette Syndrome Foundation of Canada
website: www.tourette.ca, 2001

What Makes Ryan Tick? A Family's Triumph Over Tourette Syndrome and Attention Deficit Hyperactivity Disorder
Susan Hughes
Hope Press, 1996

OBSESSIVE-COMPULSIVE DISORDER

Anxiety Disorders in Children and Adolescents: Second Revised Edition
John S. March M.D., Tracy L. Morris, Ph.D.
Guilford Publications, Inc., 2004

Blink, Blink, Clop, Clop: Why We Do We Do Things We Can't Stop? An OCD Storybook
E. Katia Morita, Ph.D.
Childwork/Childplay, 2001

The Boy Who Couldn't Stop Washing: The Experience and Treatment of Obsessive-Compulsive Disorder
Judith L. Rapoport, M.D.
E. P. Dutton, 1980

Brain Lock: Free Yourself from Obsessive-Compulsive Behavior
Jeffrey M. Schwartz, M.D., Beverly Beyette
Regan Books, 1996

Challenging Kids, Challenged Teachers (Working Title)
Leslie E. Packer, Ph.D., Sheryl K. Pruitt, M.Ed., ET/P
Woodbine House, (In Press)

Cognitive Behavioral Treatment of Childhood OCD
John Piacentini, Ph.D., Audra Langley, Ph.D., Tami Roblek, Ph.D.
Oxford University Press, 2007

Everything In Its Place: My Trials and Triumphs with Obsessive-Compulsive Disorder
Marc Summers
Jeremy P. Tarcher/Putnam, 1999

Find A Way or Make A Way: Checklists of Helpful Accommodations For Students with Attention Deficit Hyperactivity Disorder, Executive Dysfunction, Mood Disorders, Tourette's Syndrome, Obsessive-Compulsive Disorder, and Other Neurological Challenges
Leslie E. Packer, Ph.D.
Parkaire Press, 2009

Freeing Your Child from Obsessive-Compulsive Disorder: A Powerful, Practical Program for Parents of Children and Adolescents
Tamar E. Chansky, Ph.D.
Crown Publishing Group, 2001

Getting Control: Overcoming Your Obsessions and Compulsions, Revised Edition
Lee Baer, Ph.D.
Plume/Penguin Group, 2000

Section IX

Helping Your Child with OCD: A Workbook for Parents of Children with Obsessive-Compulsive Disorder
Lee Fitzgibbons, Ph.D., Cherry Pedrick, RN
New Harbinger Publications, 2003

The Imp of the Mind: Exploring the Silent Epidemic of Obsessive Bad Thoughts
Lee Baer, Ph.D.
Plume/Penguin Group, 2002

It's Only a False Alarm: A Cognitive Behavioral Treatment Program Workbook
John Piacentini, Ph.D., Audra Langley, Ph.D., Tami Roblek, Ph.D.
Oxford University Press, 2007

Kissing Doorknobs
Terry Spencer Hesser
Random House, 1998

Learning to Live with OCD (4th edition)
Barbara L. Van Noppen
OC Foundation, 1997

Obsessive-Compulsive Disorder: A Guide
J. H. Griest, M. D.
Obsessive-Compulsive Information Center, 1992

Obsessive-Compulsive Disorder: Contemporary Issues in Treatment
Wayne K. Goodman, M.D., Matthew V. Rudorfer, M.D., Jack D. Masser, M.D. (Editors)
Lawrence Erlbaum Associates, 1999

Obsessive-Compulsive Disorder in Children and Adolescents: A Guide (3rd edition)
Hugh F. Johnston, M.D., J. Jay Fruehling, M.A.
Madison Institute of Medicine, 2002

Obsessive-Compulsive Disorders: Practical Management (3rd Edition)
Michael A. Jenike, M.D., Lee Baer, Ph.D., William E. Minichiello, Ed.D. (Editors)
Mosby, 1998

OCD in Children and Adolescents: A Cognitive-Behavioral Treatment Manual
John S. March, M.D., Karen Mulle, M.S.W.
Guilford Press, 1998

Phobic and Anxiety Disorders in Children and Adolescents: A Clinician's Guide to Effective Psychosocial and Pharmacological Interventions
Thomas H. Ollendick, Ph.D., John S. March, M.D.
Oxford University Press, 2003

Stop Obsessing! How to Overcome Your Obsessions and Compulsions – Revised Edition
Edna B. Foa, Ph.D., Reid Wilson, Ph.D.
Bantam Books, 2001

Talking Back to OCD: The Program That Helps Kids and Teens Say "No Way" – and Parents say "Way to Go"
John S. March, M.D.
Guilford Press, 2007

Teaching the Tiger: A Handbook for Individuals Involved in the Education of Students with Attention Deficit Disorders, Tourette Syndrome, or Obsessive-Compulsive Disorder
Marilyn P. Dornbush, Ph.D., Sheryl K. Pruitt, M.Ed.
Hope Press, 1995

Treatment of OCD in Children and Adolescents: A Cognitive-Behavioral Therapy Manual
Aureen P. Wagner, Ph.D.
Lighthouse Press, 2003

What To Do When Your Child Has Obsessive-Compulsive Disorder: Strategies and Solutions
Aureen P. Wagner, Ph.D.
Lighthouse Press, 2002

When Once Is Not Enough
Gail Steketee, Ph.D., Kevin White, M.D.
New Harbinger Publications, 1991

Worried No More: Help and Hope for Anxious Children (2nd edition)
Aureen P. Wagner, Ph.D.
Lighthouse Press, 2005

Worry: Controlling It and Using It Wisely
Edward M. Hallowell, M.D.
Random House, 1997

CHILDREN AND ADOLESCENTS

ATTENTION DEFICIT HYPERACTIVITY DISORDER

ADHD – A Teenagers Guide
James J. Crist, Ph.D.
Childswork/Childsplay, 1996

A Bird's-Eye View of Life with ADD and ADHD: Advice from Young Survivors
Chris A. Zeigler Dendy, M.A., Alex Zeigler
Cherish the Children, 2003

A Bird's-Eye View of Life with ADD and ADHD: Advice from Young Survivors, Second Edition
Chris A. Zeigler Dendy, M.A., Alex Zeigler
Cherish the Children, 2007

Eukee The Jumpy Jumpy Elephant
Clifford L. Corman, M.D., Esther Trevino, M.F.C.C.
Specialty Press, 1995

Help 4 ADD @ High School
Kathleen G. Nadeau, Ph.D.
Advantage Books, 1998

Living with a Brother or Sister with Special Needs: A Book for Sibs, Second Edition, Revised and Expanded
Donald J. Meyer, Ph.D., Patricia Vadasy, Ph.D.
University of Washington Press, 1996

Section IX

Making the Grade: An Adolescent's Struggle with ADD
Roberta N. Parker, Ph.D., Harvey C. Parker, Ph.D.
Specialty Press, 1992

Putting on the Brakes: Young People's Guide to Understanding Attention Deficit Hyperactivity Disorder
Patricia O. Quinn, M.D., Judith M. Stern, M.A.
Magination Press, 1992

Shelley the Hyperactive Turtle
Deborah Moss
Woodbine House, 1989

Teen to Teen: The ADD Experience (video)
Chris A. Zeigler Dendy, M.A.
Cherish the Children, 2006

TOURETTE SYNDROME

Adam and the Magic Marble
Adam Buehrens
Hope Press, 1991

Hi, I'm Adam: A Child's Book about Tourette Syndrome
Adam Buehrens
Hope Press, 1990

Living with a Brother or Sister with Special Needs: A Book for Sibs, Second Edition, Revised and Expanded
Donald J. Meyer, Ph.D., Patricia Vadasy, Ph.D.
University of Washington Press, 1996

Nix Your Tics!: Eliminate Unwanted Tic Symptoms: A How-To-Guide for Young People
B. Duncan McKinlay, Ph.D., C. Psych.
Life's A Twitch! Publishing, 2008

Quit It
Marcia Byalick
Random House Children's Books, 2004

Tic Talk: Living with Tourette Syndrome: A 9-Year-Old Boy's Story in His Own Words
Dylan Peters
Little Five Star, 2007

Tiger Trails: An Unconventional Introduction to Tourette's Syndrome
Darin M. Bush
Parkaire Press, 2009

Why Do You Do That? A Book About Tourette Syndrome for Children and Young People
Uttom Chowdhury, M.D., Mary Robertson, M.D.
Jessica Kingsley Publishers, 2006

Obsessive-Compulsive Disorder

A Thought Is Just A Thought: A Story of Living With OCD
Leslie Talley
Lantern Books, 2004

Living with a Brother or Sister with Special Needs: A Book for Sibs, Second Edition, Revised and Expanded
Donald J. Meyer, Ph.D., Patricia Vadasy, Ph.D.
University of Washington Press, 1996

Mr. Worry: A Story about OCD
Holli I. Niner
Whitman & Company, 2004

Polly's Magic Games
Constance H. Foster
Dilligaf Publishing, 1994

Up & Down the Worry Hill: A Children's Book about Obsessive-Compulsive Disorder and Its Treatment
Aureen P. Wagner, Ph.D.
Lighthouse Press, 2004

 Updates to the list of books and resources can be located at www.parkairepress.com and www.tourettesyndrome.net

INDEX

INDEX

A

academic games 321
academic mentors/assistants 48
accurate perceptions, development of 336
acronyms 141, 289
acrostics 141, 289
ADD coaches. *See* coaches
Addition Facts Strategies Chart Template 392
ADHD. *See* Attention-Deficit/Hyperactivity Disorder
ADHD-C. *See* Attention-Deficit/Hyperactivity Disorder, Combined Type
ADHD-H/I. *See* Attention-Deficit/Hyperactivity Disorder, Predominately Hyperactive/Impulsive Type
ADHD-I. *See* Attention-Deficit/Hyperactivity Disorder, Predominately Inattentive Type
administrators 47
advocates 50
aggression 16, 70, 82, 83, 87, 90, 92, 308, 309. *See* storms
  and ADHD 4, 7, 10, 83
  and OCD 83
  and TS 16, 83
  change in routines 57
  storms and 83
  redirection 90
Agoraphobia 372
allocating time 121, 191, 283, 287, 299
anger 15, 23, 54, 55, 69, 82, 83, 84, 87, 90, 91, 92, 123, 275, 335, 336
  and ADHD 15
  bullying 54-55
  interventions 69
  and OCD 23
  storms 82-87
  therapy for 46
answering multiple-choice questions 300
Antisocial Personality Disorder 371
anxiety 3, 7, 8, 9, 10, 15, 16, 23, 24, 25, 26, 44, 79-81, 427
  behavioral symptoms 79
  cognitive behavioral therapy 79
  cognitive symptoms 44
  interventions 80
  physical symptoms 79
anxiety attack 82, 124, 427
Anxiety Disorders 372
  Agoraphobia 372
  Generalized Anxiety Disorder 372
  Panic Disorder 372
  Separation Anxiety 372
  Social Anxiety Disorder 373
  Social Phobia 373
  Specific Phobia 373
anxiety management 44, 427
anxiety, math 225
apologies 95, 111, 321
appropriate instructional level 100
arousal 16, 27, 72, 73, 74, 76, 77, 81, 82, 100, 125, 131, 132, 133, 144, 179, 260, 275, 293, 294, 427, 429
  arousal levels 72, 125, 133, 293
    optimal arousal 27
  overarousal 81-95
  underarousal 7, 71-73, 156, 157, 167, 179, 204, 223, 242, 260, 267, 269, 315, 316
ask for help 64, 125, 126, 193, 205, 213, 225, 231, 244, 250
assertive vs. aggressive language 320
assignment sheet/notebook 63, 116, 279
assistive technology consultants 48
association/integration of new material 141, 164
attention 28
Attention Deficit Hyperactivity Disorder 3-10 107, 133, 341, 415, 418, 422, 435
  adolescence 8
  adulthood 9
  age of onset 6
  behaviors 5
  combined type 4
  comorbid (co-occurring) disorders 6
  diagnostic criteria 3
  frequency 5
  gender 6
  prognosis 8
  predominately hyperactive/impulsive type 4
  predominately inattentive type 5
auditory memory span 163
automaticity 27, 36, 68, 136, 172, 235
awareness education 43

B

backward chaining 174, 237, 255
basic number facts 237
basic reading skills 37, 165-175
basic sight words 174, 202
bedroom environment 76
bedtime routine 75
behavioral therapy 44
behavior management 94-95
Bipolar Disorder 7, 8, 10, 372
books on tape 166, 179
brainstorm 47, 59, 111, 112, 160, 183, 207, 208, 212, 227, 246, 248, 277, 286, 288, 302, 324, 325, 328
buddy 57, 70, 84, 86, 99, 126, 181, 259, 279, 286, 311, 321, 427
bullying 54, 55, 56, 57, 81, 84, 311, 371
bus problems 86

C

calculator 223, 238, 242, 251, 253, 255
calendars 120-121, 146, 278, 283, 287
called on in class 313
capacity. *See* working memory
categorization 142
  skills 196
cause-and-effect 192
  Cause-and-Effect Template 388
CBIT. *See* Comprehensive Behavioral Intervention for Tics
CBT. *See* Cognitive-Behavioral Therapy
celsius 255
central executive. *See* working memory
change of schools 124
changing behavior, strategies for 329

Section X

charts
- Addition Facts Strategies Chart 392
- Dolch Basic Sight Vocabulary Words Chart 398
- Feeling Words Chart 402
- Math Words and Corresponding Symbols 397
- Multiplication Facts and Strategies Chart 393
- Shorthand Symbols for Notetaking Chart 401

checklists
- Proofreading 391
- For Expository Writing 390
- For Narrative Writing 389

child and adolescent psychotherapy 46
Chronic Motor Or Vocal Tic Disorder 12
clarification of communications 336
class meetings 55, 58, 84, 90, 311
Class Notes Template 400
classroom modifications/accommodations 53-59
- arrangement 58
- environment 54, 200
- materials 59
- organization 58
- routines 57
- rules/limits 57

coaches 49
Cognitive-Behavioral Therapy 44
cognitive
- cue 57, 99, 233, 229
- cue card 231
- processing speed 27
- sequencing cues 119, 146
- strategies 100-101, 108-109, 158-160, 181-183, 205-207, 225-227, 233, 244-246, 254, 272, 275-277
- strategies to edit written expression 217
- therapy 44

color code 59, 116, 117, 118, 143, 174, 194, 197, 198, 211, 224, 230, 232, 235, 244, 253, 262, 280, 282
communication log 63, 117, 279
communication with parents 62-63, 117, 278-279
community resources 49-50
- advocates 50
- coaches 49
- computer consultants 50
- educational consultants/educational therapists 49
- pediatric (child) neuropsychologists 49
- social skills trainers 50
- tutors 49

comorbid (co-occurring) disorders 6, 15, 23, 371-373
compare and contrast 192
- Compare and Contrast 3 Circle Template 385
- Compare and Contrast 2 Circle Template 384

completion of homework 282
complex tics 11
Comprehensive Behavioral Intervention for Tics 45
compulsions 19, 21, 22
computational procedures 238
computer use 69, 165, 201
computer consultants 50
Conduct Disorder 7, 8, 10, 371
consequences 4, 32, 36, 38, 43, 48, 55, 56, 58, 65, 78, 83, 87, 88, 92, 94, 95, 102, 103, 111, 125, 127, 129, 133, 136, 161, 184, 210, 228, 247, 263, 270, 274, 278, 317, 325, 335, 337, 427, 428, 429
content-specific 72, 98, 261

control of impulsive comments 319
conversations, initiating and maintaining 331
cooperative learning experiences 59, 62, 312
coprolalia 13, 15. *See also* Tourette syndrome
COPS 217
Cornell Notetaking Technique 263
cramming 287
cue words 190, 261
cueing 101, 158, 312
curbing impulsive, intrusive actions 320
Cycle of Stages/Steps/Events Template 387

D

delaying tactics 316
Depression *See* Major Depression
details in reading materials 184
Diagnostic and Statistical Manual of Mental Disorders
- Attention-Deficit/Hyperactivity Disorder 3
- Chronic Motor or Vocal Tic Disorder 12
- Obsessive-Compulsive Disorder 19
- Transient Tic Disorder 11
- Tourette syndrome 11

difficulty with
- awakening 77-78
- copying 232
- encoding/consolidating 136-144, 173-174, 197-198, 236-238, 253-255, 266
- falling asleep 75-76
- flexibility 122-125, 191-192, 230, 249-250, 327-329
- forgetting the sequence of division 233
- immediate memory 131
- initiation/execution 125-127, 171, 193, 213, 231, 250, 263-264, 283-284, 330-332
- managing time 119, 190, 212, 230, 249, 283
- metamemory 147
- organizing 114, 161, 186-189, 209-212, 228-230, 247-249, 262-263, 279-282, 326-327
- planning 111, 160, 183, 207, 227, 246, 277, 324
- prioritizing 112, 161, 184, 209, 228, 247, 261, 278, 325
- procedural memory 145
- proposing and analyzing ideas/solutions/strategies 160, 183, 207, 227, 246, 277, 324
- prospective memory 146
- remembering division sequence 233
- remembering math operations 235
- retrieval 71, 144-145, 175, 198, 220, 238-239, 255, 338
- self-correcting 130, 193-195, 214-218, 231-235, 250-251, 285, 332-336
- self-monitoring 127-129, 171, 193-195, 214-218, 231-235, 250-251, 285, 332-336
- sequencing 118-119, 170, 190, 208-212, 228-230, 247-249, 262-263, 279-282, 326-327
- setting goals 110-111, 160, 183, 227, 246, 277, 324
- strategic memory 147
- using feedback 127-129, 162, 171, 193-195, 214-218, 231-235, 251, 285-286, 332-336
- working memory 132, 163, 172, 195, 219, 235, 252, 264, 286, 337

directions/instructions 73, 98, 99, 108, 126, 128, 129, 132, 141, 153, 154, 156, 161, 162, 165, 169, 190, 193, 213, 215, 216, 224, 225, 229, 260, 279, 280, 283, 284, 285, 286, 294, 299, 301, 302, 310, 316, 327
disorganization 10, 59, 93, 108, 115, 117, 118, 326

Index

distractions 28, 62, 97, 98, 133, 280, 290, 293, 299
    external 98
    internal 62
Dolch Basic Sight Vocabulary Chart 378
Dunn and Dunn learning style preferences 65

E

echolalia 13, 15. *See also* Tourette syndrome
EDF, *See* Executive Dysfunction
editing strips
    Math Editing Cue Strip 231, 394
    Written Expression Editing Strip 217, 394
educational consultants 49
educational resources 47-48
    academic mentors/assistants 48
    administrators 47
    assistive technology consultants 48
    educational support team 47
    home-school case managers 48
    learning disability teachers 47
    occupational therapists 47
    school psychologists 48
    speech and language pathologists 47
emotional needs of student 61, 311
encoding/consolidation 38
    difficulty 136-144, 173-174, 197-198, 236-238, 266
encoding strategies 137-144, 174, 197-198, 236-238, 253-255, 288
episodic/autobiographical memory 39
errorless learning 137, 236, 173
essay questions 301
estimation 119, 121, 250, 283
execution difficulties 171, 193, 213, 231, 250, 263, 283
Executive Dysfunction 107-130
    and ADHD 107, 112, 115, 122, 124, 127
    and OCD 107, 115, 122
    and TS 107, 124
    impaired problem solving 108-121, 158-162, 181-190, 205-213, 225-230, 244-249, 275-283, 322-327
        difficult managing time 119-121, 146, 230, 299
        difficulty planning 111-120, 160-162, 183-191, 207-213, 227-230, 246-249, 277-283, 324-327
        difficulty prioritizing 112-114, 161, 184-185, 209, 228, 247, 261-262, 278, 325-326
        difficulty proposing/analyzing idea 111-112, 160-161, 183-184, 207-208, 227-228, 246-247, 277-278, 324-325
        difficulty organizing 114-118, 161-162, 186-189, 209-212, 228-230, 247-249, 262-263, 279-282, 326-327
        difficulty sequencing 118-119, 161-162, 190-191, 209-212, 228-230, 247-249, 262-263, 279-282, 326-327
        difficulty setting goals 110-111, 160, 183, 227, 246, 277, 324
    impaired self-correction 130, 162, 171, 193-195, 214-218, 231-235, 285-286, 332-336
    impaired self-monitoring 127-129, 162, 171, 193-195, 214-218, 231-235, 285-286, 332-336
    impaired use of feedback 129-130, 162, 171, 193-195, 214-218, 231-235, 285-286, 332-336
    inflexibility 122-125, 191-192, 230, 249-250, 327-329
    initiation/execution difficulties 125-127, 171, 193, 213, 231, 250, 263-264, 283-284, 330-332
executive functions 29-33, 36, 49, 50, 74, 107, 132, 133, 241, 322
    flexibility 30, 31
    goal setting 30
    initiation/execution 30, 32, 33
    intact executive functioning 33
    organization 30, 31
    planning 30
    prioritization 30
    problem solving 30
    proposal/analysis 30
    self-correction 30, 32, 33
    self-monitoring 30, 32, 33
    sequencing 30, 31
    time management 30, 31, 33
    utilization of feedback 30, 32
explicit memory 39
expository text structure 187
expository writing 210
exposure response prevention therapy 44

F

family therapy 46
feelings
    awareness of 333-334
        expression of 310
    being expressed by others, understanding of 334
    understanding and awareness of 333
Feeling Thermometer 91, 335
    Feeling Thermometer Template 403
feeling words 333
    Feeling Words Chart Template 402
figurative language 328
fill-in-the-blank tests 301
flash cards 140, 289
flexibility 30, 31
fluency 165, 167
focusing during conversational interactions 318
forgetfulness 117
Four Alarm Clock System 77
Franklin Spelling Ace 203
free recall 39, 145
frustration 29, 46, 54, 59, 69, 82, 87, 88, 89, 91, 171, 178, 193, 219, 221, 270, 272-273, 294, 308
frustration level 64, 178, 193

G

gain attention 99
Generalized Anxiety Disorder 372
generation of solutions 87, 129, 277, 328
GET A CLUE 58, 80, 88, 91, 92, 109, 110, 115, 119, 146, 158, 159, 181, 182, 205, 206, 225, 226, 244, 245, 275, 276, 277, 322, 323
    GET A CLUE Template 374
goal setting. *See* setting goals
Graceful Exit 81, 90, 123, 329
Grandma's Rule 92
graphic organizers 66, 67, 114, 115, 119, 135, 138, 142, 145, 153, 154, 155, 161, 162, 164, 177, 184, 189, 191, 196, 197, 202, 204, 210, 211, 212, 219, 220, 222, 262, 265, 266, 288, 289, 290, 295, 301, 302
graphomotor problems 68, 201, 221, 259, 294-295.
    See also handwriting problems
    and ADHD 68, 201, 221, 259
    and OCD 68, 201, 221, 259
    and TS 68, 201, 221, 259
graph paper 232

Section X

greater than/less than 253
greeting skills 330
group therapy 46

H

Hand Trick, The 254
handwriting problems 68, 221, 259
handwritten assignments 201
highlight 59, 68, 99, 116, 121, 126, 129, 135, 142, 154, 155, 156, 165, 170, 179, 180, 181, 184, 185, 188, 190, 192, 194, 197, 224, 230, 244, 247, 261, 264, 265, 266, 271, 278, 280, 287, 289, 294, 301, 302, 311
hoarding 20, 21
home-school case managers 48
home-school communications 62-63
homework 267-286
    assigning 279
    collecting 282
    completion 282
    directions 283-284
    length of assignment 270, 281
    location 280-281
    movement 272
    reason for difficulty 267
    recording 279
homework survey 268
    Homework Survey - Parent Reporting Form Template 406
Howard Gardner's theory. *See* multiple intelligences
humor 89
hyperactivity 3, 4, 97, 105, 157, 169, 180, 204, 224, 243, 261, 271, 316

I

immaturity 309
immediate memory 35
    difficulty 131-132
impaired self-correction 130, 162, 171, 193-195, 214-218, 231-235, 285-286, 332-336
impaired self-monitoring 127-129, 162, 171, 193-195, 214-218, 231-235, 285-286, 332-336
impaired use of feedback 129-130, 162, 171, 193-195, 214-218, 231-235, 285-286, 332-336
impaired sense of time 119
implicit memory 39
impulsivity 3, 4, 97, 103-104, 157, 169, 180, 204, 224, 243, 261, 271, 316, 320, 428
inattention 3, 4, 97-102, 157, 169, 180, 204, 224, 243, 261, 271, 316
increase of symptoms 69
independent instructional level 64, 166, 178, 180, 193, 272, 268-269
index cards 140, 211, 289
Individual Education Plan 293
individual interventions 61
inferences 191
inflexibility 122-125, 191-192, 230, 249-250, 327-329
Information/Description Template 382
inhibition 28
initiation/execution 30, 32, 33
    difficulty 125-127, 171, 193, 213, 231, 250, 263-264, 283-284, 330-332
in-school reinforcers 274
instructional level 64, 126, 166, 168, 171, 178, 193, 194, 224, 283, 285
    appropriate 100
internal clock 72, 120, 191
interpersonal learner 67, 153, 177
interventions 61, 72, 74, 75, 76, 77, 80, 86, 98, 103, 105, 107, 110, 111, 112, 115, 118, 120, 122, 125, 128, 129, 130, 131, 133, 137, 144, 145, 146, 147, 148, 151, 153, 156, 158, 160, 161, 162, 163, 166, 167, 169, 170, 171, 172, 173, 175, 177, 179, 180, 183, 184, 186, 190, 191, 193, 194, 196, 197, 198, 200, 204, 205, 207, 209, 212, 213, 214, 219, 220, 221, 223, 224, 227, 228, 229, 230, 231, 235, 236, 238, 241, 244, 246, 247, 248, 250, 252, 253, 255, 259, 260, 261, 262, 264, 266, 267, 270, 271, 277, 278, 279, 283, 285, 286, 307, 309, 316, 317, 322, 324, 325, 326, 327, 330, 333, 337, 338, 416, 420, 427, 428, 429, 430
intrapersonal learner 67, 153, 177
introduction of friend 331
Is It Naughty or Neurological 86
isosceles triangle 254

J

joining group conversations 331
"Just Right" Feeling 20

K

kinesthetic learner 66, 153, 177, 429
K-W-L 134

L

language that conveys respect 320
language therapy 151
learned helplessness 63-65
learning disability teachers 47
Learning Pyramid 138
learning strategies 64-65
learning style preferences 65-67, 73, 100, 134, 140, 148, 153, 166, 167, 177, 178, 198
linguistic/verbal learner 66
Liquid Measure: The Hand Trick 254
listening comprehension 37, 153-164
    after lesson 156
    before lesson 154
    during lesson 155
logical consequences 94
logical/mathematical learner 67, 100, 153, 177
long-term memory 38-39
    difficulty 136-148, 173, 197, 220, 236, 253, 266, 338
long-term reports 199
loss of behavioral control 88

M

main ideas of reading materials 184
Major Depression 7, 8, 10, 371
Manic Depression *See* Bipolar Disorder
mastery 222, 237
matching tests 300
math
    anxiety 225
    assignments, modify 221
    calculation. *See* math computation
    computation 37, 221-239
    Editing Checklist for Computations 234
    Editing Checklist for Computations Template 396

Index

Editing Checklist for Word Problems Template 251, 399
Editing Cue Strip 394
error patterns 232
folder 222, 242
Ideas/Facts Chart Template 383
Math Words and Corresponding Symbols Chart 397
notebook 222
problems, modifications for 222
reasoning 241-255
sequencing strategies 229
mathematical learner 67, 428
medication 43
medication resources 43
memory 35-39
difficulty 131, 163, 172, 173, 195, 197, 219, 220, 235, 236, 252, 253, 264, 266, 286, 337, 338
encoding/consolidation learning 38, 136, 288
episodic/autobiographical memory 39
long-term memory 38
metamemory 39, 147
procedural memory 39
prospective memory 39
retrieving (recalling) 38
rote memory 139, 236
semantic memory 39
short-term memory 35
strategic memory 39
working memory 35
metamemory 39, 147
Method of Loci 142, 289
mind maps 115, 142, 260, 265
mapping program 208
mapping strategy 289
Mind Map Template 382
minimize distractions 98
mistakes 65
mobility options 85, 105
modality-specific 98, 132, 261
monitor social interactions, teach how to 336
morning routines 77
Mother Vowel 135, 172, 376
The Story of Mother Vowel 377
motor movements 11, 12, 74, 105, 272
ignore 105
movement 72, 85, 105, 272
multiple-choice questions 300
multiple intelligences 66
Multiplication Facts Strategies Chart 393
multi-step directions, difficulty 229
music 142, 289
musical learner 67

N

narrative text structure 186
narrative writing 209
natural consequences 94. *See also* consequences
needs of the listener 335
negotiation and compromise 90
neuropsychological evaluation 153
neuropsychologists 49
non-standardized tests 296
nonverbal expression of feelings 310
nonverbal social cues 310, 334

notebook 59, 63, 100, 104, 108, 114, 116, 117, 121, 140, 201, 203, 209, 212, 222, 229, 242, 248, 249, 252, 262, 263, 272, 280, 282, 285, 320
notetaking 155, 259-266
number facts, basic 237

O

obsessions 19, 20, 23, 418, 419, 420
Obsessive-Compulsive Disorder 19-26, 107, 133, 346, 347, 416, 417, 419, 420, 421, 423, 435
adolescents 25
adulthood 26
age of onset 22
comorbid (co-occurring) disorders 23
compulsions 21
diagnostic criteria 19
frequency 22
gender 22
non-tic-related OCD 25
obsessions 20
symptom control 23, 69
tic-related OCD 24
occupational therapists 47
OCD. *See* Obsessive-Compulsive Disorder
off-task behavior interventions 101
on-task behavior reinforcement 101
opinions/facts in reading 185
Opinions/Facts Chart Template 386
Oppositional Defiant Disorder 7, 8, 10, 371
optimal arousal 27
oral expression 37, 151
organization 30, 31, 33
difficulty 114-118, 161-162, 186-189, 209-212, 228-230, 247-249, 262-263, 279-282, 326-327
organizational skills survey 118
Organizational Skills Survey - Parent Reporting Form Template 405
organizational strategies 114, 115, 124, 228, 229
organize a classroom 58
organize communications 326
overarousal 81-95
situations that produce 82

P

palilalia 13. *See also* Tourette syndrome
Panic Disorder 372
parental involvement 314
reinforcers 274
parent reporting forms
Homework Survey - Parent Reporting Form Template 406
Organizational Skills Survey - Parent Reporting Form Template 405
Sleep Survey - Parent Reporting Form Template 404
parent support groups 46
passive review 140
pediatric (child) neuropsychologists 49
peer interactions 313
pen pal 200
perseverating 122, 191
perspective-taking skills 328
phobia 373
phonemic awareness 165
phonetically-based words 202

Section X

phonics 165
PLAN 58, 80, 88, 91, 92, 109, 110, 115, 119, 146, 158, 159, 160, 181, 182, 183, 205, 206, 207, 225, 226, 227, 244, 245, 246, 275, 276, 277, 322, 323, 324, 375
    PLAN Template 375
planning 29, 30, 33, 36,
    difficulty 111-112, 160-162, 183-191, 207-213, 227-230, 246-249, 277-283, 324-327
power struggles 88
practice test booklets 296
pragmatic language 151
predictions 192
presentation of information 100
pre-storm warnings 84
prioritizing 30
    difficulty 112-114, 161, 184-185, 209, 228, 247, 261-262, 278, 325-326
problem on the bus 86
Problem/Solution Template 380
problem solving 30, 108
problem solving strategy 88, 108-109, 158, 181, 205, 225, 242, 244, 275, 322
procedural memory 39
    difficulty 145-146
processing speed 27
    difficulty 71-73, 156, 157, 167, 179, 204, 223, 242, 260, 269, 315, 316
prognosis 8, 17, 25
proofreading checklist 218
    Proofreading Checklist Template 391
proposing or generating ideas/strategies/solutions, difficulty 30, 33
    difficulty 111-112, 160-161, 183-184, 207-208, 227-228, 246-247, 277-278, 324-325
prosocial behaviors 317
prospective memory 39
    difficulty 146
public hangings 92

R

rage attack 83
reading 165-198
    after reading 187, 189
    aloud 168, 171
    basic skills 37, 165-175
    before reading 186, 187
    comprehension 37, 165, 177-198
    during reading 187, 188
    fluency 165, 167-168
    schedule/timetable 191
    tests 297
reading aloud 168
reading comprehension 37, 165, 177
    tests for 297
reading programs 165
reads too quickly 170
Ready the Plane For Math's Four C's 248, 250
    Ready the Plane For Math's Four C's Template 398
reasons for misbehavior 92-93
reasonable and fair 102
recall 38, 39, 139
recognition 145
Recordings for the Blind and Dyslexic 166, 179

redirection 101
reinforcers 274
reports, presenting 313
response prevention 44
retrieval (recalling) 38
    difficulty 71, 144-145, 175, 198, 220, 238-239, 255, 295
retrieval problems 295
return homework assignments 282
review following lessons 143
Revision Checklist for Expository Writing Template 390
Revision Checklist for Narrative Writing Template 389
revision of expository writing 216
revision of narrative writing 215
revision of writing 214
rewards 32, 64, 67, 94, 117, 129, 273, 274, 279
rhymes 141
rote memorization 139, 236
routine 19, 31, 57, 75, 79, 85, 115, 117, 122, 123, 146, 268, 279, 281, 282, 427

S

schedules, daily and weekly 120
school counselors 47
school psychologists 48
scoring criteria 296
self-awareness 39, 46, 49, 128, 162
self-correction 30, 32, 33
    difficulty 130, 162, 171, 193-195, 214-218, 231-235, 250-251, 285-286, 332-336
self-monitoring 30, 32, 33, 45
    difficulty 127-129, 162, 171, 193-195, 214-218, 231-235, 250-251, 285-286, 332-336
self-questioning 128, 162, 184, 193, 194, 249, 285
self-talk 88-89, 140, 205, 214
self-testing 290
semantic memory 39
Separation Anxiety 372
sequence communications 326
Sequence Organizer Template 381
sequencing 31
    difficulty 118-119, 161-162, 190-191, 209-212, 228-230, 247-249, 262-263, 279-282, 326-327
setting/environment 293
setting goals 30, 33
    difficulty 110-111, 160, 183, 227, 246, 277, 324
short answer tests 301
Shorthand Symbols For Notetaking Chart 401
short-term memory 29, 35-38
    difficulty 131-136, 163, 166, 172, 195, 219, 235-238, 252, 264, 286, 337
sight words, basic 174, 202
simple tics 11
sleep disorders 74
    difficulty awakening 77
    difficulty falling asleep 75
    difficulty remaining asleep 76
    general interventions 74
sleep hygiene 74, 75
Sleep Survey - Parent Reporting Form Template 404
slope 254
slow cognitive processing speed 71-73, 156, 167, 179, 204, 223, 242, 260, 269, 315
    interventions 72

Index

Social Anxiety Disorder 373
social boundaries 334
social competence 38, 305
social customs of new school 329
social deficits, interventions for 309
social disability 307
socialization group 312
social performance deficit 308
Social Phobia 373
social skills 307-338
    emotional needs of student/listener 331, 335
    game/sports activities 314, 321
    giving/accepting compliments 320
    impulsivity 319
    nonverbal expression of feelings 310
    organization/sequencing communications 326
    parental involvement 314
    perspective-taking skills 328
    social activities, arrangement of 314
    social anxiety 313, 373
    social skills group 312
    topic initiation/maintenance 327, 331
    turn-taking 318
    verbal expression of feelings 310
social skills trainers 50
solution organizer template 380
spatial learner 66
specific phobia 373
speech and language pathologists 47
speed of processing 36, 49, 71, 72, 73, 132, 166, 167, 221, 223, 243, 260, 270, 293, 316
spelling instruction 202
sport team 314
stages, manageable 213
standardized tests 296
steps for writing 211
storms 81-95
    classroom interventions 84
    implosive 83
    pre-storm warnings 84
    rage attack 83
    reasons for 92
    student interventions 86
Story of Mother Vowel. *See* Mother Vowel
Story Organizer Template 379
strategic memory 39
    difficulty 147
strategies 140
    for editing 217
strategies (trick) book 64, 229
strategy instruction 177
structure 37, 48, 53, 66, 93, 100, 109, 115, 120, 124, 136, 140, 142, 159, 165, 177, 182, 186, 195, 196, 206, 209, 210, 212, 219, 220, 226, 245, 252, 261, 271, 276, 279, 282, 312, 323
stuck 21, 22, 78, 83, 84, 85, 94, 122, 123, 137, 174, 191, 199, 203, 236, 294, 327, 429
student interventions 61-70
study
    environment 280
    group 288
    skills 197
    tests 287
stuttering 151

subvocalization 35, 244
summarization 185
sustaining attention during conversations 318

T

tactile learner 66, 100, 429
taking assignment materials home 280
teacher-prepared tests 296
teacher's attitude 61
templates
    Addition Facts Strategies Chart 392
    Cause-and-Effect 388
    Class Notes 400
    Compare and Contrast 2 Circle 384
    Compare and Contrast 3 Circle 385
    Cycle of Stages/Steps/Events 387
    Feeling Thermometer 403
    Get A Clue 374
    Homework Survey - Parent Reporting Form 406
    Information/Description 382
    Math Editing Checklist for Computations 396
    Math Editing Checklist for Word Problems 399
    Math Ideas/Facts Chart 383
    Mind Mapping 382
    Opinions/Facts 386
    Organizational Skills Survey Parent Reporting Form 405
    Plan 375
    Problem/Solution 380
    Proofreading Checklist 391
    Ready The Plane For The Math's 4 C's 398
    Revision Checklist For Expository Writing 390
    Revision Checklist For Narrative Writing 389
    Sequence Organizer 381
    Sleep Survey - Parent Reporting Form 404
    Story Organizer 379
    Venn Diagram, 2 Circle 384
    Venn Diagram, 3 Circle 385
tests 293-298
    difficulty reading the questions 298
    formats 294
    handwriting 294-295
    instructions 294
    math 297, 302
    nonstandardized 296
    reading comprehension 297
    requiring calculations 302
    retrieval problems 295
    review 302
    scheduling 294
    setting 293
    standardized 296-298
test-taking strategies 299-303
    calculation 302
    essay 301
    fill-in-the-blank 301
    multiple-choice 300
    short answer 301
    true-false 300
text structure 186
    expository 187-189, 210
    narrative 186-187, 209
The Hand Trick 254
therapeutic interventions 44-46

anxiety management 44
child/adolescent psychotherapy 44
cognitive-behavioral therapy 44
Comprehensive Behavior Intervention for Tics 45
family therapy 46
group therapy 46
parent support groups 46
thought stopping 45
tic disorders 11-17
Chronic Motor Or Vocal Tic Disorder 12
Tourette Syndrome 12-17
Transient Tic Disorder 11
timelines 115, 142, 177, 212
time management 30, 31, 33
allocation 121, 191, 283, 287, 299
and ADHD 119
difficulty with 119-121, 146, 230, 299
estimation 119, 120, 283
passage of 119, 120, 212
timer 101, 272
timing for approaching another 330
timing/scheduling 294
"To Do List" 114, 121, 278, 283
topic maintenance 327
touching rules 334
Tourette syndrome 12-17, 24, 25, 26, 43, 92, 107, 133, 345, 347, 350, 352, 435, 408, 409, 416, 417, 418, 418, 420, 422, 423
See also Tics Disorders
adolescence 17
adulthood 17
age of onset 14
co-morbid (co-occurring) disorders 16
diagnostic criteria 12
frequency 14
gender 14
motor symptoms 13
plus ADHD 16, 97
plus OCD 16, 17
symptom control 14, 69
vocal symptoms 13
tracking problems 169, 225
Transient Tic Disorder 11
transitions 31, 79, 81, 123, 124
trichotillomania 19, 24
trick book 64, 229
true-false questions 300
TS *See* Tourette syndrome
turn-taking 104, 318
tutors 49

U

underarousal 71-73, 156, 157, 167, 179, 204, 223, 242, 260, 267, 269, 315, 316
understand instructions 284
unfinished class assignments 102, 268
ungraded assignments 64
unstructured time 124
use of feedback 30, 32, 33
difficulty 129-130, 162, 171, 193-195, 214-218, 231-235, 285-286, 332-336

V

Venn diagram 115, 142, 153, 177, 189, 192, 210
Venn Diagram Template, 2 Circle 384
Venn Diagram Template, 3 Circle 385
verbal and visual cues 318
verbal expression of emotions 310
verbal/auditory learner 66, 153, 177
verbal memory strategies 141
abbreviation 141
acronyms 141
acrostics 141
music 141-142
rhymes 141
stories 141
verbal rehearsal 196
verbal social cues 310, 334
verbal strategies 141
visual aids 155
visual cue card 100, 108, 186, 235, 252
visualization 142, 196
visual memory strategies 142
visual-motor integration 259
Visual Organizer Template 374, 375
visual proofreading strategy 217
visual-spatial learner 66, 153, 177
Vocal Tic Disorder 12

W

who, what, when, where, how, and why 98
Story Organizer Template 379
work completion reinforcement 101
working memory 35-38
academic skills 37, 132
and ADHD 80, 131, 133, 137, 163
and OCD 131, 133, 137
and TS 131, 133
behavior 133
capacity 36, 134, 173, 196, 198, 219
complexity of material 134, 252
conceptualization 35
difficulty with 72, 74, 80, 119, 131, 132-136, 139, 144, 146, 151, 153, 163-164, 172-173, 186, 195-196, 201, 202, 204, 218, 219, 220, 221, 235-236, 248, 252-253, 261, 264-265, 267, 278, 286, 294, 337
executive function 36, 132
central executive (workspace) 35
phonological 35
visual-spatial 35
writing folder or notebook 201
writing steps 211
written directions 283
written expression 7, 37, 199-220
written expression checklist 215, 216, 218
Proofreading Checklist 391
Revision Checklist For Expository Writing 390
Revision Checklist For Narrative Writing 389
Written Expression Editing Strip 394
written expression time table 212

About the Authors

Marilyn P. Dornbush, Ph.D. is a school psychologist in private practice who specializes in child neuropsychology. Since she wrote her dissertation in 1984 on children with Tourette syndrome, she has been involved in the assessment, education, and behavioral management of students with neurological disorders. She has been a member of the Board of Directors of the Tourette syndrome of Georgia and served on the Scientific Advisory Board. She received her master's degree in Learning Disabilities from Emory University and her Ph.D. in School Psychology from Georgia State University. Dr. Dornbush co-authored with Sheryl K. Pruitt *Teaching the Tiger*, which addressed the education of students with Attention Deficit Hyperactivity Disorder, Tourette Syndrome, and Obsessive-Compulsive Disorder.

Sheryl K. Pruitt, M.Ed., ET/P is the Clinical Director of Parkaire Consultants, Inc., a clinic that she founded to serve neurologically impaired individuals. Prior to the founding of Parkaire Consultants, Ms. Pruitt conducted a State of Georgia Exemplary Model of Learning Disabilities Program and taught behavior disordered students in a psychoeducational setting. She served on the Board of Directors of the Tourette Syndrome Association of Georgia for six years and the National Tourette Syndrome Association's Educational Committee. Ms. Pruitt was a member of the Scientific Advisory Board of the Tourette Syndrome Association of Georgia and South Carolina as well as the Tourette Spectrum Disorder Association of California. She is a member of the Professional Advisory Board of the Tourette Syndrome Foundation of Canada and is on the Professional Advisory Board for North Atlanta and Central Georgia CHAAD. Ms. Pruitt is a writer who, in addition to co-authoring *Teaching the Tiger*, was a contributor to the Tourette Foundation of Canada's *Understanding Tourette Syndrome: A Handbook for Educators*. She speaks at local, national, and international conferences and teaches seminars and learning courses for health care professionals and educators about Attention Deficit Hyperactivity Disorder, Tourette Syndrome, and Obsessive-Compulsive Disorder. She has two sons with neurological disorders and understands the problems from a personal as well as professional point of view.

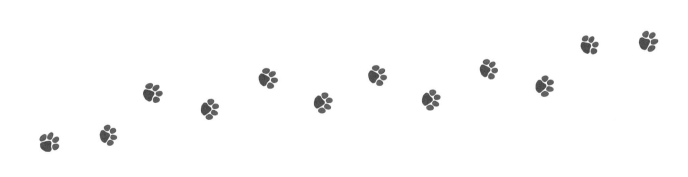